theclinics.com

SURGICAL CLINICS OF NORTH AMERICA

Esophageal Surgery

GUEST EDITOR
Rodney J. Landreneau, MD

CONSULTING EDITOR
Ronald F. Martin, MD

June 2005 • Volume 85 • Number 3

SAUNDERS

An Imprint of Elsevier, Inc.
PHILADELPHIA   LONDON   TORONTO   MONTREAL   SYDNEY   TOKYO

W.B. SAUNDERS COMPANY
A Division of Elsevier Inc.

1600 John F. Kennedy Blvd., Suite 1800, Philadelphia, PA 19103-2899

http://www.theclinics.com

SURGICAL CLINICS OF NORTH AMERICA
June 2005
Editor: Catherine Bewick

Volume 85, Number 3
ISSN 0039–6109
ISBN 1-4160-2792-0

Reprints. For copies of 100 or more of articles in this publication, please contact the commercial Reprints Department Elsevier Inc., 360 Park Avenue South, New York, New York 10010-1710. Tel. (212) 633-3813, Fax: (212) 462-1935, email: reprints@elsevier.com

The ideas and opinions expressed in *The Surgical Clinics of North America* do not necessarily reflect those of the Publisher. The Publisher does not assume any responsibility for any injury and/or damage to persons or property arising out of or related to any use of the material contained in this periodical. The reader is advised to check the appropriate medical literature and the product information currently provided by the manufacturer of each drug to be administered to verify the dosage, the method and duration of administration, or contraindications. It is the responsibility of the treating physician or other health care professional, relying on independent experience and knowledge of the patient, to determine drug dosages and the best treatment for the patient. Mention of any product in this issue should not be construed as endorsement by the contributors, editors, or the Publisher of the product or manufacturers' claims.

Surgical Clinics of North America (ISSN 0039–6109) is published bimonthly by Elsevier; Corporate and editorial Offices: 1600 John F. Kennedy Blvd., Suite 1800, Philadelphia, PA 19103-2899. Accounting and circulation offices: 6277 Sea Harbor Drive, Orlando, FL 32887-4800. Periodicals postage paid at Orlando, FL 32862, and additional mailing offices. Subscription prices are $190.00 per year for US individuals, $299.00 per year for US institutions, $95.00 per year for US students and residents, $234.00 per year for Canadian individuals, $365.00 per year for Canadian institutions, $250.00 for international individuals, $365.00 for international institutions and $125.00 per year for Canadian and foreign students/residents. To receive student/resident rate, orders must be accompanied by name of affiliated institution, date of term, and the *signature* of program/residency coordinator on institution letterhead. Orders will be billed at individual rate until proof of status is received. Foreign air speed delivery is included in all *Clinics* subscription prices. All prices are subject to change without notice. POSTMASTER: Send address changes to *The Surgical Clinics of North America*, W.B. Saunders Company, Periodicals Fulfillment, Orlando, FL 32887-4800. **Customer Service: 1-800-654-2452 (US). From outside of the US, call 1-407-345-1000.**

The Surgical Clinics of North America is also published in Spanish by McGraw-Hill Interamericana Editores S.A., P.O. Box 5-237 06500 Mexico D.F. Mexico; and in Portuguese by Interlivros Edicoes Ltda., Rua Comandante Coelho 1085, CEP 21250, Rio de Janeiro, Brazil; and in Greek by Paschalidis Medical Publications, Athens Greece.

The Surgical Clinics of North America is covered in *Index Medicus, EMBASE/Excerpta Medica, Current Contents/Clinical Medicine, Current Contents/Life Sciences, Science Citation Index*, and *ISI/BIOMED.*

Printed in the United States of America.

Your *Clinics* subscription just got better!

You can now access the FULL TEXT of this publication online at no additional cost! Activate your online subscription today and receive...

- Full text of all issues from 2002 to the present
- Photographs, tables, illustrations, and references
- Comprehensive search capabilities
- Links to MEDLINE and Elsevier journals

Activate Your Online Access Today!

Plus, you can also sign up for E-alerts of upcoming issues or articles that interest you, and take advantage of exclusive access to bonus features!

To activate your individual online subscription:

1. Visit our website at **www.TheClinics.com**.

2. Click on "Register" at the top of the page, and follow the instructions.

3. To activate your account, you will need your subscriber account number, which you can find on your mailing label (note: the number of digits in your subscriber account number varies from six to ten digits). See the sample below where the subscriber account number has been circled.

This is your subscriber account number

```
********************************************3-DIGIT 001
FEB00   J0167   C7   ( 123456-89 )  10/00   Q: 1

J.H. DOE, MD
531 MAIN ST
CENTER CITY, NY  10001-001
```

4. That's it! Your online access to the most trusted source for clinical reviews is now available.

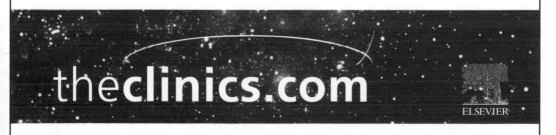

theclinics.com

ELSEVIER

CONSULTING EDITOR

RONALD F. MARTIN, MD, Staff Surgeon, Department of Surgery, Marshfield Clinic, Marshfield, Wisconsin; Clinical Associate Professor of Surgery, University of Vermont, Burlington, Vermont; Lieutenant Colonel, Medical Corps, United States Army Reserve

GUEST EDITOR

RODNEY J. LANDRENEAU, MD, Professor of Surgery, Division of Thoracic and Foregut Surgery, Shadyside Medical Center, University of Pittsburgh; Director of the Comprehensive Lung Center, University of Pittsburgh Shadyside Medical Center, Pittsburgh, Pennsylvania

CONTRIBUTORS

MARK S. ALLEN, MD, Division of General Thoracic Surgery, Mayo Clinic College of Medicine, Rochester, Minnesota

NASSER ALTORKI, MD, Professor of Cardiothoracic Surgery, Weill Medical College of Cornell University, New York, New York

PERCIVAL O. BUENAVENTURA, MD, Section of Thoracic Surgery, University of Pittsburgh Medical Center, Pittsburgh, Pennsylvania

STEPHEN D. CASSIVI, MD, Division of General Thoracic Surgery, Mayo Clinic College of Medicine, Rochester, Minnesota

NEIL A. CHRISTIE, MD, Assistant Professor of Surgery, Division of Thoracic and Foregut Surgery, Shadyside Medical Center, University of Pittsburgh, Pittsburgh, Pennsylvania

ALBERTO DE HOYOS, MD, Assistant Professor of Surgery, Director of Minimally Invasive Thoracic Surgery Center, Northwestern University, Chicago, Illinois

MARIO DEL PINO, MD, Division of Thoracic and Foregut Surgery, University of Pittsburgh Medical Center, Pittsburgh, Pennsylvania

STEVEN R. DEMEESTER, MD, Clinical Associate Professor, Department of Cardiothoracic Surgery, Keck School of Medicine, University of Southern California, Los Angeles, California

CLAUDE DESCHAMPS, MD, Division of General Thoracic Surgery, Mayo Clinic College of Medicine, Rochester, Minnesota

HIRAN C. FERNANDO, MD, FRCS, FACS, Associate Professor, Cardiothoracic Surgery, Boston University Medical Center, Boston, Massachusetts

ZIV GAMLIEL, MD, Assistant Professor of Surgery, Division of Thoracic Surgery, University of Maryland Medical Center, Baltimore, Maryland

CHUONG D. HOANG, MD, Resident, Section of General Thoracic Surgery, Division of Cardiovascular and Thoracic Surgery, University of Minnesota Medical School, Minneapolis, Minnesota

MARK D. IANNETTONI, MD, MBA, Johann L. Ehrenhaft Professor of Cardiothoracic Surgery; Chair, Department of Cardiothoracic Surgery, The University of Iowa Hospitals and Clinics, Iowa City, Iowa

PAUL S. KOH, MD, Fellow, Section of General Thoracic Surgery, Division of Cardiovascular and Thoracic Surgery, University of Minnesota Medical School, Minneapolis, Minnesota

MARK J. KRASNA, MD, Professor of Surgery; Head, Division of Thoracic Surgery, University of Maryland Medical Center, Baltimore, Maryland

KING F. KWONG, MD, FCCP, Director, Thoracic Surgery Research Laboratory, Greenebaum Cancer Center, University of Maryland School of Medicine, Baltimore, Maryland

RODNEY J. LANDRENEAU, MD, Professor of Surgery, Division of Thoracic and Foregut Surgery, Shadyside Medical Center, University of Pittsburgh; Director of the Comprehensive Lung Center, University of Pittsburgh Shadyside Medical Center, Pittsburgh, Pennsylvania

PATRICIA A. LIMPERT, MD, Division of General Surgery, Department of Surgery, St. Louis University Health Sciences Center, St. Louis, Missouri

JULES LIN, MD, General Surgery Research Fellow, Department of Surgery, Section of Thoracic Surgery, University of Michigan Medical Center, Ann Arbor, Michigan

VIRGINIA R. LITLE, MD, Assistant Professor of Surgery, Department of Cardiothoracic Surgery, Mount Sinai Medical Center, New York, New York

JAMES D. LUKETICH, MD, Professor of Surgery, Chief, Division of Thoracic and Foregut Surgery, University of Pittsburgh Medical Center, Pittsburgh, Pennsylvania

MICHAEL A. MADDAUS, MD, Professor and Chief, Section of General Thoracic Surgery, Division of Cardiovascular and Thoracic Surgery, University of Minnesota Medical School, Minneapolis, Minnesota

MARY S. MAISH, MD, Instructor in Surgery, Department of Surgery, Keck School of Medicine, University of Southern California, Los Angeles, California

KEITH S. NAUNHEIM, MD, Vallee L. and Melba Willman Professor; Chief, Division of Cardiothoracic Surgery, Department of Surgery, St. Louis University Health Sciences Center, St. Louis, Missouri

FRANCIS C. NICHOLS III, MD, Division of General Thoracic Surgery, Mayo Clinic College of Medicine, Rochester, Minnesota

BRANT K. OELSCHLAGER, MD, Director of the Center for Videoendoscopic Therapy, Director of the Swallowing Center, Assistant Professor, Department of Surgery, University of Washington, Seattle, Washington

PETER C. PAIROLERO, MD, Division of General Thoracic Surgery, Mayo Clinic College of Medicine, Rochester, Minnesota

AMIT N. PATEL, MD, MS, Resident in Thoracic Surgery, Section of Thoracic Surgery, University of Pittsburgh Medical Center, Pittsburgh, Pennsylvania

PAVLOS PAPASAVAS, MD, Assistant Professor of Surgery, Temple University School of Medicine at the Western Pennsylvania Hospital Clinical Campus, Pittsburgh, Pennsylvania

CARLOS A. PELLEGRINI, MD, Henry Harkins Professor and Chair, Department of Surgery, University of Washington, Seattle, Washington

RICARDO SANTOS, MD, Division of Thoracic and Foregut Surgery, University of Pittsburgh Medical Center, Pittsburgh, Pennsylvania

CONRAD M. VIAL, MD, Department of Cardiothoracic Surgery, Stanford University School of Medicine, Stanford, California

RICHARD I. WHYTE, MD, Department of Cardiothoracic Surgery, Stanford University School of Medicine, Stanford, California

TODD A. WOLTMAN, MD, PhD, Laparoscopic Fellow, Department of Surgery, University of Washington, Seattle, Washington

CONTENTS

treatment of choice for most patients. This article reviews the evaluation of patients who have achalasia, treatment options, and surgical techniques.

Esophageal diverticula can cause disabling symptoms. The authors describe here our preferred surgical approach for Zenker's and epiphrenic diverticula. For most patients, excision of the diverticulum and addition of a myotomy will result in a favorable functional outcome and a low recurrence rate.

This article reviews the indications and surgical techniques for esophageal replacement with a colon interposition or jejunal free graft. The advantages and disadvantages for each are examined, specific technical challenges that accompany each are highlighted, and the principles that promote a successful outcome are discussed.

Boerhaave's syndrome, or postemetic rupture of the esophagus, represents one of several etiologies of esophageal perforation. Early diagnosis, which requires both a high index of suspicion and contrast esophagography, is essential for optimal outcome. Primary repair is often possible, although other techniques, such as esophageal exclusion or diversion, may be appropriate in certain circumstances.

Functional problems following fundoplication primarily are dysphagia, gas bloat, diarrhea, and persistence or recurrence of the preoperative symptoms. These complaints can be debilitating, and may lead to reoperations and additional interventions. Prevention is the best remedy, and it can be achieved by proper patient selection and meticulous surgical technique.

the avoidance of thoracotomy and intrathoracic anastomosis. This article discusses the indications, diagnostic evaluation, and operative techniques for transhiatal esophagectomy. Potential complications as well as the results from large clinical series are also discussed.

The treatment of esophageal cancer remains controversial. Standard techniques of surgical resection are associated with a local recurrence rate of 30% to 60% and 5-year survival of 20% to 25%. The addition of induction therapy of any kind does not significantly alter these survival rates. This article examines the rationale, technique, and results of radical esophagectomy, including two-field and three-field lymph node dissection.

Cure rates in esophageal cancer remain low with surgical resection alone. Various combinations of surgery, chemotherapy, and radiotherapy have been used in an effort to improve treatment outcome. In this article, the results of various treatment modalities and of multimodality therapy are reviewed, and the importance of pre-treatment staging is discussed.

Advances in minimally invasive technology and surgical techniques have allowed surgeons to perform more complex procedures safely. Minimally invasive esophagectomy is a technically demanding operation requiring advanced laparoscopic and thoracoscopic skills.

Esophagectomy is the treatment of choice for cancer or high-grade dysplasia. Although the patients frequently experience symptoms postoperatively, their quality of life is most often comparable to that of a control population. This article provides details of post-esophagectomy symptomatology and examines how quality of life can be measured in these patients.

FORTHCOMING ISSUES

RECENT ISSUES

ELSEVIER
SAUNDERS

SURGICAL
CLINICS OF
NORTH AMERICA

Surg Clin N Am 85 (2005) xiii–xiv

Foreword

Esophageal Surgery

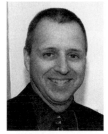

Ronald F. Martin, MD
Consulting Editor

We find ourselves at a time when surgery is undergoing tremendous change. This is happening in many specialties, but most sharply in general surgery. The nature of what constitutes a general surgical problem and who constitutes a general surgeon is evolving and morphing into a complex and sometimes difficult-to-answer question. We general surgeons represent a widely diverse population of professionals. We are found in academic centers and remote rural areas. We are young and older, male and female, full-time employees of large corporations and private practitioners. Many of us serve in administrative capacities in addition to our clinical responsibilities. We serve in civilian and military sectors. We serve those with and without resources. We serve those in need at home and abroad with tremendous volunteerism. We are all subject to the rapidly and unpredictably changing political and financial landscape of modern medicine.

The *Surgical Clinics of North America* has a long and proud tradition of providing a written mechanism for distributing knowledge to our colleagues in a format that has depth and breadth and is provided in a timely manner. It serves in that crucial position between the rapidly expanding source of individual journals and the encyclopedic nature of textbooks.

Elsevier, in its continued effort to produce the highest quality product, has requested the assistance of a Consulting Editor for this publication. The goal, as we move forward, will be to not only assure the high-quality clinical information that the *Surgical Clinics of North America* has become known for but also to assure that the materials presented are truly relevant to the practicing general surgeon. We shall also plan to incorporate some

doi:10.1016/j.suc.2005.03.001   *surgical.theclinics.com*

information that traditionally may not have found its place here; topics such as surgical training, public policy, medical litigation, and practice management. Above all, the intent of any change that we may make will be to elevate the discourse of our craft, outline the issues as they arise, and help us define a course to take during this confusing period in surgical history.

In this issue, Dr. Rodney Landreneau has assembled a collective review of esophageal disorders that should be of great interest to any surgeon who deals with diseases of the foregut. He and his fellow contributors distill a wealth of information and experience in the understanding and management of benign and malignant diseases of a potentially unforgiving organ.

As we venture into the future of general surgery, I would like to take a moment to quote the Introduction to the inaugural issue of the *Surgical Clinics of North America* (February 1921). In that introduction, Dr. William Williams Keen wrote: "It is a pleasure to survey the constantly growing medical literature by our American colleagues. ... I have seen all of this luxuriant growth from Gross' 'System of Surgery' (1859) down to the present time." Eighty-four years later, I would conclude that Dr. Keen's final wish—"May it always grow in value and be dedicated solely to the cause of Scientific Truth"—well summarizes our hopes as we move forward with this series.

Ronald F. Martin, MD
Department of Surgery
Marshfield Clinic
1000 North Oak Avenue
Marshfield, WI 54449, USA

E-mail address: martin.ronald@marshfieldclinic.org

SURGICAL
CLINICS OF
NORTH AMERICA

Surg Clin N Am 85 (2005) xv–xvi

Preface

Esophageal Surgery

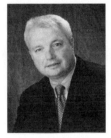

Rodney J. Landreneau, MD
Guest Editor

In this issue of the *Surgical Clinics of North America*, we explore the realm of surgery for diseases of the esophagus. Probably more than most areas of surgery, opinions range and controversy abound regarding the most appropriate management of esophageal problems.

The introduction of powerful antisecretory medications, which are possibly overprescribed for extended periods, and new endoscopic methods of "correcting" gastroesophageal reflux disease may change the nature of the patient population that is seen by esophageal surgeons. Accordingly, surgeons interested in the management of esophageal problems must keep pace with these developments and strive to improve the results of appropriate surgical treatment.

I feel fortunate to have been able to bring together the written opinions of an extremely experienced group of esophageal surgeons. I also believe that the combined independent, insightful accounts of the various problems surrounding the management of esophageal problems provided by the authorship are uniquely assimilated in this issue.

The surgical management of a variety of benign esophageal problems ranging from complex gastroesophageal reflux disease to primary motor disorders of the esophagus is discussed in this issue. In addition, special attention to the objective evaluation of the results of these surgical interventions is compared with that of medical management of these conditions. The various approaches to management of paraesophageal herniation and esophageal shortening are examined, as are the reconstructive options available to manage these problems. A detailed description of the situations in which jejunal and colonic substitutes for establishing alimentary continuity following esophageal resection are considered and the technical nuances regarding the performance of these reconstructions is provided.

This issue also contains an extensive review of the management trends for the treatment of esophageal carcinoma. The emerging concepts of molecular biologic prognostication and potential interventions are presented along with the present staging strategies for carcinoma of the esophagus. These efforts are understandably important as the use of multimodality therapy for carcinoma of the esophagus is examined elsewhere in this issue.

The various surgical strategies available for esophageal resection of esophageal carcinoma are also detailed, and the potential benefits and limitations of each surgical approach are thus made available. Finally, advances in techniques for palliation of esophageal carcinoma are provided, as is an appraisal of the quality of life following surgical treatment for carcinoma of the esophagus.

In gratitude to the contributors of this issue, it is my sincere hope that the information provided may encourage introspection and spark the inquisitive nature of present and future generations of esophageal surgeons striving to improve the treatment of patients who have esophageal disease.

Rodney J. Landreneau, MD
University of Pittsburgh
Pittsburgh, Pennsylvania
Comprehensive Lung Center
UPMC Shadyside
Shadyside Medical Center
5200 Centre Avenue, Suite 715
Pittsburgh, PA 15232, USA

E-mail address: landreneaurj@upmc.edu

ELSEVIER
SAUNDERS

Surg Clin N Am 85 (2005) 399–410

SURGICAL
CLINICS OF
NORTH AMERICA

Partial Versus Complete Fundoplication: Is There a Correct Answer?

Patricia A. Limpert, MD, Keith S. Naunheim, MD*

*Division of Cardiothoracic Surgery, Department of Surgery,
St. Louis University Health Sciences Center,
3635 Vista Avenue, St. Louis, MO 63110-0250, USA*

Gastroesophageal reflux disease (GERD) is one of the most common chronic disorders of the gastrointestinal tract, affecting an estimated 10% of the United States population [1]. Forty percent of symptomatic GERD patients develop erosive reflux esophagitis, with the potential sequelae of impaired quality of life, hemorrhage, peptic stricture formation, and Barrett's esophagus [1]. After diagnosis of GERD, patients generally require lifelong treatment. With the advent of proton pump inhibitors, some patients are able to heal esophagitis, with rare relapses. In those who cannot, laparoscopic antireflux surgery is a satisfactory maintenance therapy, and potentially the only option for patients who have medically refractory GERD.

The etiology of GERD is complex and multifactorial. Failure of the lower esophageal sphincter mechanism to protect the distal esophagus from the reflux of gastric juice is the greatest single factor in the pathogenesis of heartburn [2]. Other factors affecting the presence and severity of reflux include esophageal motility and the nature and volume of gastric contents. The symptoms of GERD are highly variable, as are the pathologic complications. Formal evaluation of symptomatic patients may be necessary to rule out cardiac and other gastroenterologic etiologies. Appreciating the presence and extent of pathologic alteration of esophageal mucosa requires endoscopic evaluation. A 24-hour pH probe records the presence and severity of acidic reflux, and esophageal manometry documents the adequacy of the lower esophageal sphincter (LES) and the propulsive ability of the esophageal body.

---

* Corresponding author.
E-mail address: naunheim@slu.edu (K.S. Naunheim).

0039-6109/05/$ - see front matter © 2005 Elsevier Inc. All rights reserved.
doi:10.1016/j.suc.2005.01.008
surgical.theclinics.com

Over the past 10 to 15 years, laparoscopic fundoplications have become the mainstay of surgical treatment for GERD. The Nissen fundoplication entails a complete 360° wrap, and is the most commonly performed procedure. Unfavorable postoperative sequelae, including gas bloat and dysphagia, have prompted the development of alternative procedures such as the partial fundoplication. The Toupet procedure is one such alternative. This article examines whether total or partial fundoplication is the better procedure for GERD. To assess relative efficacy, the results of these two procedures must be reviewed.

Nissen fundoplication

Nissen fundoplication is the most commonly used surgical procedure for the treatment of GERD. Although a circumferential wrap is employed in all Nissen procedures, there are a number of modifications reported. The procedure was originally described by Rudolf Nissen in 1956 as an open abdominal approach, but it has since been performed using laparoscopic technique. Traditionally, a 3- to 5-cm wrap was performed over a 38 to 50 French bougie. Because postoperative complaints of gas bloat and dysphagia occurred in up to 40% of patients, more recently a shorter "floppy" Nissen has been used. This entails construction of a 1.5- to 2-cm long wrap, often performed with a 52 to 60 French dilator in place. Patterson and colleagues [3] investigated the effect of using a bougie on postoperative dysphagia. In their series, 171 patients were prospectively blinded and randomized to a bougie group (56 French) versus a no-bougie group during fundoplication. After follow-up of 11 months, the bougie group reported a significant decrease in mild to moderate dysphagia (13% versus 31%) and in severe dysphagia (5% versus 14%).

Another modification from the traditional operation, which is still debated, includes division of the short gastric vessels. Watson and associates [4] enrolled 102 patients in a double-blind, randomized trial to determine the efficacy of short gastric vessel division in reducing dysphagia. They found no difference in postoperative dysphagia or overall satisfaction.

Recent studies demonstrated good results with up to 95% relief of symptoms after Nissen fundoplication. Table 1 depicts a number of recent series to evaluate mid- to long-term outcomes after laparoscopic Nissen fundoplication. Good to excellent results are reported in 85% to 90% of patients for up to 6 years following surgery. More precise outcomes have been reported by Granderath and other investigators using the Gastrointestinal Quality of Life Index (GIQLI) [5,6]. Granderath prospectively studied a cohort of 150 patients undergoing laparoscopic Nissen fundoplication. The GIQLI scores improved significantly, from preoperative scores of 90.1 ± 8.9 points to a mean of 123.7 ± 9.8 points at a 3-year follow-up. These improved scores compare with those points designated by healthy

Table 1
Clinical results of laparoscopic Nissen fundoplication

Study	Follow-up (years)	Number	Recurrence of reflux n (%)	Dysphagia n (%)	Reoperation n (%)	Flatulence n (%)	Dilation n (%)	Outcome excellent/good
Beldi [23] (2002)	3.6	55	3 (5)	13 (25)		33 (60)		
Granderath [5] (2002)	3	150		5 (3.3)	2 (1.3)	7 (4.6)		98%
Lafullarde [24] (2001)	6	166	21 (13)	18 (11)	27 (15)			90%
Anvari [25] (2003)	5	181	21 (12)	8 (4.4)	6 (3.3)		6 (3.3)	86%
Bammer [26] (2001)	5	171	11 (5.8)	(27)	3 (1.8)		12 (7)	93%

individuals, scoring 122.6 ± 8.5 points. The Granderath group [5] also documented significantly improved LES pressures.

Review of these clinical series, however, reveals that the Nissen fundoplication is a good but not perfect operation. Clinically scientific dysphagia was reported in 3% to 25% of patients (although definitions varied between reports), and reoperation occurred in up to 15% of patients. Despite these drawbacks, the Nissen procedure is performed by many surgeons across multiple continents, and it is considered the gold standard to which partial fundoplication must be compared.

Toupet fundoplication

Techniques of partial fundoplication originated in the mid 1960s as alternatives to the Nissen procedure [2]. The frequency of postoperative dysphagia and the occasional requirement for dilation or reoperation influenced surgical investigators to seek a less obstructive form of wrap that would still provide protection from reflux. Multiple techniques with an array of partial wraps have been described in the literature, but currently the most prevalent alternative appears to be the Toupet procedure. This is described as a 270° posterior fundoplication, with crural closure and fixation of the wrap to the closure. Its physiologic efficacy has been demonstrated in a prospective trial by Lindenboom and coworkers [7]. They demonstrated that the Toupet procedure significantly increases LES pressure during both fasting and postprandial periods.

Table 2 depicts recent trials evaluating the outcomes after laparoscopic Toupet fundoplication. This table represents studies from Klapow [8], Bell [9], Franzen [10], and Jobe [11] and their coauthors. All of the groups were performing the Toupet procedure routinely for GERD. Early short-term results after a partial fundoplication demonstrate good control of reflux symptoms and fewer complaints of flatulence and dysphagia; however, with longer follow-up these studies show that the control of symptoms may not be as prolonged, with recurrent reflux in 8% to 20% of patients.

Comparison of the results from the Toupet series to those of the Nissen series suggests roughly equivalent reflux control with the suggestion of lesser incidence of dysphagia in the Toupet patients; however, there also appears to be a slightly higher incidence of reoperation in the Toupet reports, which might reflect a higher incidence of wrap failure and recurrent reflux.

Unfortunately, these comparisons do not really allow for firm and definitive conclusions regarding the superiority of one procedure over the other. Multiple confounding factors, such as differing lengths of follow-up, variable surgical techniques (with or without short gastric division, routine crural closure, or dilator use), and inconstant definitions of outcome parameters (ie, recurrent reflux, dysphagia) prevent hard and fast determinations of relative efficacy.

Table 2
Clinical results of laparoscopic Toupet fundoplication

Study	Follow-up (years)	Number	Recurrence of reflux n (%)	Dysphagia n (%)	Reoperation n (%)	Regurgitation n (%)	Heartburn n (%)	Medication n (%)	Outcome good/excellent
Klapow [1] (2002)	2.9	55	11 (20)	7 (12.7)		18 (33)	27 (61%)	18 (32.7)	88%
Jobe [11] (1997)	22 months	74	10 (13.5)	7 (9)			15 (20)		
Granderath [5] (2002)	1–5	155		3 (1.9)	4 (2.6)	(5.2)	4 (2.6)	4 (2.6)	
Bell [9] (1999)	30 months	143	19 (13.3)	2 (1.4)	20 (14)		0		
Franzen [10] (1999)	10	101	7 (8)	11 (1.1)	3 (3.0)	0	0		

Perhaps the most helpful information emanates from those studies directly comparing the two procedures.

Nissen versus Toupet in patients who have normal motility

There have been several clinical trials directly comparing total and partial fundoplications. Lundell and associates [12] studied 137 patients who had GERD prospectively in a randomized clinical trial with a mean follow-up of 3 years. These patients all underwent an open abdominal operation; 65 had a Nissen-Rosetti (complete fundoplication without short gastric division) and 72 underwent a Toupet. The investigators found significantly higher LES basal pressure at 6 months in patients having a total fundic wrap, but there was no difference in the incidence of recurrent reflux that was noted in 6% and 5% of patients who had partial and total fundoplications, respectively. A bougie dilator was not used to "size" the wrap in either group, and dysphagia was more frequently reported at 3 months in patients undergoing a Nissen-Rossetti (47% versus 19%, $P < 0.01$), but this difference disappeared thereafter. Six patients required reoperation: 1 in the Toupet group secondary to severe gas bloat, and 5 patients in the Nissen-Rossetti group because of thoracic herniation. This study has been criticized because patients did not undergo a routine crural repair, an omission that may have led to the high reoperation rate.

Hagedorn and colleagues [13] published long-term results from a prospective, randomized clinical trial of 110 patients, completing a median follow-up of 11.5 years: 54 had a total wrap (Nissen-Rossetti) and 56 underwent a partial wrap (Toupet). Seven patients required reoperation, 5 in the Nissen-Rossetti group and 2 in the Toupet group. Control of heartburn was achieved in 88% and 92% in the total and partial fundoplication groups, respectively. There was no difference observed in dysphagia scoring, although there was a significant increase in the prevalence of flatulence and postprandial fullness in those undergoing a total fundoplication ($P < 0.001$ and $P < 0.03$, respectively).

Zornig and coworkers [14] reported similar findings after a prospective randomized trial comparing fundoplication procedures in 200 patients, 100 of whom had abnormal preoperative esophageal motility, and 100 of whom had normal motility. The early follow-up at 4 months for the normal motility subgroup (n = 100) is depicted in Table 3, and the abnormal motility (n = 100) subgroup is shown in Table 4. The postoperative requirement for esophageal dilatation and reoperation was not substratified to the groups who had and did not have motility disorders. Postoperative dysphagia was more frequent following Nissen fundoplication (30% versus 11%, $P < 0.001$), and dilation was required in 14 patients who had a Nissen and 5 patients who had a Toupet. Fourteen patients required reoperation, 13 after a Nissen and 1 after a Toupet. At reoperation, 10 patients were

Table 3
Results at four months in normal motility subgroup

Results	Toupet fundoplication (n = 50) n (%)	Nissen fundoplication (n = 50) n (%)	P value
Recurrent reflux	4 (8%)	2 (4%)	NS
LES resting pressure (mmHg)	17.0	16.6	NS
Dysphagia	3 (6%)	16 (32%)	P < 0.01
Patient satisfaction	46 (92%)	45 (90%)	

Abbreviation: NS, not significant.

found to have herniation of the wrap through a disrupted crural closure. Four patients required a conversion from total to partial fundoplication secondary to prolonged dysphagia. In this study, a 46 Fr stent was placed in the esophagus for calibration, and crural fixation of the wrap was only performed in the Toupet subgroup.

Farrell and colleagues [15] prospectively examined a cohort of GERD patients undergoing a Nissen (n = 465) or Toupet (n = 44) fundoplication. These patients were stratified into groups on the basis of baseline esophageal motility. Heartburn and regurgitation were similarly improved in both groups at 6 weeks follow-up, but dysphagia was more prevalent among Nissen patients (45% versus 25%, P < 0.01). After 1 year, patients in the Toupet subgroup reported more heartburn (18% versus 8%, P < 0.05) and regurgitation (20% versus 8%, P = 0.06) than the Nissen patients. The incidence of dysphagia had returned to similar values in the groups (P = 0.58). Reoperation rates in Toupet (1.3%) and Nissen (4.2%) patients were not significantly different (P = 0.35).

Fernando et al [16] also reported an increased incidence of recurrent reflux symptoms after Toupet during long-term follow-up. In their study, a Nissen cohort (n = 163) and Toupet cohort (n = 43) were followed over a mean of 19.7 months and long-term results were available in 142 patients (114 Nissen, 28 Toupet). There was a significantly larger proportion of patients in the Toupet group who had decreased esophageal motility, which was the primary indication for partial fundoplication. Early outcomes were similar between the groups, but with time, a higher incidence of heartburn, regurgitation, bloating, and flatulence were reported in the Toupet group. A significant increase of dysphagia (34.5% versus 15%, P < 0.05) and

Table 4
Results at four months in abnormal motility subgroup

Results	Toupet fundoplication (n = 50) n (%)	Nissen fundoplication (n = 50) n (%)	P value
Recurrent reflux	8 (17.4)	4 (8.7)	
LES resting pressure (mmHg)	13.4	16.5	
Dysphagia	8 (16)	14 (28)	
Patient satisfaction	44 (88)	43 (86)	

increased usage of proton pump inhibitors (38% versus 20%, $P < 0.05$) were also reported in the Toupet group. A total of 14 patients reported dissatisfaction with their procedure; 8 patients (7%) in the Nissen group and 6 patients (21%) in the Toupet group ($P < 0.05$). It is important to note that in this report there was a significant increased incidence of motility disorders in the Toupet group (37.2% versus 8.6%, $P < 0.05$); however, upon comparison of the subgroups, there were no differences in the preoperative quality of life survey scores, symptoms, and medication usage.

Kamolz and coauthors [17,18] have reported quality of life data at 1 and 5 years following fundoplication. These investigators used the GIQLI, which has become a common instrument to measure the quality of life in patients who have gastrointestinal disease. The instrument has been tested and validated as a trilingual questionnaire (German, English, and French) containing 36 questions divided into five subdimensions (gastrointestinal symptoms, general physical symptoms, emotional status, social functions, and a single item for the disease specific symptoms). This response is graded from 0 to 144 points. The GIQLI data were collected for 175 patients undergoing laparoscopic floppy Nissen (n = 107) or Toupet (n = 68) fundoplication. The analysis showed that GERD patients had a low GIQLI preoperatively in comparison with healthy individuals (mean 90.4 versus 122.6 points). The scores improved significantly 6 weeks postoperatively, continued to improve at 3 months, and remained stable at 1 year (mean 123.1 points, $P < 0.01$) postoperatively. There were no differences in the quality of life between the groups. At the 5-year publication, 104 patients were followed in the Nissen group and 65 patients in the Toupet group. At this time point, the GIQLI score remained stable, with mean scores of 121 ± 8.7 points in the Nissen group and 119.8 ± 9 points in the Toupet group. Table 5 represents general outcome assessments for these groups.

Table 5
Clinical results at five years

Results	Nissen fundoplication (n = 104) n (%)	Toupet fundoplication (n = 65) n (%)
New onset symptoms		
Mild to moderate	4 (3.8%)	2 (3.1%)
Dysphagia		
Flatulence	2 (1.9%)	2 (3.1%)
Bloating	2 (1.9%)	2 (3.1%)
Recurrent symptoms	0 (0%)	5 (7.7%)
Reoperation	1 (0.9%)	3 (4.6%)
Antireflux medication	0 (0%)	2 (3.1%)
Patient satisfaction, %		
Excellent	75.9	73.8
Good	22.1	23.1
Fair	1.9	3.1

Patients who have esophageal dysmotility

The relationship between esophageal dysmotility and outcomes after laparoscopic fundoplication continues to be studied. Although poor motility was originally thought to be an indication to do a partial fundoplication, studies continue to test this hypothesis. Prospective, randomized studies are few, with conflicting results regarding superiority of partial fundoplication over the total fundic wrap in terms of preventing dysphagia in patients who have GERD and impaired esophageal peristalsis.

Chrysos and colleagues [19] studied 33 consecutive patients who had proven GERD and poor motility, defined as low amplitude (<30 mmHg) contractions in the distal esophagus. Such patients were prospectively randomized to undergo either Toupet fundoplication (n = 19) or Nissen fundoplication (n = 14). Results at 3 months favored the Toupet group. The incidences of dysphagia (57% versus 16%) and gas-bloat syndrome (50% versus 21%) were significantly higher after Nissen than Toupet ($P <$ 0.01 and $P = 0.02$, respectively.) Also at 3 months, the Toupet group was significantly more satisfied with the operation than those after Nissen (79% versus 71%, $P < 0.04$). These outcomes changed dramatically by the 12-month follow-up, however, at which time the results were virtually identical (Table 6).

Oleynikov and associates [20] prospectively evaluated 96 patients who had defective peristalsis undergoing either partial (n = 39) or total (n = 57) fundoplication. At postoperative evaluation, heartburn scores and distal esophageal acid exposure improved significantly in both groups, although the total fundoplication group's heartburn scores were significantly better than those of the partial fundoplication group. In addition, dysphagia and distal esophageal amplitudes were significantly improved in the total fundoplication group, but not in the partial group. Two patients who had a partial fundoplication underwent reoperation and conversion to total fundoplication secondary to persistent heartburn. Therefore, Oleynikov and associates suggest that total, not partial, fundoplication should be the treatment of choice in patients who have GERD and defective peristalsis.

Table 6
Clinical results at one year

Results	Toupet fundoplication (n = 19)	Nissen fundoplication (n = 14)	P value
Patient satisfaction n (%)			
Excellent	14 (73.6)	10 (71.4)	NS
Good	3 (15.8)	3 (21.4)	NS
Fair	1 (5.3)	0 (0)	NS
Poor	1 (5.3)	1 (7.1)	NS
Recurrent reflux	0	0	NS
Dysphagia	16%	14%	NS
LES mmHg	39 ± 12	38 ± 12	NS

In agreement with Oleynikov, Goss and coworkers [21] reported a retrospective case-control study of 22 patients who had poor esophageal motility and underwent a complete fundoplication compared with patients who had normal motility. The preoperative mean esophageal body pressures were 42.1 and 87.5 mmHg in the study and control groups, respectively ($P <$ 0.05). The patients were then followed postoperatively with a quality-of-life questionnaire. Average time to resolution of dysphagia was 10.1 weeks in the study group and 12 weeks in the control group. All patients but 1 in the control group graded their life quality improvement as good to excellent. Thus, these investigators concluded that complete fundoplication is a good option, even in patients who have impaired motility.

Fibbe and colleagues [22] investigated the postoperative effects of fundoplication on esophageal motor function. Two hundred patients were stratified in accordance with presence or absence of esophageal dysmotility and randomized to either a Nissen or Toupet fundoplication. At a 4-month follow-up, reflux recurrence was similar between the abnormal and normal motility groups (21% versus 14%.) Esophageal motility remained unchanged in 85% of patients and changed from pathologic to normal in 20 (10 Nissen/10 Toupet) patients, and from normal to pathologic in 9 (8 Nissen/1 Toupet) patients. Fibbe concluded that in patients who have GERD, esophageal dysmotility does not consistently affect clinical outcome and may be either improved or instigated as a result of fundoplication.

Summary

Gastroesophageal reflux disease is a common disorder, and patients diagnosed with GERD face a lifelong treatment requirement. A surgical antireflux procedure may be offered as an alternative to lifelong treatment with proton-pump inhibitors. Many investigations have been performed to help discover the best surgical alternative to medical management. An ideal antireflux procedure should be safe, effective, durable, and result in minimal complications.

Total fundoplication in the form of Nissen fundoplication is the most widely used antireflux operation worldwide. Although its efficacy is well documented, the clinical success rate in terms of reflux control is occasionally compromised by troublesome mechanical side effects. Because of these unsatisfactory symptoms and continued hindered quality of life, the Nissen fundoplication has undergone many modifications. The current standard appears to be the 2 cm floppy Nissen; however, the alternative approach has been the use of a partial fundoplication, most frequently the Toupet procedure. Both the Nissen and Toupet fundoplications have proven to provide relief in the majority of patients, but each has its own drawback. Patients undergoing Nissen fundoplication have a higher incidence of dysphagia early after operation, although this appears to resolve

in most. The Toupet, on the other hand, may not be as durable, and may lead to the early re-emergence of symptoms.

The problem of post-Nissen dysphagia led many surgeons to believe that the Nissen night be contraindicated in patients who have dysmotility, because it would cause even greater dysphagia; however, recent articles have not demonstrated this to be the case. It seems that the floppy Nissen performed over a large bougie (56–60 Fr) with division of short gastrics and crural closure is an acceptable operation for reflux in both those who have normal motility and those who have mild to moderate dysmotility. Thus, for most patients who have GERD and normal motility, either procedure appears effective in the majority of patients; however, those patients who have severe dysmotilty disorders and who require an antireflux procedure (ie, scleroderma, postmyotomy achalasia) are likely best served with a partial fundoplication.

References

[1] Klapow JC, Wilcox CM, et al. Characterization of long-term outcomes after Toupet fundoplication: symptoms, medication use, and health status. J Clin Gastroenterol 2002;34: 509–15.

[2] Swanstrom LL. Partial fundoplications for gastroesophageal reflux disease: indications and current status. J Clin Gastroenterol 1999;29:127–32.

[3] Patterson EJ, Herron DM, Hansen PD, et al. Effect of an esophageal bougie on the incidence of dysphagia following Nissen fundoplication: a prospective blinded randomized clinical trial. Arch Surg 2000;135:1055–61.

[4] Watson DI, Pike GR, Baigrie RJ, et al. Prospective double-blind randomized trial of laparoscopic Nissen fundoplication with division and without division of short gastric vessels. Ann Surg 1997;173:242–55.

[5] Granderath FA, Kamolz T, Schweiger UM, et al. Quality of life, surgical outcome, and patient satisfaction three years after laparoscopic Nissen fundoplication. World J Surg 2002;26:1234–8.

[6] Eypasch E, Williams JI, Wood-Dauphinee S, et al. Gastrointestinal quality of life index: development, validation, and application of a new instrument. Br J Surg 1995;82:216–22.

[7] Lindeboom MA, Ringers J, Straathof JWA, et al. Effect of laparoscopic partial fundoplication on reflux mechanisms. Am J Gastroenterol 2003;98:29–34.

[8] Klapow JC, Wilcox CM, Mallinger AP, et al. Characterization of long-term outcomes after Toupet fundoplication. J Clin Gastroenterol 2002;34:509–15.

[9] Bell RC, Hanna P, Mills MR, et al. Patterns of success and failure with laparoscopic Toupet fundoplication. Surg Endosc 1999;13:1189–94.

[10] Franzen T, Bostrom J, Tiggling G, et al. Prospective study of symptoms and gastroesophageal reflux 10 years after posterior partial fundoplication. Br J Surg 1999;86:956–60.

[11] Jobe BA, Wallace J, Hansen PD, et al. Evaluation of laparoscopic Toupet fundoplication as a primary repair for all patients with medically-resistant gastroesophageal reflux. Surg Endosc 1997;11:1080–3.

[12] Lundell L, Abramsson H, Ruth M, et al. Long-term results of a prospective randomized comparison of total fundic wrap (Nissen-Rossetti) or semifundoplication (Toupet) for gastro-oesophageal reflux. Br J Surg 1996;83:830–5.

[13] Hagedorn L, Lonroth H, Rydberg L, et al. Long term efficacy of total (Nissen-Rossetti) and posterior partial (Toupet) fundoplication: results of randomized clinical trial. J Gastrointest Surg 2002;6:540–5.

[14] Zornig C, Strate U, Emmermann A, et al. Nissen vs. Toupet laparoscopic fundoplication. Surg Endosc 2002;16:758–66.

[15] Farrell TM, Archer SB, Galloway KD, et al. Heartburn is more likely to recur after Toupet fundoplication than Nissen fundoplication. Ann Surg 2000;66:229–37.

[16] Fernando HC, Luketich JD, Christie NA, et al. Outcomes of laparoscopic Toupet compared to laparoscopic Nissen fundoplication. Surg Endosc 2002;16:905–8.

[17] Kamolz T, Bammer T, Wykypiel H, et al. Quality of life and surgical outcome after laparoscopic Nissen and Toupet fundoplication: one-year follow-up. Endoscopy 2000;32: 363–8.

[18] Kamolz T, Granderath FA, Bammer T, et al. "Floppy" Nissen vs. Toupet laparoscopic fundoplication: quality of life assessment in a 5-year follow-up. Endoscopy 2002;34:917–22.

[19] Chrysos E, Tsiaoussis J, Zoras OJ, et al. Laparoscopic surgery for gastroesophageal reflux disease patients with impaired esophageal peristalsis: total or partial fundoplication? J Am Coll Surg 2003;197:8–19.

[20] Oleynikov D, Eubanks TR, Szold A. Total fundoplication is the operation of choice for patients with gastroesophageal reflux and defective peristalsis. Surg Endosc 2002;16:909–13.

[21] Goss B, Shacham Y, Szold A. Complete fundoplication has similar long-term results in patients with and without esophageal body dysmotility. Surg Endosc 2003;17:567–70.

[22] Fibbe C, Layer P, Keller J, et al. Esophageal motility in reflux disease before and after fundoplication: a prospective randomized clinical and manometric study. Gastroenterology 2001;121:5–14.

[23] Beldi G, Glattli A. Long-term gastrointestinal symptoms after laparoscopic nissen fundoplication. Surg Laparosc Endosc Percutan Tech 2002;12:316–9.

[24] Lafullarde T, Watson DI, Jamieson GG, et al. Laparoscopic Nissen fundoplication: five-year results and beyond. Arch Surg 2001;136(2):180–4.

[25] Anvari M, Allen C. Five-year comprehensive outcomes evaluation in 181 patients after laparoscopic Nissen fundoplication. J Am Coll Surg 2003;196:51–7.

[26] Bammer T, Hinder RA, Klaus A, et al. Five- to eight-year outcome of the first laparoscopic Nissen fundoplications. J Gastrointest Surg 2001;5:42–8.

SURGICAL
CLINICS OF
NORTH AMERICA

ELSEVIER
SAUNDERS

Surg Clin N Am 85 (2005) 411–432

Management of Paraesophageal Hernias

Rodney J. Landreneau, MD*, Mario Del Pino, MD,
Ricardo Santos, MD

*Division of Thoracic and Foregut Surgery, University of Pittsburgh Medical Center,
Shadyside Medical Center, 5200 Centre Avenue, Pittsburgh, PA 15232, USA*

Paraesophageal hernias are relatively uncommon problems of the esophageal hiatus that deserve specific attention by surgeons and attending medical physicians caring for the patient who has this disorder. The recommendations for management of this problem depend on a variety of patient-related and hernia-related factors [1–4]. Appreciation of the unique nature of paraesophageal hernias, in contrast to the much more clinically common sliding hiatal hernia, is the first hurdle that must be overcome. To do so, an understanding of the anatomic and pathophysiologic nature of paraesophageal herniation is critical [3]. In this article, the authors delineate the unique clinical characteristics of paraesophageal hernias and review the clinical management arguments of interest today.

Anatomic/physiologic distinction of paraesophageal herniation

Paraesophageal hernias are truly extreme forms of hiatal herniation. A primary argument is whether paraesophageal hernias represent an exaggerated manifestation of the more common sliding hiatal, or a primary pathophysiologic process in itself. To better understand this argument, we must review the present anatomic classifications of hiatal hernias.

Type I: sliding hiatal hernias

These are by far the most common hiatal hernias, accounting for over 95% of patients who have this diagnosis. The sliding hiatal hernia is characterized by weakness and elongation of the phrenoesophageal ligamentous structures that are important in maintaining the normal intra-abdominal location of the

* Corresponding author.
E-mail address: landreneaurj@upmc.edu (R.J. Landreneau).

0039-6109/05/$ - see front matter © 2005 Elsevier Inc. All rights reserved.
doi:10.1016/j.suc.2005.01.006

gastroesophageal junction. This laxity of ligamentous support results in a variable migration of the gastroesophageal junction through a hiatal aperture that is variably widened (Fig. 1). In this scenario, there is no peritoneal lined "pocket," but merely an advancement of the gastroesophageal junction through the hiatus. In this respect, the sliding hiatal hernia is similar to the "direct" inguinal hernia, through which the retroperioneal aspect of the urinary bladder bulges forward because of a general weakness in the lower abdominal wall.

The driving force leading to progression of the hiatal hernia is increased intra-abdominal positive pressure, combined with the negative pressure normally present within the thoracic cavity. Sliding hernias are therefore more likely to progress or become symptomatic in obese patients and the pregnant patient, because of increased intra-abdominal pressure. Patients who have chronic cough are also prone to symptoms or progression of their sliding hiatal hernia, for similar reasons of increased intra-abdominal pressure. Sliding inguinal hernias are also prone to progression, as a result of increased intra-abdominal pressure related to the above factors, and the inability to freely void because of prostatic obstruction of the urethra.

The loss of phrenoesophageal ligament integrity with sliding hiatal hernias also leads to dysfunction in the lower esophageal sphincter. Accordingly, sliding hiatal hernias are primarily associated with functional gastrointestinal problems and the esophageal mucosal injury related to abnormal exposure of gastric refluxate.

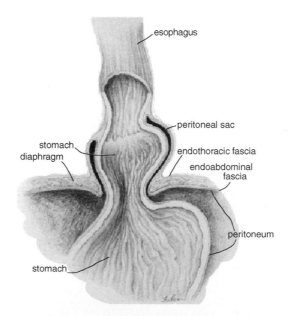

Fig. 1. Illustration of sliding hiatal hernia (Type I).

Type II: paraesophageal hernias

True Type II paraesophageal hernias are relatively uncommon, representing fewer than 5% of hiatal hernias in many clinical series [1]. These hiatal hernias are characterized by a relative preservation of the posterolateral component of the phrenoesophageal ligament, allowing for stabilization of the position of the gastroesophageal junction within the abdomen. A variably large peritoneal lined hernia sac anterior to a relatively normal position of the gastroesophageal junction is characteristic of Type II paraesophageal hernias (Fig. 2A, B). These hiatal hernias can be likened to the indirect inguinal hernia, in which a true hernia sac is present through an abdominal communication with the anatomic inguinal canal. As with indirect inguinal hernias, the important problems associated with paraesophageal hernias are physical and mechanical in nature. The usual organ affected by the paraesophageal hernia is the stomach, the fundic portion of which tends to herniated into this anteriorly located hernia sac and assume an "upside-down" relationship to the lower aspect of the stomach (Fig. 3). This anatomic derangement can lead to mechanical problems of gastric obstruction, chest pain, gastric incarceration, and possible gastric strangulation. These mechanical problems are similar to those of indirect inguinal and other true hernias of the abdominal cavity. Additionally, pulmonary dysfunction related to chronic aspiration and the intrathoracic space-occupying sequelae of the gastric displacement is also associated with paraesophageal herniation [5–7]. Occult gastric ulceration within the intrathoracic stomach or chronic

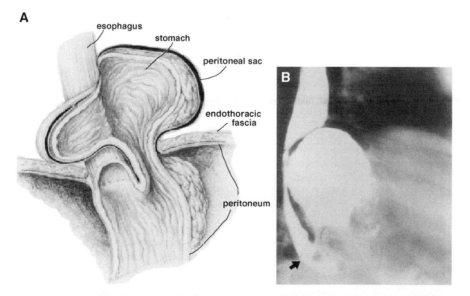

Fig. 2. (*A*) Illustration of true paraesophageal hernia (Type II). (*B*) Lateral contrast radiograph of Type II paraesophageal hernia, black arrow depicts location of gastroesophageal junction.

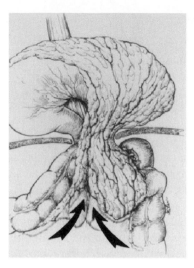

Fig. 3. Illustration of "upside down" stomach associated with intrathoracic fundic incarceration. Black arrows aid in understanding direction of ascent of abdominal organs through the enlarged esophageal hiatus.

mucosal venous engorgement can also result in anemia [8]. Finally, acute chest pain syndromes and syncope have been reported in association with giant paraesophageal herniation [9,10]. Notably, classic gastroesophageal reflex disease (GERD) symptoms of heartburn and regurgitation are less important complaints among Type II paraesophageal hernia patients. Some authors believe that this classification of Type II paraesophageal hernia is incorrect. They believe that such hernias merely reflect a more radical, chronic extension of the general sliding hiatal hernia process. The preservation of the normal location of the gastroesophageal junction speaks against this, as does the infrequently reported occurrence of this paraesophageal anatomic defect in newborns. It is speculated that developmental abnormality, combined with a basic defect in the collagen/elastin integrity of these individuals, may lead to the development of Type II paraesophageal hernias [11,12]. Interestingly, the authors have noted a more common occurrence of other "true" abdominal hernias (ie, umbilical, indirect inguinal) among our patients who have paraesophageal hernias compared with our patients who have sliding hiatal hernias referred for surgical correction. This leads us to believe that these patients who have true paraesophageal hernias may have a more general derangement in their connective tissue integrity than those who have sliding hiatal hernias.

Type III: combined sliding and paraesophageal hiatal hernias

This anatomic classification possibly represents the largest grouping of patients classified with paraesophageal hernias. These patients have migration of the gastroesophageal junction cephalad through the esophageal hiatus as the sliding component of the pathology, and a large true hernia sac anterior to this sliding component associated with the gastric herniation typical of Type II hiatal hernias (Fig. 4). Although these patients commonly complain of typical GERD symptoms, it remains clear that the most important symptoms and potentially adverse consequences are related to the mechanical aspects of the patient's paraesophageal herniation. Management of these patients' problems should be directed toward relief of GERD symptoms and correction of the mechanical aberrations inherent to the paraesophageal herniation.

Type IV: complex paraesophageal hiatal hernias

Type IV paraesophageal hernias are defined by the intrathoracic herniation of other organs, such as the colon, omentum, small bowel, spleen, and liver, into the true anterior hernia sac of the paraesophageal hernia (Fig. 5A, B). As with the Type III or II paraesophageal hernia, this pathologic process may or may not be associated with a sliding hiatal hernia. The uniqueness of the Type IV hernia relates to the extent of the process and the unusual complications that may be associated with the process [13].

Parahiatal hernias

These are extremely uncommon hiatal hernias defined by the presence of a normal hiatus and gastroesophageal junction with the presence of a "true" hernia defect through the diaphragm lateral to the hiatal crura. Although this problem had been described in earlier reports of surgical management of hiatal hernia problems, many surgeons were skeptical of their true existence.

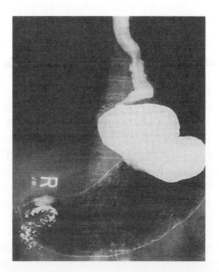

Fig. 4. Contrast radiograph of combined sliding and paraesophageal herniation (Type III).

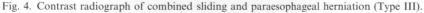

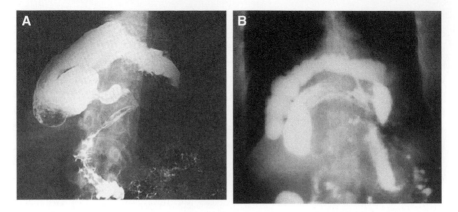

Fig. 5. (*A*) Complex paraesophageal hernia (Type IV). (*B*) Contrast radiograph demonstrating stomach and colon within paraesophageal hernia.

These skeptics felt that this hernia defect was a misinterpretation of the anatomic situation encountered by the reporting investigators. Documentation of the validity of this pathologic hiatal defect has recently occurred as a consequence of videoscopic approaches to hiatal hernia problems [14].

For the purposes of this article, the authors focus attention on those hiatal hernias with important paraesophageal components—Types II through IV.

Clinical features of paraesophageal hernias

Surgical series reporting the management of primary paraesophageal herniation usually reveal a patient population older than GERD patients who have sliding hiatal hernias that are undergoing surgical management. Some investigators have reported their belief that paraesophageal hernias are merely a natural extension of the more common sliding hiatal hernias. If a direct association between sliding and paraesophageal hernias exists, why is it that these older patients who have paraesophageal hernias usually deny medically recalcitrant GERD symptoms? Although many of these patients describe a remote a history of some GERD symptoms, most of them consider their GERD symptoms as insignificant. This fact is particularly perplexing when one considers that the anatomic derangement around the esophageal hiatus is considerably more extreme among paraesophageal hernia patients than among patients who have sliding hiatal hernias. Although the authors do not completely accept this concept, those favoring a direct association with sliding hiatal hernias argue that the paucity or loss of significant GERD symptoms among paraesophageal hernia patients relates to progressive obstruction of the esophagogastric junction by the displaced gastric fundus. Their conception is that this obstruction ultimately converts the patient's primary symptoms from regurgitation and heartburn to symptoms of dysphagia and chest pain. Indeed, most patients presenting for surgical management of paraesophageal herniation do have a long history of "hiatal hernia" that has been observed and treated medically for several years. The authors do admit that this pathophysiologic scenario may be of importance among patients who have combined sliding and paraesophageal hiatal hernias (Type III).

The authors believe that the key feature distinguishing the primary paraesophageal hiatal hernia variants described from sliding hiatal hernias involves the relative preservation of the posterolateral phrenoesophageal attachments around the gastroesophageal junction among paraesophageal hernia patients. The absence of significant GERD symptoms early in life, and the development of primarily mechanical problems later in life from herniation of the gastric fundus into a large "true" hernia sac through the enlarged diaphragmatic hiatus support the notion of the unique nature of paraesophageal hernias. Indeed, the primary presenting complaints of patients who have paraesophageal hernias usually relate to the space-occupying nature of the herniation within the chest, causing dyspnea or chest pain. Obstruction of the stomach resulting in dysphagia, gastric ulceration, pulmonary aspiration risk, and possible vascular compromise of the organo-axially rotated stomach within the hernia sac are other important clinical features of paraesophageal hernias.

Most patients who have paraesophageal hernias are symptomatic; however, a minority of patients may be minimally symptomatic, and the condition may go unnoticed until an incidental radiological evaluation reveals an unexplained air-fluid level behind the cardiac silhouette (Fig. 6A, B). This air-fluid level is representative of the herniated upside-down gastric fundus within the posterior mediastinum. In support of this clinical appraisal, an insightful clinical series reporting the management of massive paraesophageal hernias [15] revealed that only 5% of patients in the series were asymptomatic. The primary symptoms of the patients in this series related to organo-axial malrotation of the herniated stomach, with resultant incarceration or obstruction. The clinical symptoms of these patients were in accordance with those described earlier (ie, postprandial fullness, epigastric/substernal chest pain, dysphagia, iron deficiency anemia, and regurgitation with aspiration). Most of the patients in this series who have iron deficiency anemia reported no history of hematemesis or melena; however; patients who have a paraesophageal hernia may infrequently complain of hematemesis secondary to ulceration or ischemia of the herniated gastric mucosa.

The physical examination of paraesophageal hernia patients is usually unrevealing, unless significant complications have occurred. At presentation, a clinical finding of significant chest or upper abdominal pain with an inability to vomit is classic for gastric incarceration within the paraesophageal hernia sac. The presence of a large retrocardiac air-fluid level in association with these primary complaints is worrisome for gastric incarceration. The inability to

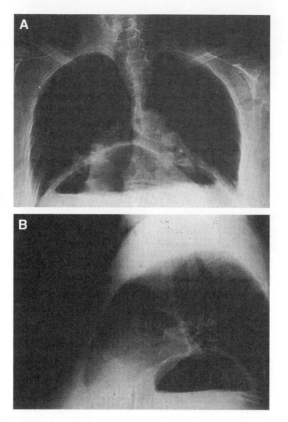

Fig. 6. (A) Typical chest roentgenogram demonstrating retrocardiac air-fluid level related to paraesophageal herniation. (B) Lateral chest roentgenogram demonstrating retrocardiac air-fluid level within incarcerated extrathoracic stomach.

pass a nasogastric tube to decompress the stomach also supports a diagnosis of gastric incarceration. This clinical triad is known as the Borchardt triad, after the individual who first described it in 1904 [15,16]. This constellation of symptoms and findings should lead to an urgent surgical consultation, because a clinical transition from incarceration to gastric strangulation is possible [17–20]. Prompt surgical exploration, and surgical reduction of the incarcerated stomach and repair of the paraesophageal hernia process are generally recommended in this circumstance. The reported greater-than-40% likelihood of developing significant complications related to the patient's paraesophageal hernia has led many to recommend elective surgical management in all but the most physiologically impaired patients [21–23].

Evaluation of the patient who has paraesophageal herniation

As mentioned, most patients who have paraesophageal herniation come to a diagnosis of this problem serendipitously. The paraesophageal hernia patient is almost universally misdiagnosed for some time as having an "ordinary" but large hiatal hernia, until the patient develops important symptoms, or until a discerning physician investigates in greater detail the patient's abnormal chest roentgenographic findings characteristic of para-esophageal herniation. Most medical physicians and gastrointestinal special-ists poorly understand the clinical importance and pathophysiologic nature of paraesophageal hernias. With these thoughts in mind, it is common for the authors to note that the patient who has a paraesophageal hernia comes to us after undergoing a negative cardiac work-up for chest pain, or an inconclusive investigation of recurrent respiratory problems. The occult anemia associated with the above complaints is noted to have confounded the diagnostic puzzle further. The medical team has ultimately been faced with evaluating the "funny-looking" hiatal hernia that has been ignored for some time.

The authors believe that barium contrast study of the upper gastroin-testinal tract is the most important diagnostic tool in evaluating the patient who has a presumed paraesophageal hernia. The barium esophagram can demonstrate the paraesophageal hernia in virtually all patients. In patients who have large paraesophageal hernia, an organo-axial volvulus was present in 50% to 97% [1,15,22]. The barium contrast study can also give important information regarding the location of the gastroesophageal junction suggestive of a pure (Type II) or combined (Type III) paraesophageal hernia. Although the actual determination of esophageal "shortening" is difficult in most circumstances, the barium esophagram can identify the more obvious instances of this problem. Additionally, the barium contrast study can give some indication of esophageal motor dysfunction, as evidenced by uncoordinated contractility of the esophageal body and poor esophageal clearance of contrast material. Occasionally, the barium study demonstrates the ominous finding of the "figure-of-8" incarceration of the upside down stomach (Fig. 7) [3,20]. This represents the partial descent of the gastric fundus out of the intrathoracic hernia sac and back into the abdomen. This phenomenon is associated with a twisting of the gastric blood supply to this area of the stomach. Unless rapid decompression of the stomach is accomplished, the possibility of strangulation of this incarcerated segment of the stomach is imminent. Urgent surgical management may be necessary if the situation is not remedied with nasogastric tube or endoscopic decompression.

Endoscopic evaluation is an important consideration before surgical repair. Variable degrees of esophageal mucosal inflammation may be found in 16% to 36% of patients [24], with Grade III or IV esophagitis reported in 29% of patients in one clinical series [15]. Identification of other associated pathology, such as esophageal stricture and cancer, is not uncommon. Indeed, approximately 3% of the authors' patients who have carcinoma of the gastroesophageal junction are found to have an associated large para-esophageal hernia. Many of these patients had their carcinomas identified

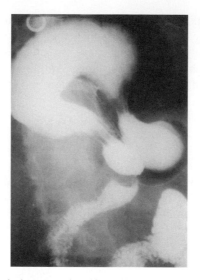

Fig. 7. Contrast radiograph demonstrating "figure-of-8 stomach" suggestive of incarceration with vascular compromise of the herniated stomach.

during the evaluation of what were considered recalcitrant symptoms from their paraesophageal hernias.

Standard catheter-based esophageal function testing is difficult to accomplish in paraesophageal hernia patients. Passage of the catheter through the gastroesophageal junction for assessment of lower esophageal sphincter function is usually unsuccessful. The primary indication for manometric testing in this setting is for the assessment of esophageal body peristaltic activity. Prolonged intraesophageal acid reflux monitoring is also of questionable importance among these patients, because acid reflux resulting from mechanical gastric antrum and fundic obstruction makes interpretation of the studies difficult, and certainly disqualifies any interpretation of this acid exposure as being related to a primarily defective lower esophageal sphincter mechanism. Accordingly, the authors have come to rely primarily on esophagogastric nuclear scintigraphy as our primary means of assessing esophagogastric motor function in this setting of paraesophageal herniation. These scintigraphic techniques are known as "esophageal transit" and "gastric emptying" nuclear studies. We use a semisolid transfer medium (scrambled eggs, Cream of Wheat, or grits) laced with a radioactive isotope. The patient swallows a bolus of the medium and is placed in front of a standard nuclear camera, and the time for transit and emptying are recorded and compared with accepted standard values. We have found these nuclear scintigraphic methods of assessment of esophageal function to be acceptable, particularly when the method of surgical repair involves the use of a partial fundoplication or "floppy" total fundoplication.

The recent work of Low and Simchuk [5] has demonstrated the salutary benefit on pulmonary function of surgical repair among patients who had paraesophageal hernia. Because of these important findings, we are now included pulmonary function testing as part of our standard preoperative assessment of paraesophageal hernia patients.

Treatment

There are several points of controversy regarding the most appropriate approach to management of paraesophageal herniation. Endoscopic reduction and percutaneous gastrostomy techniques have been described, but are certainly out of the realm of the standard of care [25]. Surgical correction of paraesophageal hernia correction remains the gold standard. Several basic surgical management concepts are generally accepted: reduction of the herniated abdominal viscera from the thorax, hernia sac excision, diaphragmatic crural repair, and gastropexy to prevent recurrence of the gastric herniation. Points of management controversy include the preference for a transthoracic versus a transabdominal approach, and the effectiveness of minimally invasive surgical approaches compared with standard open surgical approaches to repair. Additionally, the necessity of performing a fundoplication as part of basic repair of paraesophageal hernias has been argued. A further argument among advocates of fundoplication involves the question of the selection of a total or partial fundoplication following repair of the paraesophageal hernia. Prosthetic patch repair of the large hiatal hernia defect has also been both advocated and condemned in the literature. Finally, the use of an esophageal lengthening procedure as part of the standard surgical repair is debated. The authors have described the basic surgical concepts of repair in detail [1,3]. In this section of this review, we discuss each of these areas of management.

Transabdominal versus transthoracic repair

The argument over a transabdominal versus transthoracic approach to repair appears to be primarily colloquial in nature. It appears that the experience of the esophageal surgeon in the management of complex esophageal problems is the most important factor determining operative outcome. The authors have long held the belief that a slip of respiratory muscle should not be the territorial boundary determining the best approach to management of paraesophageal hernias, or decisive in determining which surgeon should perform a given procedure. We believe that the esophageal surgeon should be well-versed in both transabdominal and transthoracic approaches to management, in order to offer patients the opportunity for the best care.

Generally speaking, the acute and chronic discomfort associated with a thoracotomy approach is greater than that of an upper celiotomy [26]. The liberal use of perioperative epidural analgesia and the growing trend toward smaller lateral thoracotomy incisions among thoracic surgeons choosing transthoracic repair has reduced these pain-related differences in paraesophageal hernia repair.

Reviewing the literature, the authors find that excellent results have been obtained with both strategies. The abdominal approach to repair has been shown to have an effectiveness approaching 90% [20,21,27–29]. The central principles of repair described earlier are routinely applied. Authors variously support the addition of an antireflux procedure with the paraesophageal hernia management. Several investigators believe that most paraesophageal hernia patients are free of significant GERD symptoms, have minimal evidence of esophagitis, and lack impairment of the lower esophageal sphincter mechanism on manometric testing. They also report a much lower estimate of esophageal shortening than that of patients managed with a transthoracic approach to repair. These authors also believe that the performance of fundoplication goes beyond the effort for control of GERD, but also is a means of accomplishing gastropexy within the abdomen. When fundoplication is not performed, it is commonly recommended to include a pexing Stamm gastrostomy in these patients, as a means of maintaining gastric decompression and reducing the likelihood of gastric herniation after repair [3,23,27,28].

Those favoring a transthoracic approach also report excellent long-term results in the management of paraesophageal hernias [15,22,24,26,30,31]. They argue that greater mobilization of the esophagus can be accomplished with the transthoracic approach, to insure a tension-free return of the stomach and gastroesophageal junction into the abdomen. An antireflux procedure is necessary after the transthoracic approach, because the phrenoesophageal attachments are routinely disrupted during the dissection and mobilization of the stomach and esophagus. The inclusion of an antireflux procedure to the thoracic approach was felt necessary, because symptomatic reflux was commonly seen after primary repair only, as described by Allison [32]. In contrast to most reports of open abdominal repair of paraesophageal hernia, many surgeons using the transthoracic approach include a Collis esophageal lengthening procedure, because of their belief that esophageal shortening is associated with most paraesophageal hernias.

The authors frequently used either the abdominal or thoracic open approaches during our experience in surgically managing paraesophageal herniation before the laparoscopic surgical era [33]. The decision to choose one approach over the other was based on previous surgery in one cavity or another, associated pathologies needing to be addressed, or the presence of severe esophageal stricture and shortening documented by barium contrast studies. We generally believe that the visibility of the paraesophageal hernia through the chest during the course of mobilization and dissection of the esophagus tends to enhance the impression that esophageal shortening is present. The converse impression of associated esophageal shortening is true when one uses the transabdominal approach to repair paraesophageal hernias. The truth regarding important esophageal shortening and the need for gastroplasty is probably somewhere between these two impressions. Further discussion of this issue of esophageal shortening follows.

Antireflux procedure or not?

The argument regarding the use of an antireflux procedure as part of the surgical management of paraesophageal hernias has largely subsided. This is a result of the growing popularity of minimally invasive, laparoscopic approaches to this problem, in which some form of fundoplication has generally been included. It has resulted from the fact that the overwhelming preponderance of surgeons performing laparoscopic paraesophageal hernia surgery today have been primarily influenced by esophageal surgeons who believed an antireflux procedure was a vital aspect of the repair. It is, however, interesting to review this topic, which was heatedly debated in the not-too-distant past [34].

Investigators performing primarily transabdominal management of paraesophageal hernias have reported a low incidence of GERD symptoms and preoperative esophagitis among paraesophageal hernia patients (less than 20%) [27,28,34]. They reported successful management with reduction of the hernia, hernia sac excision, and repair of the hernia defect in over 90% of patients. Fundoplication was selectively used in that minority of patients who had significant GERD symptoms.

Most reports of a transthoracic approach to paraesophageal hernia repair include an antireflux procedure, although objective evidence indicates that esophagitis and important GERD symptoms are uncommon. This is best documented in the report by Allen et al [24], in which the primary complaints in over 90% of their 147 patients who had paraesophageal hernia undergoing repair were obstructive in nature. Only 23 (16% of their patients) had significant GERD complaints. Esophagitis was noted in only 4 of these 23 patients. Nevertheless, 98% of patients underwent fundoplication as part of their repair. Again, this inclusion of fundoplication is primarily related to the necessary disruption of phrenoesophageal attachments occurring with the thoracic approach, which does not necessarily occur with a transabdominal repair approach.

The most compelling objective evidence for the inclusion of an antireflux procedure with the paraesophageal hernia repair comes from the work of Walther and associates [35]. These investigators compared the manometric and 24-hour pH results of paraesophageal hernia patients and sliding hiatal hernia patients with a group of normal volunteers. There were fewer than 20 patients in each group. They found that 60% of paraesophageal hernia patients had abnormal 24-hour pH readings, compared with 70% of sliding hiatal hernia patients. The primary manometric finding among the paraesophageal hernia patients was the interpretation of a less-than-normal length of lower esophageal sphincter under the influence of intra-abdominal pressure. The other manometric findings were generally normal in nature among this small group of paraesophageal hernia patients. There was no specific account of the presence of esophagitis in the group. These authors concluded from their data that, "When urgent surgery is necessary, repair should include an anti-reflux procedure. If facilities and time permit, more specific evaluation of the cardia can be performed, and if competent, the repair should be limited to reduction of the stomach and closure of the defect" [35].

The authors generally agree with the conclusions of Walther and his colleagues; however, we must cast doubt on their interpretation of primary incompetence of the lower esophageal sphincter mechanism in their paraesophageal hernia patients. Certainly, the manometric abnormalities found were minimal in nature, and gastric outlet obstruction related to the mechanical derangement of the stomach within the hernia sac could account for the abnormal reflux seen. Additionally, it is erroneous to assume that the manometric and pH study analysis in this paraesophageal hernia patient population can be compared with the results of studies aiming to validate the utility of these parameters among patients who had simple sliding hiatal hernias and pathologic GERD [36,37]. It is not unreasonable to speculate that reduction of the hernia contents and repair of the hiatal hernia could restore relatively normal antireflux function for many of the paraesophageal patients in their study.

Total fundoplication or partial fundoplication?

Due to the difficulty in evaluating the esophageal function of para-esophageal patients with standard manometric techniques, and the common preoperative complaint of dysphagia, many esophageal surgeons have chosen to create a partial fundoplication, rather than undertake total fundoplication as part of their operative management. There has been little objective evidence to support this trend. In a review of the available literature, it does appear that the partial Toupet procedure may be associated with fewer functional problems than the total Nissen fundoplication among patients who have GERD and impaired esophageal motility; however, the overall durability of the Toupet procedure regarding control of acid reflux exposure may be slightly less reliable that the total Nissen fundoplication procedure [38–43].

The authors' concern with the potential for postoperative esophageal dysfunction among patients who have paraesophageal hernias leads us to use a partial fundoplication procedure in lieu of a total fundoplication in those patients without objective documentation of adequate esophageal peristalsis.

Open versus minimally invasive repair

There have been few comparisons between open and laparoscopic approaches to surgical correction of paraesophageal herniation. The most commonly noted comparison is that of Hashemi and coauthors [44]. This group reviewed the outcomes of 54 patients who had paraesophageal hernias managed by laparotomy, thoracotomy, or laparoscopic approaches. Half of these patients underwent laparoscopic repair, and the results of this group were compared with the open surgical cohorts, which were generally operated at an earlier date in the period of study, from 1985 through 1998. At a mean follow-up of 17 months, 42% of the laparoscopically managed patients had some evidence of hiatal herniation, compared with 15% of the patients who had open repairs, and who were followed on average for 35 months. The symptomatic outcomes of the open and laparoscopically treated patients were similar. Most of the hiatal hernia recurrences were small and sliding in nature.

This experience contrasts with that of more recent reports of laparoscopic management of paraesophageal hernias. Although the postoperative hernia rate was not evaluated, Schauer and coworkers [45] retrospectively compared the perioperative morbidity of paraesophageal hernia patients undergoing open and laparoscopic repair. These investigators noted a significant reduction in blood loss, intensive care unit stay, ileus, hospital stay, and overall morbidity when the laparoscopic approach was used, compared with open surgical approaches. Others have also come to appreciate the value of the laparoscopic approach to paraesophageal herniation. It is, however, commonly stated that this is a technically demanding intervention, requiring significant laparoscopic surgical experience. A strong fund of knowledge of the pathophysiology of hiatal hernia and GERD is also important for improved results, as is mature surgical judgment regarding the management of such complex disorders of the esophagus.

It appears that the hiatal hernia recurrence following laparoscopic repair of large paraesophageal hernias may be improving as experience with these approaches expands (Fig. 8). A recent report of laparoscopic management of 166 patients who had large paraesophageal hernias by Andugar et al [46] revealed symptomatic improvement in 93% of patients at a mean interval of 24 months. The radiographic evidence of some abnormality about the hiatus was seen in 20% of patients at a mean interval of 15 months. The vast majority of these hiatal hernias were small sliding hernias. Only 6 patients had radiographic evidence of a recurrent paraesophageal hernia. Two of these patients required reoperation. The results of this study appear to represent the trend in operative results among centers with extensive experience in the laparoscopic management of paraesophageal hernia and other complex esophageal pathologic conditions [47–53]. This trend is reflected further in the recent review of paraesophageal hernia management by Oelschlager and Pellegrini [54].

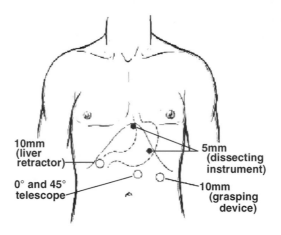

Fig. 8. Usual trocar positioning for laparoscopic management of paraesophageal hernia.

Prosthetic patch repair of hiatal hernia or not?

The hiatal hernia defect associated with paraesophageal hernias is large, and often difficult to repair. Repair of the hiatal hernia, or the failure thereof, is the defining point for success or failure in the management of paraesophageal hernias. Tension on the repair and postoperative stressors related to repair tension are primary etiologies for repair failure [55]. Although some have reported success with prosthetic mesh repair of the hiatal defect [56,57], the authors have avoided prosthetic mesh insertion favor of primary repair in nearly all of our patients. This appears to be the practice of most esophageal surgeons approaching repair of paraesophageal hernias. Although the risk may be small, esophagogastric erosion by the mesh is a potentially serious problem that we look to avoid by relying upon primary repair of the hernia.

Esophageal lengthening procedure or not?

The determination of clinically important esophageal shortening associated with the paraesophageal hernia process is difficult [58]. As mentioned, the perception of esophageal shortening may have a lot to do with the surgical approach chosen for paraesophageal repair. Thoracotomy series are dominated by the use of the Collis procedure [15,22,24,26,30,31], yet it is used in only a minority of series approaching paraesophageal hernias through the abdomen. Although there are laparoscopic surgical teams aggressively using Collis gastroplasty [59], for the most part this lengthening procedure is reported as a component of paraesophageal hernia repair in fewer than 5% of patients managed laparoscopically [43,44,46–51,53,54,60,61].

Although some investigators have stressed the importance of pre-operative barium contrast studies and manometric findings in predicting the clinical significance of esophageal shorting [15,22,30], Mittal and associates [62] have recently analyzed these parameters and the endoscopic findings of patients who had paraesophageal hernias being considered for surgical repair, and have found conflicting results. These investigators noted that esophagogastric barium contrast studies and manometry had positive predictive values for determining short esophagus of 37% and 25%, respectively. The most accurate preoperative determination for the need for an esophageal lengthening procedure was the endoscopic determination of esophageal stricture or Barrett's esophagus.

In accordance with these observations, O'Rourke and colleagues [63] reported that the need for gastric lengthening procedures could be significantly reduced by using an approach of "extended mediastinal dissection" during the operative management of large hiatal hernias. These investigators compared the recurrence rate among patients who had smaller hernias, in whom a limited mediastinal dissection (less than 5 cm) was performed, to that of patients who had large hernias, for whom an extended (greater than 5 cm) mediastinal dissection/mobilization was performed. A similar hiatal hernia recurrence of approximately 10% was noted in both groups. The study's authors concluded that, "This finding suggests that aggressive application of laparoscopic transmediastinal dissection to obtain adequate esophageal length may reduce fundoplication failure in patients with esophageal shortening and provide a success rate similar to that of patients with normal esophageal length. More liberal application of Collis gastroplasty in these patients is not warranted."

Symptomatic improvement among paraesophageal patients undergoing Collis gastroplasty for presumed short esophagus has been excellent; however, the confounding issue is that the reported symptomatic improvement among patients undergoing repair without gastroplasty is equally good. There is a significant lack of objective data regarding hiatal hernia recurrence and acid reflux control in both surgical treatment groups (Collis versus no Collis). Indeed, Lin and coauthors [64] recently reported an objective analysis of the intermediate-term outcomes of their patients undergoing an esophageal lengthening procedure for "short esophagus" in the setting of paraesophageal herniation. At a mean follow-up of 30 months, these investigators reported significant improvement in nearly 90% of their patients with regard to GERD and obstructive symptoms. Eighty-four percent of their patients were off medicines related to their esophagogastric complaints. Interestingly, among those patients undergoing physiologic follow-studies, 17% of patients had recurrent hernias, and 80% had evidence of pathologic esophageal acid exposure documented by endoscopy and pH testing. Of further note is that 65% of the patients who have these abnormalities identified on objective testing reported improvement in their preoperative symptoms. Lin and his associates concluded by stating, "Distal esophageal injury can persist after esophagogastric fundoplication (EGF) with Collis gastroplasty, despite significant symptomatic improvements. Appropriate follow-up in these patients requires objective surveillance, which should eventuate in further treatment if esophageal acid is not completely controlled. Although the Collis gastroplasty is conceptually appealing, these results call into question the liberal application of this technique during esophagogastric fundoplication."

Certainly, there is a subset of paraesophageal hernia patient who have esophageal shorting, estimated by preoperative work-up and confirmed at surgery, who will require an esophageal lengthening procedure. In the authors' opinion and that of others, this subgroup of patients is small. Accordingly, it is our belief that the perioperative risk of gastroplasty leak, and the longer-term issues related to an acid producing neoesophageal segment with poor peristaltic function, are important considerations limiting the more liberal use of Collis gastroplasty in the setting of paraesophageal hernia repair [65]. This issue will persist until objective comparisons between surgical approaches to paraesophageal hernia with and without Collis gastroplasty are conducted.

Observation versus elective repair versus urgent repair

The elective management of patients who have asymptomatic or minimally symptomatic paraesophageal hernia continues to be debated. Earlier studies have identified a significant risk (greater than 40% of patients) for the development of important symptoms among individuals managed without surgical repair [15,20,21,24,66]. A high mortality has also been reported among patients managed medically for mechanical problems from the paraesophageal hernia [2]. A recent report of the impact of surgical management of "asymptomatic " paraesophageal hernia patients compared with a "watchful waiting" approach was of made by Stylopoulos et al [67]. These authors developed a relative risk assessment for treatment of a hypothetical cohort of patients who had paraesophageal hernias, based on review of the operative results from 20 reports of elective repair of paraesophageal hernias. They compared these outcomes to those of the Health Care Cost and Use Project (HCUP) Nationwide Inpatient Sample (NIS) and the published results of emergency surgery for paraesophageal surgery from 1964 to 2000. This analysis reported an annual probability of developing acute symptoms requiring emergency surgery of 1.16% per year, ranging from 0.69% to 1.93%, and a lifetime risk of 18% for developing urgent acute symptoms among patients older than 65. The analysis also reported that the estimate for operative mortality for emergency surgery is generally overstated, and estimated it at around 5%. The elective surgical mortality was estimated at approximately 1%.

Accordingly, the authors state that, "The model predicted that watchful waiting was the optimal treatment strategy in 83% of patients and elective hernia repair in the remaining 17%. The model was sensitive only to alterations of the mortality rates of elective hernia repair (ELHR) and emergency surgery."

The authors do question the hypothetical patient outcome analysis reported in this study; however, it does appear reasonable to closely follow the patient who has significant medical comorbidities and who has minimal symptoms from their paraesophageal hernia. This is echoed in the report previously cited by Allen and associates [24], in which surgery was required in only 4 of 23 patients (17%) followed medically over a median interval of 78 months.

The results of the Stylopoulos study do draw attention to the need for experienced surgical management of paraesophageal hernias. Operative mortality rates below 2% can be difficult to obtain if patients who have significant comorbidities suffer important technical mishaps during the course of their paraesophageal hernia repair.

Summary

A tailored approach to the management of patients who have paraesophageal herniation appears to be the best policy. No one approach can universally apply to this patient population if optimal therapy, quality of life, and overall survival are to be optimized.

References

[1] Landreneau RJ, Johnson JA, Marshall JB, et al. Clinical spectrum of paraesophageal herniation. Dig Dis Sci 1992;37:537–44.

[2] Skinner DB, Belsey RHR, Russell PS. Surgical management of esophageal reflux and hiatus hernia: long term results with 1030 patients. J Thorac Cardiovasc Surg 1967;53:33–44.

[3] Landreneau RJ. Surgical management of paraesophageal herniation. In: Nyhus LM, Baker RJ, Fischer JE, editors. Mastery of surgery. Boston: Little, Brown and Company; 1996. p. 694–707.

[4] Landreneau RJ. Gastroesophageal reflux disease. Identification and management of the surgical patient. Postgrad Med 1989;85:117–26.

[5] Low DE, Simchuk EJ. Effect of paraesophageal hernia repair on pulmonary function. Ann Thorac Surg 2002;74(2):333–7 [discussion: 337].

[6] Ueda T, Mizushige K. Large hiatus hernia compressing the heart and impairing the respiratory function. J Cardiol 2003;41(4):211 [author reply: 211–2].

[7] Greub G, Liaudet L, Wiesel P, et al. Respiratory complications of gastroesophageal reflux associated with paraesophageal hiatal hernia. J Clin Gastroenterol 2003;37(2):129–31.

[8] Cameron AJ, Higgins JA. Linear gastric erosion: a lesion associated with large diaphragmatic hernia and chronic blood loss anaemia. Gastroenterology 1986;91:338–42.

[9] Maekawa T, Suematsu M, Shimada T, et al. Unusual swallow syncope caused by huge hiatal hernia. Intern Med 2002;41(3):199–201.

[10] Akdemir I, Davutoglu V, Aktaran S. Giant hiatal hernia presenting with stable angina pectoris and syncope—a case report. Angiology 2001;52(12):863–5.

[11] Shiihara T, Kato M, Honma T, et al. Progressive sliding hiatal hernia as a complication of Menkes' syndrome. J Child Neurol 2002;17(5):401–2.

[12] Petersons A, Liepina M, Spitz L. Neonatal intrathoracic stomach in Marfan's syndrome: report of two cases. J Pediatr Surg 2003;38(11):1663–4.

[13] Szwerc MF, Landreneau RJ. Splenic rupture as a consequence of giant paraesophageal hernia. Ann Thorac Surg 2000;70:1727–8.

[14] Scheidler MG, Keenan RJ, Maley RH Jr, et al. "True" parahiatal hernia—a rare entity: radiologic presentation and clinical management. Ann Thorac Surg 2002;73:416–9.

[15] Maziak DE, Todd TRJ, Pearson FG. Massive hiatus hernia: evaluation and surgical management. J Thorac Cardiovasc Surg 1998;115(1):53–62.

[16] Landreneau RJ, Hazelrigg SR, Johnson JA, et al. The giant paraesophageal hernia: a particularly morbid condition of the esophageal hiatus. Mo Med 1990;87:884–8.

[17] Larson NE, Larson RH, Dorsey JM. Mechanisms of obstruction and strangulation in hernias of the esophageal hiatus. Surg Gynecol Obstet 1964;119:835–41.

[18] Ozdemir IA, Burke WA, Ikins PM. Paraesophageal hernia: a life-threatening disease. Ann Thorac Surg 1973;16:547–54.

[19] Deitel M. Chronic or recurring organoaxial rotation of the stomach. Can J Surg 1973;10: 195–205.

[20] Hill LD. Incarcerated paraesophageal hernia: a surgical emergency. Am J Surg 1973;126: 286–91.

[21] Treacy PJ, Jamieson GG. An approach to the management of para-oesophageal hiatus hernias. Aust N Z J Surg 1987;57:813–7.

[22] Pearson FG, Cooper JD, Patterson GA, et al. Gastroplasty and fundoplication for complex reflux problems. Long-term results. Ann Surg 1987;206(4):473–81.

[23] Wichterman K, Geha AS, Cahow CE, et al. Giant paraesophageal hiatus hernia with intrathoracic stomach and colon: the case for early repair. Surgery 1979;86(3):497–506.

[24] Allen MS, Trastek VF, Deschamps C, et al. Intrathoracic stomach. Presentation and results of operation. J Thorac Cardiovasc Surg 1993;105:253–9.

[25] Tabo T, Hayashi H, Umeyama S, et al. Balloon repositioning of intrathoracic upside-down stomach and fixation by percutaneous endoscopic gastrostomy. J Am Coll Surg 2003;197(5): 868–71.

[26] Stirling MC, Orringer MB. Continued assessment of the combined Collis-Nissen operation. Ann Thorac Surg 1989;47:224–30.

[27] Geha AS, Massad MG, Snow NJ, et al. A 32-year experience in 100 patients with giant paraesophageal hernia: the case for abdominal approach and selective antireflux repair. Surgery 2000;128:623–30.

[28] Ellis FH, Crozier RE, Shea JA. Paraesophageal hiatus hernia. Arch Surg 1986;121:416–20.

[29] Herrington JL, Ellis FH. Paraesophageal hernia. In: Schwartz SI, editor. Current modalities in surgery, #14. West Berlin (NJ): Innovative Publishing Inc; 1985. p. 1–16.

[30] Pearson FG, Cooper JD, Ilves R, et al. Massive hiatal hernia with incarceration: a report of 53 cases. Ann Thorac Surg 1983;35:45–51.

[31] Nguyen NT, Schauer PR, Hutson W, et al. Preliminary results of thoracoscopic Belsey Mark IV antireflux procedure. Surg Laparosc Endosc 1998;8:185–8.

[32] Read RC. The contribution of Allison and Nissen to the evolution of hiatus herniorrhaphy. Hernia 2001;5:200–3.

[33] Landreneau RJ, Marshall JB, Johnson JA, et al. A new balanced operation for complex gastroesophageal reflux disease. Ann Thorac Surg 1991;52:325–6.

[34] Williamson WA, Ellis FH Jr, Streitz JM Jr, et al. Paraesophageal hiatal hernia: is an antireflux procedure necessary? Ann Thorac Surg 1993;56:447–52.

[35] Walther B, Demeester TR, Lafontaine E, et al. Effect of paraesophageal hernia on sphincter function and its implication on surgical therapy. Am J Surg 1984;147:111–6.

[36] Demeester TR, Wernly JA, Bryant GH, et al. Clinical and in vitro analysis of determinants of gastroesophageal competence: a study of the principles of antireflux surgery. Am J Surg 1979;137:39–46.

[37] Zaninotto G, DeMeester TR, Schwizer W, et al. The lower esophageal sphincter in health and disease. Am J Surg 1988;155:104–11.

[38] Swanstrom LL, Jobe BA, Kinzie LR, et al. Esophageal motility and outcomes following laparoscopic paraesophageal hernia repair and fundoplication. Am J Surg 1999;177(5): 359–63.

[39] Ottignon Y, Pelissier EP, Mantion G, et al. Gastroesophageal reflux. Comparison of clinical, pH-metric and manometric results of Nissen's and of Toupet's procedures. Gastroenterol Clin Biol 1994;18:920–6.

[40] Thor KB, Silander T. A long-term randomized prospective trial of the Nissen procedure versus a modified Toupet technique. Ann Surg 1989;210:719–24.

[41] Lundell L, Abrahamsson H, Ruth M, et al. Long-term results of a prospective randomized comparison of total fundic wrap (Nissen-Rossetti) or semifundoplication (Toupet) for gastro-oesophageal reflux. Br J Surg 1996;83:830–5.

[42] Chrysos E, Tsiaoussis J, Zoras OJ, et al. Laparoscopic surgery for gastroesophageal reflux disease patients with impaired esophageal peristalsis: total or partial fundoplication? J Am Coll Surg 2003;197:8–15.

[43] Erenoglu C, Miller A, Schirmer B. Laparoscopic toupet versus nissen fundoplication for the treatment of gastroesophageal reflux disease. Int Surg 2003;88:219–25.

[44] Hashemi M, Peters JH, DeMeester TR, et al. Laparoscopic repair of large Type III hiatal hernia: objective followup reveals high recurrence rate. J Am Coll Surg 2000;190:553–60 [discussion: 560–1].

[45] Schauer PR, Ikramuddin S, McLaughlin RH, et al. Comparison of laparoscopic versus open repair of paraesophageal hernia. Am J Surg 1998;176:659–65.

[46] Andujar J, Birdas T, Papasavas P, et al. Laparoscopic repair of large paraesophageal hernia is associated with a low incidence of recurrence and reoperation. Surg Endosc 2004;18:444–7.

[47] Mattar SG, Bowers SP, Galloway KD, et al. Long-term outcome of laparoscopic repair of paraesophageal hernia. Surg Endosc 2002;16:745–9.

[48] Gantert WA, Patti MG, Arcerito M, et al. Laparoscopic repair of paraesophageal hiatal hernias. J Am Coll Surg 1998;186:428–32 [discussion: 432–3].

[49] Diaz S, Brunt LM, Klingensmith ME, et al. Laparoscopic paraesophageal hernia repair, a challenging operation: medium-term outcome of 116 patients. J Gastrointest Surg 2003;7: 59–66 [discussion: 66–7].

[50] Wiechmann RJ, Ferguson MK, Naunheim KS, et al. Laparoscopic management of giant paraesophageal herniation. Ann Thorac Surg 2001;71:1080–7.

[51] Soper NJ, Dunnegan D. Anatomic fundoplication failure after laparoscopic antireflux surgery. Ann Surg 1999;229:669–76.

[52] Pierre AF, Luketich JD, Fernando HC, et al. Results of laparoscopic repair of giant paraesophageal hernias: 200 consecutive patients. Ann Thorac Surg 2002;74:1909–15 [discussion: 1915–6].

[53] Livingston CD, Jones HL Jr, Askew RE Jr, et al. Laparoscopic hiatal hernia repair in patients with poor esophageal motility or paraesophageal herniation. Am Surg 2001;67: 987–91.

[54] Oelschlager BK, Pellegrini CA. Paraesophageal hernias: open, laparoscopic, or thoracic repair? Chest Surg Clin N Am 2001;11:589–603.

[55] Kakarlapudi GV, Awad ZT, Haynatzki G, et al. The effect of diaphragmatic stressors on recurrent hiatal hernia. Hernia 2002;6:163–6.

[56] Champion JK, Rock D. Laparoscopic mesh cruroplasty for large paraesophageal hernias. Surg Endosc 2003;17:551–3.

[57] Keidar A, Szold A. Laparoscopic repair of paraesophageal hernia with selective use of mesh. Surg Laparosc Endosc Percutan Tech 2003;13:149–54.

[58] Collis JL. An operation for hiatus hernia with short esophagus. J Thoracic Surg 1957;34: 767–78.

[59] Luketich JD, Grondin SC, Pearson FG. Minimally invasive approaches to acquired shortening of the esophagus: laparoscopic Collis-Nissen gastroplasty. Semin Thorac Cardiovasc Surg 2000;12:173–8.

[60] Johnson AB, Oddsdottir M, Hunter JG. Laparoscopic Collis gastroplasty and Nissen fundoplication. A new technique for the management of esophageal foreshortening. Surg Endosc 1998;12:1055–60.

[61] Jobe BA, Aye RW, Deveney CW, et al. Laparoscopic management of giant Type III hiatal hernia and short esophagus. Objective follow-up at three years J Gastrointest Surg 2002;6: 181–8 [discussion: 188].

[62] Mittal SK, Awad ZT, Tasset M, et al. The preoperative predictability of the short esophagus in patients with stricture or paraesophageal hernia. Endoscopy 2000;14:464–8.

[63] O'Rourke RW, Khajanchee YS, Urbach DR, et al. Extended transmediastinal dissection: an alternative to gastroplasty for short esophagus. Arch Surg 2003;138:735–40.

[64] Lin E, Swafford V, Chadalavada R, et al. Disparity between symptomatic and physiologic outcomes following esophageal lengthening procedures for antireflux surgery. J Gastrointest Surg 2004;8:31–9.

[65] Jobe BA, Horvath KD, Swanstrom LL. Postoperative function following laparoscopic collis gastroplasty for shortened esophagus. Arch Surg 1998;133:867–74.

[66] Wichterman K, Geha AS, Cahow CE, et al. Giant paraesophageal hiatus hernia with intrathoracic stomach and colon: the case for early repair. Surgery 1979;86:497–506.

[67] Stylopoulos N, Gazelle GS, Rattner DW. Paraesophageal hernias: operation or observation? Ann Surg 2002;236:492–500 [discussion: 500–1].

SURGICAL
CLINICS OF
NORTH AMERICA

Surg Clin N Am 85 (2005) 433–451

Short Esophagus and Esophageal Stricture

Chuong D. Hoang, MD, Paul S. Koh, MD,
Michael A. Maddaus, MD*

*Section of General Thoracic Surgery, Division of Cardiovascular and Thoracic Surgery,
University of Minnesota Medical School, 420 Delaware Street SE, Minneapolis,
MN 55455, USA*

Gastroesophageal reflux disease (GERD) is a common disorder. Surveys indicate that about 7% of the US population experiences heartburn, regurgitation, or both on a daily basis [1]. Most patients who have GERD have a benign course characterized by intermittent symptoms of heartburn and acid regurgitation; however, a subset of patients (up to 40%) may eventually, for reasons that are not completely understood, develop complications of GERD such as esophagitis, Barrett's esophagus, peptic esophageal stricture, or acquired short esophagus [2–4]. Esophageal stricture due to localized transmural scarring is one of the most frequent sequelae of longstanding severe esophagitis; in that patient subgroup, the incidence is 1% to 5% [5,6]. Short esophagus is thought to be the result of similar pathogenic processes, but may occur in the absence of esophageal stricture and inflammation. Although the existence of acquired short esophagus is disputed, evidence of its more widespread acceptance continues to gradually appear in the literature. This article reviews the pathophysiology of short esophagus and esophageal stricture, and includes an update on minimally invasive surgical approaches to their treatment.

Short esophagus

Definition

The presence of short esophagus is determined surgically. In patients who do not have GERD or hiatal hernia, the inbtra-abdominal esophagus

---

* Corresponding author.
E-mail address: madda001@tc.umn.edu (M.A. Maddaus).

0039-6109/05/$ - see front matter © 2005 Elsevier Inc. All rights reserved.
doi:10.1016/j.suc.2005.01.019

measures 3 to 4 cm. An accepted tenet of a properly performed antireflux procedure is to restore a minimum of 2.5 to 3 cm of distal esophagus to an intra-abdominal location. The inability to achieve this goal intraoperatively defines the presence of short esophagus. This clinical entity of short esophagus was first described by Barrett in 1950 [7]. Lortat-Jacob [8] first proposed in 1957 that acquired esophageal shortening was a complication of advanced reflux disease. Despite this long history and numerous studies, debate continues regarding the prevalence and even the very existence of this entity.

Influential arguments against the existence of short esophagus were advanced by Hill and coworkers [9] in 1970. Their original report described 36 patients undergoing esophagogastropexy for complicated GERD. They concluded that, because the gastroesophageal junction (GEJ) could routinely be brought to an intra-abdominal position and anchored after esophageal mobilization, the term "acquired short esophagus" should be eliminated. Korn and associates [10] recently conducted a manometric study comparing patients at different stages of GERD (n = 180) versus healthy controls (n = 190). Their objective was to determine the prevalence and degree of short esophagus. They could not demonstrate significant differences in esophageal length among their patient groups, and so concluded that short esophagus did not exist in their patient population.

A substantial body of literature [11–18] supports the concept of acquired short esophagus, however. Its presence can be suggested by objective studies (barium esophagram, endoscopy, and manometry) that are integral to the complete preoperative evaluation of patients who have suspected GERD (see the Diagnosis section below), but definitive diagnosis can only be made intraoperatively. Precise criteria for short esophagus differ slightly among reported surgical series [12,14,15,17–20]. In general, after complete esophageal mobilization, at least 2 to 3 cm of intra-abdominal esophagus must be visually confirmed under tension-free conditions in order to exclude the diagnosis of short esophagus.

Horvath and coworkers [21] defined three subcategories of short esophagus: (1) apparent short esophagus, (2) true, reducible short esophagus, and (3) true, nonreducible short esophagus. Patients who have apparent short esophagus actually have a normal-length esophagus, but it is accordioned into the distal mediastinum. Both of the true types of short esophagus imply that some intrinsic shortening has occurred. In the case of true, reducible short esophagus, extensive mediastinal dissection (>5 cm) can be used to restore the GEJ to a subdiaphragmatic position 2 to 3 cm below the diaphragm. In contrast, in the case of true, nonreducible short esophagus, an esophageal lengthening procedure is required.

Epidemiology

Estimates of the prevalence of short esophagus vary widely. Pearson and colleagues [22] reported a prevalence as high as 60% in a series of open antireflux procedures; at the other end of the spectrum, Hill and coauthors [9] reported a 0% prevalence. Variability and subjectivity in the definition of short esophagus undoubtedly contribute to the ongoing debate. If open surgical series are reexamined using the definition of short esophagus as the intraoperative requirement for an extensive mediastinal mobilization or a Collis gastroplasty, then a prevalence of 8% to 10% of all patients undergoing fundoplication for GERD is observed [23,24].

Large series of patients undergoing laparoscopic antireflux surgery show a comparable prevalence of short esophagus. Using the same definition of short esophagus that was applied retrospectively to the series of open antireflux procedures, Awad and colleagues [25] observed a frequency of 7% in 260 patients; Swanstrom and associates [15], a frequency of 10% in 238 patients; and O'Rourke and coworkers [26], a frequency of 19% in 487 patients. Perhaps the most unequivocal measure of short esophagus prevalence is the percentage of patients who have surgically treated reflux and who require a Collis gastroplasty: in general—only 1% to 5% of all patients undergoing surgery for GERD [27,28].

Pathogenesis

A prerequisite for acquired short esophagus is the presence of chronic GERD. The squamous epithelium of the esophagus is a poor barrier to gastrointestinal refluxate. Previous experimental data from an animal model [29,30] and from an in-vivo human study [31] demonstrated that gastroesophageal reflux (composed of gastric, biliary, and pancreatic secretions) permits penetration of hydrogen ions into the deeper layers of the esophageal wall. An acute, local inflammatory reaction is initiated by the release of kinins, complement factors, and prostaglandins. The result is tissue edema, then infiltration by neutrophils, then infiltration by macrophages. This acute process is followed by stages of healing: fibroblasts, which produce collagen, and keratinocytes, which restore epithelial integrity, are recruited. The entire process in chronic GERD may eventually extend transmurally. After repeated cycles of injury and repair, irreversible functional damage, manifesting as scar formation from disorganized collagen deposition and remodeling, ultimately occurs. Fibrosis and scar contraction in the longitudinal muscular layer causes intrinsic shortening.

Preoperative diagnosis

Multiple investigations have been conducted [12,25,32,33], all aimed at identifying preoperative criteria that reliably and accurately predict short esophagus, but their cumulative results suggest that no single criterion exists. Upright barium esophagram demonstration of a large, nonreducing Type I (≥5 cm) hiatal hernia, or of a Type III hiatal hernia is considered to be highly predictive of the presence of short esophagus [34]; however,

Horvath and coworkers [21], in an objective assessment of that test in a masked review of 15 patients requiring Collis gastroplasty, found only a 50% positive predictive value. Frequently cited endoscopic criteria include identification of the GEJ greater than or equal to 5 cm above the crural impression, Savary-Miller Grades III–IV esophagitis, peptic stricture, and Barrett's esophagus. Awad and coworkers [25], in a study of 260 patients undergoing laparoscopic primary antireflux surgery, reported that esophago-scopy had a sensitivity of 61%, and a low positive predictive value of only 27%. The third common preoperative diagnostic technique is esophageal manometry, which measures the mean esophageal length (the distance between the upper and lower esophageal sphincters) normalized for patient height. Mittal and colleagues [32], in a retrospective analysis of 39 patients undergoing esophageal mobilization with intraoperative length assessment, documented a sensitivity of 43% and a low positive predictive value of 25% for preoperative manometry.

When these three preoperative techniques (esophagraphy, endoscopy, and manometry) were combined and tested in trials, the results were similarly disappointing. Gastal and coauthors [12] used univariate and multivariate analyses to assess 236 primary antireflux surgery patients tested by all three techniques. Manometric esophageal length below the fifth percentile of normal (determined in 95 asymptomatic volunteers) was associated with short esophagus, but no minimal threshold length could be identified with certainty, given wide individual measurement variability. On multivariate analysis, only the presence of peptic stricture had significant predictive value for a diagnosis of short esophagus and a need for Collis gastroplasty. Awad and coauthors [25] systematically assessed the effectiveness of all three predictive techniques, used individually and in multiple combinations. The combination of radiologic, endoscopic, and manometric preoperative tests yielded 100% specificity, but at the sacrifice of sufficient sensitivity (28%). Manometry, as an individual test, had the best positive predictive value (but only 36.3%); correspondingly, esophag-raphy and manometry, used in combination, had a positive predictive value of 75%, but a low sensitivity of 42%. Thus, in general, preoperative findings are most useful to increase the index of suspicion for short esophagus and to alert the surgeon to the potential need for a lengthening procedure.

Intraoperative diagnosis

As already discussed, the most accurate method to assess esophageal length is direct, intraoperative visualization. In the vast majority of cases where a short esophagus may exist, a large hiatal hernia is present. Following hernia sac mobilization and division of the short gastric vessels, the mediastinal esophagus is mobilized up to 8 cm or more, as defined by Johnson and associates [14]. The first assessment of esophageal length is made at this point in the surgical procedure. An important consideration here is that there must be no tension or traction on the esophagus and stomach; the nasogastric tube or bougie should be removed from the esophagus, because they tend to stent or exert downward pressure, artificially displacing the GEJ. If the GEJ can be easily visualized, the distance from the crura to the GEJ is measured. In a laparoscopic procedure, the end of a grasper is placed at the crura, parallel to the esophagus and the level of the GEJ along the side of the grasper is noted (Fig. 1). This distance is measured, and if it is less than 2.5 cm, short esophagus is diagnosed.

In many cases, however, the exact location of the GEJ is very difficult to ascertain. The distance of intra-abdominal esophagus being searched for is a mere 2.5 cm—slightly more than one inch. In larger hernias, a redundant sac and large amount of fat around the GEJ ("fat-pad") can completely obscure this anatomic landmark and make accurate determination of the true GEJ difficult, if not impossible. In addition, with upward displacement of the esophagus as occurs in hiatal hernias, a phenomenon of "gastric tubularization" is observed, with the stomach just below the GEJ developing a tubular appearance that may be mistaken for esophagus. With dissection of the fat-pad, the junction of the stomach and esophagus can be clearly seen, and is best observed by viewing the junction at the angle of His (Fig. 2).

Maziak and coworkers [35], using a left thoracotomy approach in 94 patients who had giant hiatal hernia repair, performed extensive esophageal mobilization combined with fat-pad dissection of the GEJ area. With this level of meticulous mobilization and delineation of the exact location of the

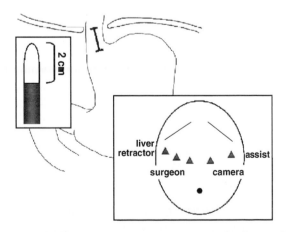

Fig. 1. Laparoscopic method of esophageal length assessment. The distance from crus to GEJ is determined after esophageal mobilization using the longitudinal length of a laparoscopic grasper placed parallel to the esophagus (left inset). The authors' laparoscopic port placement for performing a Collis-Nissen procedure is depicted in the right inset, and the relative positions of the surgical team are as indicated (see text under Treatment).

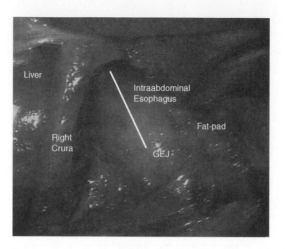

Fig. 2. Intraoperative measurement of esophageal length. The normal orientation of critical anatomic landmarks that must be clearly identified to ensure accurate determination of intra-abdominal esophageal length is depicted. The fat-pad has been dissected and pushed laterally to expose the location of the true GEJ. White line depicts the intra-abdominal segment of esophagus.

GEJ and its relationship to the crura, they found an 80% incidence of short esophagus. Using Collis gastroplasty, they documented a long-term recurrence rate of only 2%. Pierre and colleagues [36], using the equivalent laparoscopic approach, determined that a short esophagus was present in 56% of patients undergoing surgical repair of a giant hiatal hernia. These methods of esophageal shortening assessment and their recurrence rates should serve as benchmarks for past and future studies of open and laparoscopic giant hiatal hernia repair.

Intraoperative endoscopy can also help to accurately assess the location of the GEJ in equivocal circumstances. The position of the GEJ relative to the crura is identified after advancement of an esophageal endoscope, combined with visual confirmation of the lighted endoscope tip trans-illuminating through the esophageal wall. Mittal and coauthors [32] used intraoperative endoscopy to accurately locate the GEJ after extensive mobilization; then they measured the distance between the endoscope tip and the crural arch. They diagnosed short esophagus if a minimum of 2 cm (a later criterion that they changed to 3 cm) of tension-free intra-abdominal esophagus was not measurable.

In contrast, to prevent potential overestimation of short esophagus, O'Rourke et al [26] recently demonstrated that additional esophageal mobilization up to 10 cm was feasible through a laparoscopic abdominal approach; they stressed that extensive mediastinal dissection is necessary to accurately determine length. Using that approach, they diagnosed short esophagus in 4.3% of patients (n = 487) undergoing laparoscopic antireflux surgery.

Treatment

An esophageal lengthening procedure (Collis gastroplasty) is performed if all intraoperative diagnostic maneuvers fail to establish a 2-cm segment of intra-abdominal esophagus. If short esophagus is unrecognized, a tension-free surgical repair is precluded, thereby increasing the risk of mechanical failure of the fundoplication, or crural disruption with mediastinal wrap herniation [37]. High rates (20% to 33%) of failure after open or laparoscopic repair of giant hiatal hernia have been partly attributed to unrecognized or untreated short esophagus [38–40].

The Collis gastroplasty [41] has become the most widely accepted method of lengthening the esophagus. This procedure was originally performed through a left thoracoabdominal incision, and included mobilization of the esophagus to the level of the aortic arch. Two clamps from the left aspect of the cardia were placed parallel to a dilator lying along the lesser curve; the stomach was divided; and the resection lines were oversewn. This technique reliably created a connecting tubular segment of stomach ("neoesophagus"), allowing for tension-free intra-abdominal placement of the GEJ. Combined with a standard antireflux procedure, the transthoracic Collis gastroplasty has been validated clinically, with excellent long-term results (up to 88% symptomatic reflux control at 10 years) [42,43].

With increasing recognition of short esophagus during minimally invasive antireflux procedures, techniques have evolved to allow laparoscopic application of the Collis gastroplasty. In 1996, Jobe and colleagues [13] and Swanstrom and coworkers [15] detailed a combined thoracoscopic-assisted laparoscopic gastroplasty and Nissen fundoplication procedure (Fig. 3A). Formation of the neoesophagus was accomplished with an endoscopic linear stapler applied parallel to the lesser curve of the stomach with a bougie in place. The stapler was introduced through the right chest, then moved across the right mediastinal pleura, and then transhiatally into the abdomen. In 2000, Awad and colleagues [25,44] described a similar approach, using left-sided thoracoscopic access to perform the lengthening (Fig. 3B).

Johnson and coauthors [14] introduced a minimally invasive, totally intra-abdominal Collis gastroplasty (Fig. 3C). They used an end-to-end anastomosis (EEA) circular stapling device to create a sealed, transgastric window in the fundus. A linear cutting stapling device was then introduced from the caudal aspect through the window and fired parallel to an esophageal dilator, forming the neoesophagus. This method is more technically demanding and necessitates a higher learning curve compared with other minimally invasive approaches. A potential pitfall is the addition of a circular staple line created by the EEA stapler. Unlike performance of an end-to-end anastomosis with the EEA, in which a pursestring is used to ensure complete "ring" development, no pursestring is used in this method. This heightens the possibility of incomplete "rings" of the anterior and

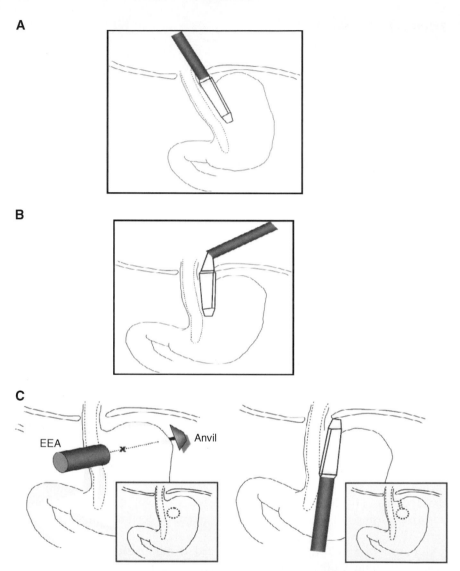

Fig. 3. Laparoscopic Collis techniques. (*A*) The thoracoscopic/laparoscopic Collis gastroplasty procedure is depicted. Access for the linear endoscopic GIA stapler is through the right chest cavity. (*B*) A variation of the thoracoscopic/laparoscopic Collis gastroplasty performed via a left chest-cavity access. An articulating linear endoscopic GIA stapler is required. (*C*) The double-stapled, totally intra-abdominal laparoscopic gastroplasty. An anvil is placed from anterior to posterior through the stomach walls. A sealed transgastric window is created with a circular EEA stapler (left inset). A linear endoscopic Endo Gia stapler is fired parallel to the bougie to create a 3- to 4-cm neoesophagus.

posterior gastric wall and predisposes to a staple line leak, an event seen in 3% of the Collis gastroplasty series reported by Pierre and associates [36].

The authors' group at the University of Minnesota uses a totally intra-abdominal laparoscopic technique described as wedge Collis gastroplasty (Fig. 4). Champion [45] originated this method in 1995 for use in laparoscopic vertical banded gastroplasty. In this technique, a 48 F bougie is placed and pushed snug against the lesser curve. With the fundus held in a taut fashion antero-inferiorly, a linear Endo GIA stapler (US Surgical, Norwalk, Connecticut) is applied and fired from the left upper quadrant (LUQ), with the tip of the articulating stapler aimed almost perpendicular to the esophagus. Usually a second firing with the stapler tip positioned up against the bougie is necessary, allowing the staple line to be brought as close as possible to the bougie. Next, the stapler is placed superiorly from a right upper quadrant (RUQ) port (assistant grasping the tip of the previous staple line), snug against the bougie on top of the developing neoesophagus, and fired, thereby excising a 2 to 3 cm wedge of stomach.

For most laparoscopic Collis patients, the early results were satisfactory (Table 1), and compared favorably with previous open studies. Mean operative time for Hunter's series was 294 minutes [14]; for Swanstrom's, 257 minutes [13]. Average length of stay was 2 and 3 days, respectively. Both groups reported no deaths and no major postoperative complications. Postoperative functional assessment at 12 months for Hunter's series revealed that 11% of patients complained of reflux symptoms and 11% had dysphagia. For Swanstrom's series, after 14 months of follow-up, 14% of patients complained of reflux symptoms and 14% had dysphagia. Importantly, Swanstrom and associates objectively documented 0% wrap failures and 0% mediastinal herniations using upper endoscopy. Awad and coworkers reported similar outcome measures at a mean follow-up of 17 months: 9% of patients complained of reflux symptoms and 9% had dysphagia [25]. They objectively documented a 9% wrap failure rate and a 9% mediastinal herniation rate.

Most recently, Pierre and colleagues [36] described 200 patients who had giant paraesophageal hernia and underwent laparoscopic repair, including a subgroup of 112 patients who underwent a Collis-Nissen procedure. At a median of 18 months of follow-up, the satisfaction rate was 93% according to a standardized questionnaire. About 16% of patients required, at least occasionally, H_2-blockers or proton-pump inhibitors, and 6% had dysphagia warranting dilation. Only 2.7% of Collis-Nissen patients had recurrent hiatal hernia.

Other authors have described similar series of patients undergoing laparoscopic fundoplication, but without an esophageal lengthening procedure. Overall, the wrap disruption or mediastinal herniation rates are higher in such series than in those using the Collis gastroplasty. Hashemi and coauthors [46], after a median of 27 months of follow-up, found a statistically significant difference in recurrence rates of laparoscopic Type III

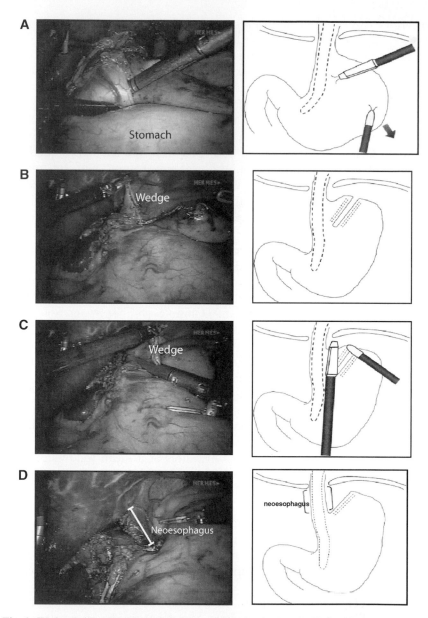

Fig. 4. Wedge Collis gastroplasty technique. (*A*) The fundus is pulled inferolateral to expose the angle of His. A linear endoscopic Endo GIA stapler is positioned with the tip perpendicular to and upon the bougie, then fired across the stomach. (*B*) A small wedge of stomach, approximating a triangle is created. (*C*) The wedge segment is held up and second linear Endo GIA stapler is placed parallel to the bougie and fired. (*D*) The completed wedge Collis gastroplasty with stapled gastric tube neoesophagus (*white line*).

Table 1
Postoperative functional results of laparoscopic Collis procedure

Study	Type	n	Follow-up(range)	Anti reflux procedure	Reflux symptoms	Dysphagia	Objective recurrence	Objective reflux
Pearson et al [22]	Open	214	1–15 years	Toupet	6 (3%)	24 (11%)	6 (3%)	NA
Stirling, Orringer [42]	Open	261	44 months	Nissen	65 (25%)	44 (17%)	26 (10%)	24 (9%)
Swanstrom et al [13,15]	Lap	15	14 months	Nissen or Toupet	2 (14%)	2 (14%)	0	7 (50%)
Johnson et al [14]	Lap	9	12 months	Nissen	1 (11%)	1 (11%)	NA	NA
Awad et al [25,44]	Lap	11	17 months (5–35 months)	Nissen or Toupet	1 (9%)	0	2 (18%)	NA
Pierre et al [36]	Lap	112	18 months (1–78 months)	Nissen	NA[a]	NA[a]	3 (3%)	NA

[a] A standardized questionnaire was used to gather data and composite results were reported.

hiatal hernia repairs (42%) compared with open repairs (15%). Likewise, after a mean of 25 months of follow-up, Khaitan and colleagues [47] found that 40% of laparoscopic paraesophageal hernia repair patients had a recurrent hiatal hernia or mediastinal migration of the wrap. Jobe and associates [48] evaluated the effectiveness of the laparoscopic Hill repair (no esophageal lengthening included) in 52 patients who had Type III hiatal hernia. At a mean follow-up of 37 months, they found that 32% of patients had hiatal recurrence on video esophagram. Multiple authors have suggested that such disappointing objective outcomes (high recurrence rates) are mostly related to the failure to recognize acquired short esophagus and perform a lengthening procedure [36,38–40].

Despite the technical success of the Collis gastroplasty, certain theoretical concerns temper enthusiasm for a policy of very liberal use. The neoesophageal segment lacks motility, and thus may predispose to eventual esophageal dilation or contribute to postoperative dysphagia. Although overall satisfaction is high, 6% to 9% [13,14,25,36] of patients report some degree of postoperative swallowing problems. Of more potential concern is the ongoing acid secretion within the neoesophagus, from translocated gastric mucosa causing localized esophagitis. Jobe and coworkers [13] found that 50% (n = 7) of their thoracoscopic-assisted laparoscopic Collis-Toupet fundoplication patients had abnormal 24-hour pH testing (mean DeMeester score = 100). Of those seven patients, five had histologic evidence of persistent esophagitis. These findings prompted the researchers to recommend chronic maintenance acid-suppression therapy and close objective follow-up. The long-term consequences of this neoesophageal inflammation are unknown.

Each of the minimally invasive approaches to the Collis gastroplasty has its proponents, and satisfactory outcomes have been reported for each (see above). Criticisms of the totally intra-abdominal EEA approach include the need for a larger access port for the EEA stapler and technical difficulties with manipulating and properly positioning the two-component stapling mechanism. The major disadvantage of the transthoracic approach is the need to enter an additional body cavity, thereby increasing the risk of injury to intrathoracic structures (especially at the level of the hiatus, where thoracoscopic visualization may be limited). In the authors' current experience (n = 33), the wedge gastroplasty is a simple and reliable method of esophageal lengthening, without the intrinsic disadvantages of the other approaches. It requires only a single type of linear stapler, introduced via standard ports, and affords excellent visualization. Our wedge gastroplasty patients have satisfactory postoperative swallowing and a low incidence of recurrent reflux symptoms. We have not yet encountered a recurrent hiatal hernia. Overall, 96% of our patients are satisfied with the surgical outcome.

Currently, it is unknown which minimally invasive approach is optimal, and formal randomized trials are unlikely to be completed to settle this issue. Practically, the comfort level and training of the individual surgeon currently determine which laparoscopic technique is used.

Esophageal stricture

Nearly 80% of benign esophageal strictures are peptic strictures [49]. A peptic esophageal stricture is a cicatricial narrowing of the esophagus resulting from chronic severe reflux esophagitis [50]. The prevalence of peptic stricture among patients who have GERD is about 10% to 25% [51–53]. The Veterans Affairs cooperative group trial [53] comparing medical versus surgical therapy for complicated GERD, objectively documented, just before randomization, an established esophageal stricture in 13.8% of 247 enrolled patients who had a reflux disorder not previously treated by surgery. During that study, patients in the medical therapy group had a rate as high as 8% of spontaneous peptic stricture appearance. Malignancy (for which the therapeutic approach would be entirely different) must be excluded in all instances of esophageal stricture.

Pathogenesis

The pathophysiology responsible for peptic stricture formation is similar to that for short esophagus. Longstanding GERD is a prerequisite, and mechanisms that prolong acid (or alkaline) refluxate contact time, such as esophageal motility disorders, are particularly important [54]. In the initial stages, esophageal narrowing is mostly attributed to edema and muscle spasm; therefore, early stages of stricture formation are reversible with appropriate acid control [55]. Repetitive reflux damage leads to progressive circumferential tissue destruction that may extend transmurally across the deep muscle-wall layers. The end result is fibrosis with deposition of Type I collagen, which then matures into typical scar tissue with consequent irreversible narrowing [56]. In addition, the involved esophagus segment is usually thickened, noncompliant, and shortened (due to scar tissue contraction). These similar processes account for the frequent observation that short esophagus is accompanied by peptic stricture. The stricturing process usually begins at the squamocolumnar junction, the area exposed to the greatest amount of acid [57]. Strictures are typically less than 1 cm long, but may extend to 8 cm [3].

Diagnosis

Dysphagia of insidious onset is the most common presenting symptom. Patients have difficulty initially with solids, but this difficulty may progress to liquids as well [3,50]. Those who have chronic peptic stricture tend to alter their diets to avoid foods that cause difficulty with swallowing, and consequently may no longer complain of significant dysphagia unless specifically questioned. More than 75% of patients have a history of heartburn symptoms [49]. Such symptoms may gradually attenuate as the fibrotic process advances, evolving to dysphagia as a primary complaint. Atypical presentations include chronic cough and asthma exacerbations (due to aspiration of acid or food into the lungs) [50]. Patients may complain of chest pain due to esophagitis, esophageal spasm, or food impaction at the level of the stricture. Weight loss is uncommon, because such patients can adapt by eating softer foods or liquids that pass through the stricture. Significant weight loss, especially in a patient who has had recent dysphagia onset, suggests malignancy.

The primary purposes of diagnostic studies are to confirm the clinical diagnosis and to define the etiology and anatomic extent of the stricture. Again, definitive exclusion of an underlying malignancy is paramount. A barium esophagram is the recommended initial study of choice. It is highly sensitive in detecting anatomic abnormalities [58], and can provide information on the location, diameter, and length of the lesion. Esophago-scopy permits direct visualization of the stricture, and enables endoscopic biopsies with brush cytology to assess for malignancy. A peptic stricture typically appears as a concentric narrowing of the distal esophageal lumen immediately proximal to the squamocolumnar junction. In 50% of patients, the stenotic area is associated with areas of esophagitis [3]. Other sequelae of severe GERD, such as Barrett's esophagus, pseudodiverticula, and fibrous bands, may also be identified by endoscopy.

Treatment

Stricture dilation

Initial management of peptic strictures focuses on establishing an adequate esophageal opening to restore swallowing. Per oral dilation has been performed for over 400 years; it has evolved from using crude instruments such as a whalebone to using a wide array of flexible thermoplastic bougies and balloons [59,60]. Several randomized, controlled studies comparing the efficacy of bougies versus balloons documented no overall significant differences [61,62]. Detailed descriptions of instruments and techniques have been discussed elsewhere [60]. The esophagus is dilated, if possible, to a 15-mm diameter (45 F) or larger, the size necessary for a regular diet [3]. Tight, complicated strictures not allowing passage of an endoscope should be dilated either with wire-guided bougies or with through-the-scope balloons to minimize risk of inadvertent esophageal injury [60].

Marks and Richter [63] reported that esophageal dilation relieved dysphagia, with an initial response rate of more than 80%. Several large studies documented a stricture recurrence rate between 12% and 65% (mean, 45%) after dilation [63,64]. Such patients thus require regular surveillance and potential repeat dilations. Intralesional steroid injection after stricture dilation has been advocated by some investigators, who cite the theoretical benefits of antifibrotic agents [65]; however, studies to date have involved small numbers of patients and have been nonrandomized and uncontrolled, rendering the significance of results unclear [66,67]. It is now well-recognized that mechanical dilation must be combined with acid-suppression therapy to prevent ongoing esophagitis, and therefore frequent stricture recurrence [55]. Randomized trials with proton-pump inhibitors established that aggressive acid suppression can heal esophagitis and decrease the need for repeated peptic stricture dilation [52,68].

Antireflux surgery

Despite optimal medical therapy, about 30% to 40% of patients who have peptic strictures require repeat dilation for stricture symptoms within 1 year [52,68,69]. The need for repetitive dilations is an indication for surgical intervention. Stricture dilation combined with an antireflux procedure results in durable treatment of the stenosis by effectively addressing the underlying chronic severe GERD. Antireflux surgery for peptic strictures in open series resulted in good to excellent results in 77% of patients (range, 43% to 90%) [70–72]. Up to 43% of patients required repeat dilation postoperatively, usually limited to only 1 or 2 sessions. Overall mortality rates were 0.5%; morbidity, less than 20%. Similar good outcomes were reported in minimally invasive antireflux surgical series. Spivak and coauthors [73] compared 40 GERD patients who had varying degrees of dysphagia and stricture with 121 GERD patients who did not. All patients underwent laparoscopic antireflux procedures (Nissen, Toupet, or Collis-Nissen, as indicated). At a mean follow-up of 1.5 years, the overall satisfaction rate was high (88%), and none of the stricture patients required secondary medical treatment or esophageal dilations. Klingler and coauthors [74] also reported similar statistics in a group of 102 patients who underwent laparoscopic antireflux surgery for GERD complicated by peptic stricture.

Good outcomes with minimally invasive surgery have led some investigators to advocate it as a primary treatment option for patients who are otherwise acceptable antireflux surgery candidates [73]. Support for this notion depends on the recognition that peptic esophageal stricture is a complication of GERD, and in itself warrants surgical correction of the reflux. This issue remains controversial, however. To date, no randomized, controlled trials have compared antireflux surgery versus medical management and serial bougienage. Watson [75] retrospectively compared a cohort of antireflux surgery patients with a control group of medically treated (H_2-blockers and bougienage) patients over a 3-year period. In the medical therapy group, 59% required an average of 3.1 subsequent dilations; in the surgery group, 29% required an average of 1.6 subsequent dilations.

The authors recommend that most patients who have peptic esophageal stricture initially undergo endoscopic dilation therapy and long-term treatment with proton-pump inhibitors. We routinely use a wire-guided technique (ie, Savary-Gilliard dilators). If conservative therapy fails, we use minimally invasive techniques to perform a standard antireflux procedure.

Intraoperative assessment for short esophagus should be conducted in every patient; if short esophagus is present, it should be addressed by adding a laparoscopic Collis gastroplasty.

Esophageal resection

Patients who have intractable esophagitis and an undilatable stricture, or for whom multiple antireflux procedures have failed [76], should be considered for esophageal resection and reconstruction. In general, resection is very uncommon for benign disease.

Summary

Short esophagus and peptic esophageal stricture are complications of chronic severe GERD. Short esophagus is properly diagnosed by an objective, intraoperative assessment after appropriate dissection of the GEJ. A laparoscopic Collis gastroplasty combined with an antireflux procedure comprises effective therapy. Peptic stricture should be addressed with an initial course of dilator therapy and optimization of antiacid medication. Consideration is given to an antireflux procedure if conservative therapy fails. Laparoscopic techniques have proven to be safe and effective in treating short esophagus and peptic stricture.

References

[1] Spechler SJ. Epidemiology and natural history of gastro-oesophageal reflux disease. Digestion 1992;51(Suppl 1):24–9.

[2] Stein HJ, Barlow AP, DeMeester TR, et al. Complications of gastroesophageal reflux disease. Role of the lower esophageal sphincter, esophageal acid and acid/alkaline exposure, and duodenogastric reflux. Ann Surg 1992;216:35–43.

[3] Richter JE. Peptic strictures of the esophagus. Gastroenterol Clin North Am 1999;28: 875–91.

[4] Bremner RM, Crookes PF, DeMeester TR, et al. Concentration of refluxed acid and esophageal mucosal injury. Am J Surg 1992;164:522–6 [discussion: 526–7].

[5] Ben Rejeb M, Bouche O, Zeitoun P. Study of 47 consecutive patients with peptic esophageal stricture compared with 3880 cases of reflux esophagitis. Dig Dis Sci 1992;37:733–6.

[6] Loof L, Gotell P, Elfberg B. The incidence of reflux oesophagitis. A study of endoscopy reports from a defined catchment area in Sweden. Scand J Gastroenterol 1993;28:113–8.

[7] Spechler SJ, Goyal RK. The columnar-lined esophagus, intestinal metaplasia, and Norman Barrett. Gastroenterology 1996;110:614–21.

[8] Lortat-Jacob JL. L'endo-brachyesophage [Barrett's esophagus]. Ann Chir 1957;11:1247 [in French].

[9] Hill LD, Gelfand M, Bauermeister D. Simplified management of reflux esophagitis with stricture. Ann Surg 1970;172:638–51.

[10] Korn O, Csendes A, Burdiles P, et al. Length of the esophagus in patients with gastro-esophageal reflux disease and Barrett's esophagus compared to controls. Surgery 2003;133: 358–63.

[11] Ellis FH Jr, Leonardi HK, Dabuzhsky L, et al. Surgery for short esophagus with stricture: an experimental and clinical manometric study. Ann Surg 1978;188:341–50.

[12] Gastal OL, Hagen JA, Peters JH, et al. Short esophagus: analysis of predictors and clinical implications. Arch Surg 1999;134:633–6 [discussion: 637–8].

[13] Jobe BA, Horvath KD, Swanstrom LL. Postoperative function following laparoscopic collis gastroplasty for shortened esophagus. Arch Surg 1998;133:867–74.

[14] Johnson AB, Oddsdottir M, Hunter JG. Laparoscopic Collis gastroplasty and Nissen fundoplication. A new technique for the management of esophageal foreshortening. Surg Endosc 1998;12:1055–60.

[15] Swanstrom LL, Marcus DR, Galloway GQ. Laparoscopic Collis gastroplasty is the treatment of choice for the shortened esophagus. Am J Surg 1996;171:477–81.

[16] Pearson FG, Henderson RD. Experimental and clinical studies of gastroplasty in the management of acquired short esophagus. Surg Gynecol Obstet 1973;136:737–44.

[17] Peters JH, Heimbucher J, Kauer WK, et al. Clinical and physiologic comparison of laparoscopic and open Nissen fundoplication. J Am Coll Surg 1995;180:385–93.

[18] Hinder RA, Filipi CJ, Wetscher G, et al. Laparoscopic Nissen fundoplication is an effective treatment for gastroesophageal reflux disease. Ann Surg 1994;220:472–81 [discussion: 481–3].

[19] Luketich JD, Grondin SC, Pearson FG. Minimally invasive approaches to acquired shortening of the esophagus: laparoscopic Collis-Nissen gastroplasty. Semin Thorac Cardiovasc Surg 2000;12:173–8.

[20] Cadiere GB, Houben JJ, Bruyns J, et al. Laparoscopic Nissen fundoplication: technique and preliminary results. Br J Surg 1994;81:400–3.

[21] Horvath KD, Swanstrom LL, Jobe BA. The short esophagus: pathophysiology, incidence, presentation, and treatment in the era of laparoscopic antireflux surgery. Ann Surg 2000;232:630–40.

[22] Pearson FG, Cooper JD, Patterson GA, et al. Gastroplasty and fundoplication for complex reflux problems. Long-term results. Ann Surg 1987;206:473–81.

[23] Kauer WK, Peters JH, DeMeester TR, et al. A tailored approach to antireflux surgery. J Thorac Cardiovasc Surg 1995;110:141–6 [discussion: 146–7].

[24] Polk HC Jr. Fundoplication for reflux esophagitis: misadventures with the operation of choice. Ann Surg 1976;183:645–52.

[25] Awad ZT, Mittal SK, Roth TA, et al. Esophageal shortening during the era of laparoscopic surgery. World J Surg 2001;25:558–61.

[26] O'Rourke RW, Khajanchee YS, Urbach DR, et al. Extended transmediastinal dissection: an alternative to gastroplasty for short esophagus. Arch Surg 2003;138:735–40.

[27] Terry M, Smith CD, Branum GD, et al. Outcomes of laparoscopic fundoplication for gastroesophageal reflux disease and paraesophageal hernia. Surg Endosc 2001;15:691–9.

[28] Richardson JD, Richardson RL. Collis-Nissen gastroplasty for shortened esophagus: long-term evaluation. Ann Surg 1998;227:735–40 [discussion: 740–2].

[29] Lillemoe KD, Johnson LF, Harmon JW. Role of the components of the gastroduodenal contents in experimental acid esophagitis. Surgery 1982;92:276–84.

[30] Lillemoe KD, Johnson LF, Harmon JW. Taurodeoxycholate modulates the effects of pepsin and trypsin in experimental esophagitis. Surgery 1985;97:662–7.

[31] Gozzetti G, Pilotti V, Spangaro M, et al. Pathophysiology and natural history of acquired short esophagus. Surgery 1987;102:507–14.

[32] Mittal SK, Awad ZT, Tasset M, et al. The preoperative predictability of the short esophagus in patients with stricture or paraesophageal hernia. Surg Endosc 2000;14:464–8.

[33] Yau P, Watson DI, Jamieson GG, et al. The influence of esophageal length on outcomes after laparoscopic fundoplication. J Am Coll Surg 2000;191:360–5.

[34] Bremner RM, Bremner CG, Peters JH. Fundamentals of antireflux surgery. In: Peters JH, DeMeester TR, editors. Minimally invasive surgery of the foregut. 1st edition. St. Louis (MO): Quality Medical Publishing; 1994. p. 119–243.

[35] Maziak DE, Todd TR, Pearson FG. Massive hiatus hernia: evaluation and surgical management. J Thorac Cardiovasc Surg 1998;115:53–60 [discussion: 61–2].

[36] Pierre AF, Luketich JD, Fernando HC, et al. Results of laparoscopic repair of giant paraesophageal hernias: 200 consecutive patients. Ann Thorac Surg 2002;74:1909–15 [discussion: 1915–6].

[37] Peters JH, DeMeester TR. The lessons of failed antireflux repairs. In: Peters JH, DeMeester TR, editors. Minimally invasive therapy of the foregut. 1st edition. St. Louis (MO): Quality Medical Publishing; 1994. p. 190–200.

[38] Siewert JR, Isolauri J, Feussner H. Reoperation following failed fundoplication. World J Surg 1989;13:791–6 [discussion: 796–7].

[39] Ellis FH Jr, Gibb SP, Heatley GJ. Reoperation after failed antireflux surgery. Review of 101 cases. Eur J Cardiothorac Surg 1996;10:225–31 [discussion: 231–2].

[40] DePaula AL, Hashiba K, Bafutto M, et al. Laparoscopic reoperations after failed and complicated antireflux operations. Surg Endosc 1995;9:681–6.

[41] Collis JL. An operation for hiatus hernia with short esophagus. Thorax 1957;12:181–8.

[42] Stirling MC, Orringer MB. Continued assessment of the combined Collis-Nissen operation. Ann Thorac Surg 1989;47:224–30.

[43] Orringer MB, Sloan H. Combined Collis-Nissen reconstruction of the esophagogastric junction. Ann Thorac Surg 1978;25:16–21.

[44] Awad ZT, Filipi CJ, Mittal SK, et al. Left side thoracoscopically assisted gastroplasty: a new technique for managing the shortened esophagus. Surg Endosc 2000;14:508–12.

[45] Champion JK. Laparoscopic vertical banded gastroplasty with wedge resection of gastric fundus [author reply]. Obes Surg 2003;13:465.

[46] Hashemi M, Peters JH, DeMeester TR, et al. Laparoscopic repair of large Type III hiatal hernia: objective followup reveals high recurrence rate. J Am Coll Surg 2000;190:553–60 [discussion: 560–1].

[47] Khaitan L, Houston H, Sharp K, et al. Laparoscopic paraesophageal hernia repair has an acceptable recurrence rate. Am Surg 2002;68:546–51 [discussion: 551–2].

[48] Jobe BA, Aye RW, Deveney CW, et al. Laparoscopic management of giant Type III hiatal hernia and short esophagus. Objective follow-up at three years. J Gastrointest Surg 2002;6: 181–8 [discussion: 188].

[49] Patterson DJ, Graham DY, Smith JL, et al. Natural history of benign esophageal stricture treated by dilatation. Gastroenterology 1983;85:346–50.

[50] Jeyasingham K. Benign strictures of the esophagus. In: Shields TW, LoCicero J III, Ponn RB, editors. General thoracic surgery. 5th edition. Philadelphia: Lippincott Williams & Wilkins; 2000. p. 1865–80.

[51] Spechler SJ. Complications of gastroesophageal reflux disease. In: Castell DO, editor. The esophagus. 1st edition. Boston: Little, Brown and Company; 1992. p. 543–56.

[52] Smith PM, Kerr GD, Cockel R, et al. A comparison of omeprazole and ranitidine in the prevention of recurrence of benign esophageal stricture. Restore Investigator Group. Gastroenterology 1994;107:1312–8.

[53] Spechler SJ. Comparison of medical and surgical therapy for complicated gastroesophageal reflux disease in veterans. The Department of Veterans Affairs Gastroesophageal Reflux Disease Study Group. N Engl J Med 1992;326:786–92.

[54] Ahtaridis G, Snape WJ Jr, Cohen S. Clinical and manometric findings in benign peptic strictures of the esophagus. Dig Dis Sci 1979;24:858–61.

[55] Dakkak M, Hoare RC, Maslin SC, et al. Oesophagitis is as important as oesophageal stricture diameter in determining dysphagia. Gut 1993;34:152–5.

[56] Jeyasingham K. What is the histology of an esophageal stricture before and after dilation? In: Giuli R, Tytgat GNJ, DeMeester TR, editors. The esophageal mucosa: 300 questions, 300 answers. 1st edition. Amsterdam (Netherlands): Elsevier Science; 1994. p. 335.

[57] Ferguson MK. Medical and surgical management of peptic esophageal strictures. Chest Surg Clin N Am 1994;4:673–95.

[58] Halpert RD, Feczko PJ, Spickler EM, et al. Radiological assessment of dysphagia with endoscopic correlation. Radiology 1985;157:599–602.

[59] Spiess AE, Kahrilas PJ. Treating achalasia: from whalebone to laparoscope. JAMA 1998; 280:638–42.

[60] Lew RJ, Kochman ML. A review of endoscopic methods of esophageal dilation. J Clin Gastroenterol 2002;35:117–26.

[61] Cox JG, Winter RK, Maslin SC, et al. Balloon or bougie for dilatation of benign esophageal stricture? Dig Dis Sci 1994;39:776–81.

[62] Saeed ZA, Winchester CB, Ferro PS, et al. Prospective randomized comparison of polyvinyl bougies and through-the-scope balloons for dilation of peptic strictures of the esophagus. Gastrointest Endosc 1995;41:189–95.

[63] Marks RD, Richter JE. Peptic strictures of the esophagus. Am J Gastroenterol 1993;88: 1160–73.

[64] Wesdorp IC, Bartelsman JF, den Hartog Jager FC, et al. Results of conservative treatment of benign esophageal strictures: a follow-up study in 100 patients. Gastroenterology 1982;82: 487–93.

[65] Kirsch M, Blue M, Desai RK, et al. Intralesional steroid injections for peptic esophageal strictures. Gastrointest Endosc 1991;37:180–2.

[66] Lee M, Kubik CM, Polhamus CD, et al. Preliminary experience with endoscopic intralesional steroid injection therapy for refractory upper gastrointestinal strictures. Gastrointest Endosc 1995;41:598–601.

[67] Zein NN, Greseth JM, Perrault J. Endoscopic intralesional steroid injections in the management of refractory esophageal strictures. Gastrointest Endosc 1995;41:596–8.

[68] Marks RD, Richter JE, Rizzo J, et al. Omeprazole versus H2-receptor antagonists in treating patients with peptic stricture and esophagitis. Gastroenterology 1994;106:907–15.

[69] Saeed ZA, Ramirez FC, Hepps KS, et al. An objective end point for dilation improves outcome of peptic esophageal strictures: a prospective randomized trial. Gastrointest Endosc 1997;45:354–9.

[70] Bender EM, Walbaum PR. Esophagogastrectomy for benign esophageal stricture. Fate of the esophagogastric anastomosis. Ann Surg 1987;205:385–8.

[71] Little AG, Naunheim KS, Ferguson MK, et al. Surgical management of esophageal strictures. Ann Thorac Surg 1988;45:144–7.

[72] Payne WS. Surgical management of reflux-induced oesophageal stenoses: results in 101 patients. Br J Surg 1984;71:971–3.

[73] Spivak H, Farrell TM, Trus TL, et al. Laparoscopic fundoplication for dysphagia and peptic esophageal stricture. J Gastrointest Surg 1998;2:555–60.

[74] Klingler PJ, Hinder RA, Cina RA, et al. Laparoscopic antireflux surgery for the treatment of esophageal strictures refractory to medical therapy. Am J Gastroenterol 1999;94:632–6.

[75] Watson A. Reflux stricture of the oesophagus. Br J Surg 1987;74:443–8.

[76] Stirling MC, Orringer MB. Surgical treatment after the failed antireflux operation. J Thorac Cardiovasc Surg 1986;92:667–72.

ELSEVIER
SAUNDERS

SURGICAL
CLINICS OF
NORTH AMERICA

Surg Clin N Am 85 (2005) 453–463

Quality of Life Measurement in the Management of Gastroesophageal Reflux Disease

Hiran C. Fernando, MD, FRCS, FACS[a,*],
Alberto de Hoyos, MD[b]

[a]Cardiothoracic Surgery, Boston University Medical Center, 88 East Newton Street,
Robinson B-402, Boston, MA 02118-2983, USA
[b]Cardiothoracic Surgery, Northwestern Memorial Hospital, 215 East Huron 10-105,
Chicago, IL 60611, USA

Gastroesophageal reflux disease (GERD) is a significant health problem, with approximately 44% of surveyed adults reporting heartburn to some degree and nearly 18% using nonprescription drugs [1]. Although GERD may be associated with significant complications such as bleeding, esophageal strictures, Barrett's disease, and potentially, esophageal cancer [2], the primary goal of treatment in most patients is to improve symptoms and ultimately quality of life (QOL). Despite the importance of QOL, this outcome measure is rarely measured in surgical practice, with most surgical publications typically reporting more standard outcomes such as mortality and morbidity. This can in part be explained by the lack of a gold standard instrument to measure QOL, and the perception that QOL measurement is difficult and too time-consuming to collect.

One of the oldest instruments to measure QOL is the Karnofsky index [3,4]. This venerable tool has been most useful to measure performance status and predict ability to tolerate therapy in oncology patients; however, it is insufficient in many aspects because it exclusively evaluates physical functioning and does not give significant weight to other domains of QOL. Another disadvantage of the Karnofsky index is its reliance on an observer's assessment of a patient's level of independence and activity rather than the patient's own assessment of his QOL.

* Corresponding author. Boston University Medical Center, 88 East Newton Street, Robinson B-402, Boston, MA 02118-2983.
E-mail address: hiran.fernando@bmc.org (H.C. Fernando).

0039-6109/05/$ - see front matter © 2005 Elsevier Inc. All rights reserved.
doi:10.1016/j.suc.2005.01.015
surgical.theclinics.com

Recently, a number of newer instruments have been developed to measure QOL. These include the Sickness Impact Profile [5], the Functional Living Index in Cancer [6], and the MOS-SF36 [7]. These newer instruments all rely on subjective assessment by the patient, rather than assessment by a potentially biased observer.

New technology continues to be introduced into surgical practice. Often these new techniques are adopted by surgeons and sought by patients before objective evidence of improved outcomes is available. Because GERD is a disease that primarily affects QOL, it is vital that QOL assessment becomes incorporated into the evaluation of new GERD treatments as they are introduced into everyday clinical practice.

This article provides an overview of instruments used to measure QOL, and their increasing application and usefulness in the management of GERD.

Measuring quality of life

Quality of life is a concept that is easy to grasp intuitively, but difficult to measure reliably. In the everyday sense of the phrase, QOL can include such aspects as personal income, location of residence, leisure time and activities, interpersonal relationships, meaningful work, and spiritual fulfillment, among other nonmedical aspects of life. In medicine, however, what we attempt to assess is health-related QOL, which measures the impact of disease on physical, psychological, and social health. The World Health Organization previously defined QOL as an absence of infirmity and a state of physical, social, and mental well being [8]. Although these definitions may be obvious, their measurement may not be.

Instruments to evaluate QOL have essentially one or more of three purposes. First, they can be used as a discriminative index. That is, the instrument used separates groups of patients based on their QOL. For example, in GERD, it is important to discriminate between patients who are satisfied with their present level of symptoms and those who are not. Another function is to be a predictive index. That is, using an instrument to assess outcomes as a result of an intervention; for example, to help separate patients who have GERD into those who would be best served by medical treatment and those who would be best served by an operation. Finally, QOL instruments can be used as an evaluative index. The instrument is used to measure the magnitude in change over time of an individual patient or group of patients, addressing, in GERD for example, whether the intervention (either medical or surgical) improves QOL.

QOL instruments have internal characteristics that should be more rigorously assessed. These qualities include reliability, validity, responsiveness, appropriateness, practicality, and interpretability. Reliability implies that the instrument must produce the same result on repeated assessment of the same level of QOL. Validity implies that the instrument measures what it is purported to measure. Responsiveness (or sensitivity to change) is the ability of the instrument to detect clinically important changes in QOL as a result of treatment or over time. The appropriateness of an instrument depends on how well the instrument measures the relevant aspects of QOL for a given health problem. Practicality reflects the ease with which the instrument can be used by health care professional and patients. Interpretability is how well the result of the questionnaire can be understood by the clinician using the results. All of these factors should be considered when selecting a QOL instrument for use in clinical practice or research.

QOL instruments can generally be categorized as generic or disease-specific. Generic instruments measure global QOL and are broadly applicable across several diseases, whereas disease-specific instruments assess specific diagnostic groups to measure clinically important changes within these diseases. This sensitivity to change (responsiveness) may be one of the most important characteristics of instruments used to evaluate the effects of treatments. The advantages of a generic instrument are that a single instrument can be used in several settings, it can detect differential effects on the various aspects of health status, and comparisons after interventions for different diseases are possible. Additionally, generic instruments allow comparisons with normal populations and patients who have other chronic diseases. The disadvantages of generic instruments are that they may not focus adequately on an area of interest (such as severity of symptoms), and they may not be responsive enough (ie, may not measure changes as a result of an intervention), which may be important for a study on the effects of a particular treatment. Disease-targeted instruments focus on a specific condition and its related symptoms. The specificity of condition-specific instruments can increase their responsiveness to detect small treatment changes over time; however, many of these instruments have not been as extensively validated by longitudinal studies as generic instruments. Additionally, many practitioners are reluctant to use a multitude of instruments for a several disease types (eg, a specific questionnaire for each digestive disease).

A third group of QOL instruments includes those that measure specific symptoms. These instruments do not take into consideration other QOL issues, such as social interactions or psychological stresses. These are still of value, however, if a primary end point of treatment or a common major complication of treatment is the symptom being evaluated. We have previously used symptom specific instruments to evaluate dysphagia after esophagectomy [9], or photodynamic therapy [10] and pain severity after thoracotomy [11].

Generic quality of life instruments

Probably the most well-known generic instrument is the Medical Outcomes Study Short Form 36 (SF36) [7]. This instrument was originally developed by John Ware and the Medical Outcomes Trust, and has gained increasing popularity in several clinical settings. This 36-item questionnaire has been extensively validated, and normal values for various populations have been well-defined. When this instrument was originally developed, scores were expressed as eight domains of QOL. These include physical functioning, role-physical, bodily pain, general health, vitality, social functioning, role-emotional, and mental health. Subsequently, these eight domain scores have been combined into two scores [12], namely a physical component summary (PCS) and mental component summary (MCS) score.

The SF36 has become one of the most popular and widely used QOL instrument in the United States and worldwide, with several foreign translation versions available.

The Psychological General Well-Being Index (PGWB) was developed to measure subjective well-being or distress [13]. Since its introduction in 1984, it has been used in many studies, including the evaluation of QOL in upper gastrointestinal diseases [14]. It assesses six dimensions of QOL: anxiety, depressed mood, positive well-being, self-control, general health, and vitality. These are then combined to give an overall score. This instrument has been popular in several European studies of GERD.

Disease-specific instruments used to evaluate gastroesophageal reflux disease

The Gastrointestinal Symptom Rating Scale (GSRS) was initially constructed to measure severity of symptoms in peptic ulcer disease and irritable bowel syndrome [14]. It is a seven-grade Likert scale questionnaire that contains 15 items. It has been found to be satisfactory with respect to internal consistency, validity, and responsiveness. It has been used to assess GERD and seems adequate for this purpose [15].

The Gastroesophageal Reflux Disease-Health Related Quality of Life Scale (HRQOL) was developed by Velanovich and colleagues to assess GERD severity [16]. The HRQOL is a disease-specific instrument that consists of 10 questions. Nine questions relate to different aspects of GERD, with each response scored from 0 to 5. The best possible score is 0 (no symptoms) and the worst possible score is 45 (most severe symptoms). The tenth question relates to an overall assessment of satisfaction. In a study comparing the HRQOL to the SF36 performed in 43 patients who had GERD [17], 59% of patients preferred the HRQOL, 62% felt it was easier to understand, and 86% felt it was more reflective of their symptoms. The authors' group [18] has preferred to use the HRQOL in combination with the SF36 in our studies of GERD, because we feel that the combination of a disease-specific and generic instrument is advantageous. The Reflux-Related Visual Analogue Scale (RVAS) has recently been developed. Data about its validity and reliability have yet to be published, although

Blomqvist et al [19] showed that there is a good correlation with specific symptoms of GERD, assessed both preoperatively and after antireflux surgery.

Quality of life measurement in untreated gastroesophageal reflux disease

There have been a number of studies evaluating the HRQOL of persons who have untreated GERD. All studies generally demonstrate impaired QOL. Revicki and coauthors [20] studied 533 patients who had moderate to severe heartburn symptoms for at least 6 months. SF36 scores were seen to be worse than those of the general population in all eight domains of the SF36. Additionally, emotional well-being was seen to be worse than in patients who have diabetes or hypertension. In another study, Dimenas and colleagues [21] used the PGWB to evaluate QOL in persons undergoing upper endoscopy for suspected peptic ulcer disease. In a cohort of more than 1500 patients, 192 had endoscopic evidence of erosive esophagitis. This group's QOL was significantly worse than that of patients who had mild heart failure, angina, or untreated peptic ulcer disease. Although GERD can in many aspects be regarded as a benign disease, these two studies illustrate the significant impact that this common disorder can have on QOL.

Quality of life measurement after medical treatment of gastroesophageal reflux disease

The primary goal of therapy in GERD is to relieve symptoms. Secondarily, therapy can heal esophageal injury if present, possibly prevent complications, and maintain remission of symptoms. Several studies have addressed QOL with different medical therapies for GERD. Currently, the most effective medical therapy is with high-dose proton pump inhibitors (PPIs). Before the introduction and regular usage of PPIs, histamine-2 receptor antagonists (H2As) were the principal therapy for GERD, and are still used in many settings, particularly for milder GERD. In one study of 354 patients in the primary care setting treated with H2A [22], QOL scores were seen to improve in all eight scales of the SF36. Similarly, QOL studies in patients who have GERD have been performed using PPIs. A Scandinavian study of 163 patients [23] used the PGWB and GSRS before and after treatment with omeprazole and placebo. In the omeprazole group, QOL scores using both the generic and disease-specific instruments were seen to improve. A prospective, randomized, double-blind study from Canada [24] compared pantoprazole with nizatidine in 208 patients. QOL measurements included the SF36 and the GSRS. Baseline scores were similar between the groups, but at 28 days the PPI group had significantly better scores in four of the eight SF36 domains and in the GSRS reflux score.

An interesting finding from some studies has been the relationship between esophagitis and QOL. A study by McDougall and coworkers [25] compared patients who had Grade II/III esophagitis treated with PPIs to non-GERD controls. Before PPI treatment, SF36 scores were significantly lower in three domains in the GERD patients compared with controls. After PPI treatment, scores improved in seven of the eight SF36 domains in the GERD patients. Surprisingly, there were no differences in scores between patients who had healed esophagitis and those who did not. In two other studies [26,27], patients who had GERD-like symptoms but no esophagitis were treated with placebo or antisecretory medications. In the groups treated with antisecretary medications, QOL was improved. These results imply that symptoms are not necessarily related to the degree or presence of esophagitis, and that if typical GERD symptoms are present, treatment is appropriate and beneficial. On the other hand, if esophagitis is noted before treatment is initiated, follow-up endoscopy should still be performed, despite symptomatic improvement, to ensure that there is no progression of adverse mucosal changes within the esophagus.

Quality of life measurement after surgical therapy of gastroesophageal reflux disease

Since the first Nissen fundoplication was performed laparoscopically in 1991 [28], the number antireflux operations performed has increased exponentially. Laparoscopic fundoplication has been shown to be a safe procedure that can be performed with acceptable early results. Despite this, the role of operation remains controversial and continues to be debated in the literature. Before the routine use of laparoscopic fundoplication, a study by Pope [29] discussed the benefits of open fundoplication on QOL. Over the last 12 years, larger and larger series of laparoscopic fundoplication are being reported using QOL measures. In an earlier study [30], QOL measurements using the PGWB index (generic) and the GSRS (disease-specific) were reported in 40 patients and demonstrated improvement after operation. More recently, reports of 300 patients (using the SF36) [31] and 500 patients using another disease-specific instrument [32], the Gastrointes-tinal Quality of Life Index, have been reported. Both of these single-center studies demonstrated improved QOL after operation. A study from Pittsburgh [33] used a disease-specific GERD score, symptom-specific heartburn scores, and dysphagia scores in 297 patients before and after operation. At a mean follow-up of 31.4 months, symptom-specific and disease-specific scores improved, with only 10% of patients requiring PPIs for typical GERD symptoms.

Other studies have compared open and laparoscopic approaches. In one nonrandomized study, Bloomqvist and associates [19] compared open and minimally invasive approaches with similar outcomes demonstrated between groups. In another study, Velanovich [34] compared open and laparoscopic antireflux operation and found superior physical function and bodily pain scores at 6 weeks in the laparoscopic group, indicating that these patients had a quicker recovery compared with those who had open operation. The group from the University of Southern California [35] used the SF36 to compare 72 patients who had a laparoscopic Nissen fundoplication with 33 patients who had more complex hiatal hernias and strictures and who underwent transthoracic Nissen fundoplication. Although the laparoscopic group recovered quicker, with less postoperative discomfort at long-term follow-up, QOL scores were similar and were only significantly decreased for those patients who, not surprisingly, had recurrent reflux symptoms. The laparoscopic group, however, were more likely to use acid suppression medications and tended to be less satisfied, arguing that at least for patients who have advanced gastroesophageal reflux disease, an open operation is preferred.

Our group [36] has previously reported our experience with 200 giant hiatal hernia repairs performed laparoscopically. All these complex hiatal hernias had at least 30% of the stomach within the mediastinum. In most cases in the later part of the series, a laparoscopic Collis gastroplasty was performed, because we believe that this helps prevent problems with recurrence of the hernia when a shortened esophagus is present [37]. The HRQOL was used to evaluate patients in follow-up, with mean scores of 2.4 and scores felt to be in the excellent or good range in 92% of patients.

Another group of patients who have complex GERD are those patients who have previously undergone antireflux operation. It is often argued that these complex operations should be approached using open techniques, because results will be worse than with primary repair and have been reported ranging from 66% to 76% [38]. If, however, the same principals as open surgery are employed (full work-up of the patient preoperatively, complete takedown of the previous repair, assessment for the presence of a shortened esophagus with appropriate use of a Collis gastroplasty), results will be as good as with those with open operation. Our own series of 80 laparoscopic reoperations [39] included the use of the SF36, HRQOL, and a dysphagia score ranging from 1 (no dysphagia) to 5 (severe dysphagia—unable to tolerate saliva). At a mean follow-up of 18 months SF36 PCS and MCS scores were similar to normal values and mean HRQOL score was 6, which is within the normal range. Dysphagia scores improved significantly from 2 to 1.3, and only 18% of patients reported that they were dissatisfied.

Other controversial aspects of laparoscopic fundoplication include the continued debate over a partial versus a complete wrap. It should be emphasized again that the primary role of antireflux operation is to relieve symptoms and improve QOL. Complete wraps such as a laparoscopic Nissen fundoplication are effective in relieving symptoms of GERD, but may be associated with side effects such as dysphagia, gas bloat, inability to belch, early satiety, and flatulence. The creation of new symptoms, such as these following operation, have the potential to adversely impact on QOL. This concern has led some surgeons to favor partial fundoplication operations such as the laparoscopic Toupet [40]. On the other hand, other reports [41] have suggested that although partial fundoplications may be associated with fewer side effects such as bloating or dysphagia, there may be an unacceptable rate of recurrent symptoms of GERD as longer follow-up becomes available. The authors' own experience favors the use of a Nissen over a Toupet fundoplication. In our series comparing 163 Nissen to 43 Toupet fundoplications [42], we found that SF36 physical function scores were significantly better in the Nissen group. Additionally, significantly more Toupet patients complained of dysphagia. These differences did not appear to be related to differences in esophageal motility between the two groups.

Age is sometimes felt to be a contraindication to laparoscopic antireflux surgery. Again, it should be emphasized that GERD primarily affects QOL, and that operation may have a significant positive effect, even in the elderly higher surgical risk patient who has severe GERD. Recently, our group compared outcomes between an older and younger group of patients, all of whom had complete fundoplications [43]. Despite a longer length of stay in the older population, follow-up HRQOL, SF36 scores, and dysphagia scores were excellent and similar between the two groups of patients, supporting the role of operation for the older patient.

Medical versus surgical therapy: how does quality of life compare?

This continues to be an area of intense discussion, particularly with the introduction of newer medications and the increasing availability of laparoscopic antireflux operation. In one of the few randomized studies that have been reported [44], open fundoplication was compared with medical therapy using H2A in a multicenter Veterans Administration (VA) setting. Patients in this study maintained a diary of symptoms to construct a gastroesophageal reflux-disease activity index (GRACI). In the initial report from this study, with 2-year follow-up, the mean activity index and grade of esophagitis were better in the surgical group. A follow-up study on these patients was recently published [45]. The median follow-up was 7.3 years for the medical group and 6.3 years for the surgical group, with follow-up available in 91 medical and 38 surgical patients. Follow-up included use of the SF36 and the GRACI. Surprisingly, a large number of the surgical patients (62%) required antireflux medications; however, this was still significantly lower than the proportion of medical patients requiring antireflux medications (92%). Additionally, GRACI scores and SF36 bodily pain scores were significantly better in the surgical group. Another randomized study from Sweden [46] compared open fundoplication to PPI, with 5-year follow-up. In this study, the PWGB (generic instrument) and the GSRS (disease-specific) were used. QOL scores were found to be similar between the groups. There were more treatment failures in the medical group, although when higher-dose omeprazole was used this difference did not reach statistical significance.

Our group compared patients undergoing medical therapy to patients undergoing laparoscopic antireflux operation [18]. The study population included all patients presenting with a primary diagnosis of reflux to the gastoenterology or surgical clinic during a 1-year period. Despite the surgical group demonstrating more severe reflux (based on greater usage of PPI and propulsid) before therapy, results were better in the surgical cohort. Reflux severity using the HRQOL was 4 in the surgical group versus 21 in the medical group. SF 36 scores were significantly better in six of the eight domains of QOL in the surgical group.

Summary

QOL measurement is being reported with increasing frequency in the surgical literature. The authors have found, as have others, that the use of a generic instrument such as the SF36 in combination with a disease-specific instrument will provide the most comprehensive information. GERD is a significant health problem that primarily affects the QOL of a large segment of the population. New therapies for GERD continue to be developed and introduced into clinical practice. QOL assessment should be an important part of the evaluation of these new therapies.

References

[1] Society of American Gastrointestinal Endoscopic Surgeons guidelines for surgical treatment of gastroesophageal reflux disease (GERD). Surg Endosc 1998;12:186–8.
[2] Lagergren J, Bergstrom R, Lindgren A, et al. Symptomatic gastroesophageal reflux as a risk factor for esophageal adenocarcinoma. N Engl J Med 1999;340:825–31.
[3] Karnofsky DA, Abelmann WH, Craver LF, et al. The use of the nitrogen mustards; in the palliative treatment of carcinoma. With particular reference to bronchogenic cancer. Cancer 1948;1:634–56.
[4] Ganz PA, Lee JJ, Siau J. Quality of life assessment. An independent prognostic variable for survival in lung cancer. Cancer 1991;67:3131–5.
[5] Selby PJ, Chapman JAW, Etazdi-Amoli J, et al. The development of a method for assessing the quality of life in cancer patients. Br J Cancer 1984;50:13–22.
[6] Shipper H, Clinch J, McMurry A, et al. Measuring the quality of life of cancer patients: The Functional Living Index—Cancer: development and validation. J Clin Oncol 1984;2:472–83.
[7] Ware JE, Sherbourne CD. The MOS 36-item short-form health survey (SF-36). Med Care 1992;30:473–83.
[8] World Health Organization. The constitution of the WHO. WHO Chron 1947;1:29.
[9] Luketich JD, Alvelo-Rivera M, Buenaventura PO, et al. Minimally invasive esophagectomy: outcomes in 222 patients. Ann Surg 2003;238:486–94.

[10] Litle VR, Luketich JD, Christie NA, et al. Photodynamic therapy as palliation for esophageal cancer: experience in 215 patients. Ann Thorac Surg 2003;76:1687–92.

[11] Luketich JD, Land SR, Sullivan SR, et al. Thoracic epidural versus intercostal nerve catheter plus patient controlled analgesia: a randomized prospective study. Ann Thorac Surg, in press.

[12] Ware JE Jr, Kosinski M, Keller SD. SF-36 physical and mental health summary scales: a users manual. Boston: The Health Institute, New England Medical Center; 1994.

[13] Dupuy HJ. The Psychological General Well-being Index (PGWG). In: Wenger NK, Mattson ME, Furberg CF, et al, editors. Assesments of quality of life in clinical trials of cardiovascular therapies. New York: Le Jacq Publishing; 1984. p. 170–83.

[14] Svedlund J, Sjodin I, Dotevall G. GSRS—a clinical rating scale for gastrointestinal symptoms in patients with irritable bowel syndrome and peptic ulcer disease. Dig Dis Sci 1988;33:129–34.

[15] Dimenas E, Glise H, Hallerback B, et al. Quality of life in patients with upper gastrointestinal symptoms. An improved evaluation of treatment regimens? Scan J Gastroenterol 1993;28:681–7.

[16] Velanovich V, Vallance SR, Gusz JR, et al. Quality of life scale for gastroesophageal reflux disease. J Am Coll Surg 1996;183:217–24.

[17] Velanovich V. Comparison of generic (SF36) vs disease-specefic (GERD-HRQOL) quality of life scales for gastroesophageal reflux disease. J Gastrointest Surg 1998;2:141–5.

[18] Fernando HC, Schauer PR, Rosenblatt M, et al. Quality of life after antireflux surgery compared with non-operative management for severe gastroesophageal reflux disease. J Am Coll Surg 2002;194:23–7.

[19] Blomqvist A, Lonroth H, Dalenback J, et al. Quality of life assessment after laparoscopic and open fundoplications: result of a prospective, clinical study. Scan J Gastroenterol 1996;31:1052–8.

[20] Revicki DA, Wood M, Maton PN, et al. The impact of gastroesophageal reflux disease on health-related quality of life. Am J Med 1998;104:252–8.

[21] Dimenas E, Glise H, Hallerback B, et al. Well-being and gastrointestinal symptoms among patients referred to endoscopy owing to suspected duodenal ulcer. Scan J Gastroenterol 1995;11:1046–52.

[22] Chal KL, Stacey JH, Sacks GE. The effects of ranitidine on symptom relief and quality of life of patients with gastroesophageal reflux disease. Br J Clin Pract 1995;49:73–7.

[23] Havelund T, Lind T, Wiklund I, et al. Quality of life in patients with heartburn but without esophagitis: effects of treatment with omeprazole. Am J Gastroenterol 1999;94:1782–9.

[24] Pare P, Armstrong D, Pericak D, et al. Pantoprazole rapidly improves health-related quality of life in patients with heartburn: a prospective, randomized, double blind comparative study with nizatidine. J Clin Gastroenterol 2003;37:132–8.

[25] McDougall NI, Collins JS, McFarland RJ, et al. The effect of treating reflux esophagitis with omeprazole on quality of life. Eu J Gastroenterol Hepatol 1998;10:451–4.

[26] Watson RGP, Tham TCK, Johnston BT, et al. Double blind cross-over placebo controlled study of patients with reflux symptoms and physiological levels of acid-reflux—the "sensitive esophagus." Gut 1997;40:587–90.

[27] Mathias SD, Colwell HH, Miller DP, et al. Health-related quality of life and quality days incrementally gained in symptomatic nonerosive GERD patients treated with lansoprazole or ranitidine. Dig Dis Sci 2001;46:2416–23.

[28] Dallemagne B, Weerts JM, Jehaes C, et al. Laparoscopic Nissen fundoplication; preliminary report. Surg Endosc 1991;3:138–43.

[29] Pope CE II. The quality of life following antireflux surgery. World J Surg 1992;6:335–58.

[30] Glise H, Hallerback B, Johannon B. Quality of life assessments in evaluation of laparoscopic Rosetti fundoplication. Surg Endosc 1995;9:183–9.

[31] Hunter JG, Trus TL, Branum GD, et al. A physiological approach to laparoscopic fundoplication for gastroesophageal reflux disease. Ann Surg 1996;223:673–87.

[32] Kamolz T, Granderath FA, Bammer T, et al. Mid and long-term quality of life assessments after laparoscopic fundoplication and refundoplication: a single unit review of more than 500 antireflux procedures. Dig Liver Dis 2002;34:470–6.

[33] Papasavas PK, Keenan RJ, Yeaney WW, et al. Effectiveness of laparoscopic fundoplication in relieving the symptoms of gastroesophageal reflux disease (GERD) and eliminating antireflux medical therapy. Surg Endosc 2003;17:1200–5.

[34] Velanovich V. Comparison of symptomatic and quality of life outcomes of laparoscopic versus open antireflux surgery. Surgery 1999;126:782–9.

[35] Streets CG, DeMeester SR, DeMeester TR, et al. Excellent quality of life after Nissen fundoplication depends on successful elimination of reflux symptoms and not the invasiveness of the surgical approach. Ann Thorac Surg 2002;74:1019–25.

[36] Pierre AF, Luketich JD, Fernando HC, et al. Results of laparoscopic repair of giant paraesophageal hernias: 200 consecutive patients. Ann Thorac Surg 2002;74(6):1909–15.

[37] Luketich JD, Grondin SC, Pearson FG. Minimally invasive approaches to acquired shortening of the esophagus: laparoscopic Collis-Nissen gastroplasty. Semin Thorac Cardiovasc Surg 2000;(12):173–8.

[38] Siewert JR, Isolauri J, Feussner H. Reoperation following failed fundoplication. World J Surg 1989;13:791–7.

[39] Luketich JD, Fernando HC, Christie NA, et al. Outcomes after minimally invasive reoperation for gastroesophageal reflux disease. Ann Thorac Surg 2002;74(2):328–31.

[40] Rydberg L, Ruth M, Lundell L. Mechanism of action of antireflux procedures. Br J Surg 1999;86:405–10.

[41] Jobe BA, Wallace J, Hansen PD, et al. Evaluation of laparoscopic Toupet fundoplication as a primary repair for all patients with medically resistant gastroesphageal reflux. Surg Endosc 1997;11:1080–3.

[42] Fernando HC, Luketich JD, Christie NA, et al. Outcomes of laparoscopic Toupet compared to Nissen fundoplication. Surg Endosc 2002;16:905–8.

[43] Fernando HC, Schauer PR, Buenaventura PO, et al. Outcomes of minimally invasive antireflux operations in the elderly: a comparative review. JSLS 2003;7(4):311–5.

[44] Spechlar SJ. Comparison of medical and surgical therapy for complicated gastroesophageal reflux disease in veterans. N Engl J Med 1992;326:786–92.

[45] Spechlar SJ, Lee E, Ahnen D, et al. Long-term outcome of medical and surgical therapies for gastroesophageal reflux disease. Follow-up of a randomized controlled trial. JAMA 2001; 285:2331–8.

[46] Lundell L, Miettinen P, Myrvold HE, et al. Continued (5-year) follow-up of a randomized clinical study comparing antireflux surgery and omeprazole in gastroesophageal reflux disease. J Am Coll Surg 2001;192:172–81.

ELSEVIER
SAUNDERS

SURGICAL
CLINICS OF
NORTH AMERICA

Surg Clin N Am 85 (2005) 465–481

Endoscopic Therapies
For Gastroesophageal Reflux Disease

Alberto de Hoyos, MD[a],
Hiran C. Fernando, FRCS, FACS[b],*

[a]Cardiothoracic Surgery, Northwestern Memorial Hospital, 215 East Huron 10-105,
Chicago, IL 60611, USA
[b]Cardiothoracic Surgery, Boston University Medical Center, 88 East Newton Street,
Robinson B-402, Boston, MA 02118-2983, USA

Gastroesophageal reflux disease (GERD) is a chronic recurrent condition that affects over 7% of individuals on a daily basis in the United States. The primary objective of antireflux therapy is relief of symptoms, with secondary goals to heal esophagitis, prevent reflux-related complications, and maintain remission. Over the past few years, several endoscopic therapies (ETs) have emerged for the treatment of GERD. These new techniques have generated considerable interest among gastroenterologists, surgeons, and patients alike. The possibility of an outpatient procedure, performed without an abdominal incision and general anesthesia, is attractive to patients and is leading to the rapid development and introduction of these alternative therapies into clinical practice, despite the lack of long-term follow-up and well-designed randomized trials. These endoscopic interventions may be considered "bridge" therapy, because patients who undergo these treatments can still elect to be treated with chronic medications or operation if the endoscopic therapy does not provide symptom relief or if symptoms recur. In this article, the authors review the endoscopic procedures that have been introduced to treat GERD. Technical aspects, mechanisms of action, safety, efficacy, and tolerability of these ETs are discussed. Patient selection and relevant human studies are reviewed in an effort to clarify advantages and disadvantages of ETs over conventional surgical procedures.

* Corresponding author.
E-mail address: hiran.fernando@bmc.org (H.C. Fernando).

0039-6109/05/$ - see front matter © 2005 Elsevier Inc. All rights reserved.
doi:10.1016/j.suc.2005.01.017   *surgical.theclinics.com*

Rationale for endoscopic antireflux therapies

Unlike medical therapy that treats only the symptoms of GERD, surgical and endoscopic approaches provide relief by targeting the disturbed physiologic antireflux barrier. Repair of a failed barrier, whether through an open surgical incision, a laparoscope or potentially, an endoscope, corrects the cause of GERD and can alter the progression of the disease. In contrast, acid suppression therapy alters the pH of the gastric juice refluxed through the defective barrier in an effort to control the symptoms of the disease, but is ineffective at correcting the cause of the disease. It is postulated that ETs modulate the function of the lower esophogeal sphincter (LES) by decreasing its compliance (all ET approaches), by creating a vale-flap mechanism (endosuturing methods) or by decreasing the incidence of transient lower esophageal sphincter relaxations (TLESRs) through a neural mechanism (radiofrequency energy), resulting in a decrease in gastroesophageal reflux. The major advantages of these ETs are as follows: (1) they do not disturb the delicate anatomic arrangements of the gastroesophageal junction (GEJ); (2) they can be performed as outpatient procedures; (3) they do not interfere with future medical or surgical therapies; (4) they decrease esophageal acid exposure, potentially allowing patients to discontinue antisecretory medications; and (5) they are appealing to patients. On the other hand, disadvantages include: (1) incomplete control of reflux or failure to normalize esophageal acid exposure; (2) failure to heal esophagitis; (3) they are technically demanding procedures; (4) limited follow-up with unknown long-term outcomes; (5) the small size or the absence of randomized studies, precluding direct comparison with other well established treatment modalities.

Endoscopic therapies for GERD can be classified into three major categories: (1) endoscopic suturing or placation of gastric folds at the gastric cardia, (2) thermal remodeling and neurolysis of the LES zone by radiofrequency energy (RFe) delivery, and (3) bulking or reinforcing of the LES zone by injection of inert material. Table 1 summarizes the different procedures currently undergoing clinical trials which will also be described in more detail below.

Endoscopic suturing

Endoscopic suturing techniques were initiated by Swain and Mills in the 1980s [1]. They developed a miniature sewing machine that attached to the end of a standard upper gastrointestinal endoscope. The first Food and Drug Administration (FDA)-approved method for treating GERD was an endoscopic suturing method introduced by Bard (Murray Hill, New Jersey) under the name EndoCinch. This method is the commercial version of the miniature sewing machine as developed by Swain and associates [2] in London. Of the three approaches used for ET, endoscopic suturing is probably the most technically demanding.

Table 1
Endoscopic-based therapies for treatment of GERD

Method	Manufacturer	Technique	FDA approval	Clinical trials
Endoscopic suturing				
Endocinch	BARD	Partial plicature	Yes	Yes
ESD	Wilson-Cook	Partial plicature	No	Yes
Plicator	NDO	Transmural plicature	No	Yes
Radiofrequency				
Stretta	Curon Medical	Thermal energy	Yes	Yes
Bulking techniques				
Enteryx	Boston Scientific	Polymer injection	Yes	Yes
PAMMA		Microsphere injection	No	Yes
Gatekeeper	Medtronic	Prosthesis implantation	No	Yes

The mechanism of action of this technique is not clear. Although no animal or human studies have examined in detail the precise mechanism by which endosuturing achieves its beneficial effect in GERD, endoscopic suturing has the potential to alter the angle of His, lengthen or tighten the sphincter mechanism, or refashion the valvular mechanism at the GEJ. Experiments in dogs have shown that distension of the cardiac region of the stomach is the site where TLESRs are elicited at the highest frequency. By improving the function of the LES, both volume and frequency of acid reflux events which occur during periods of TLESRs, decrease. A recent study on 10 patients [3] showed a significant reduction in TLESRs 6 months after endoluminal gastric plication (ELGP).

In an animal study of ELGP [4], median lower esophageal sphincter pressure increased from 4.6 mmgHg to 13.3 mmHg ($P = 0.008$). The median gastric yield pressure (GYP) of the cardia (ie, the gastric pressure required to overcome the competency of the LES, resulting in a common cavity event) increased from 10 mmHg to 19 mmHg ($P = 0.007$). Diminution of the sphincter pressure was noted over time, but it remained above initial sphincter pressure. In this study, there was also a significant increase in the length of the intra-abdominal segment of LES, from 1 cm preoperatively to 2 cm after the procedure ($P = 0.02$). In another study [5], ambulatory pH monitoring demonstrated that the time pH was less than 4 decreased from 9.3% to 0.2%, with reflux events dropping from 19 to 2. These animal studies have also demonstrated that the majority of endoscopically placed stitches are located at a mean depth of 2.8 mm (ie, in the submucosa) with occasional transmural stitches seen.

Technique of endoluminal gastric plication

Bard EndoCinch

The EndoCinch system requires two videoendoscopes, a 9 mm by 32 mm capsule suturing system, and accessories that include an overtube, needle pusher, knot pusher, and suture cutter. The first endoscope carries the metal sewing machine capsule on its tip. The second endoscope cinches the sutures through a catheter device that deploys a ceramic plug and ring, through which the sutures are threaded. An overtube allows for repeated intubations. The optimal orientation and number of plications is as yet unknown. Numerous orientations of the plications have been described (circular, linear, helical), but the most common approach has been a linear orientation, with the plications placed approximately 1 to 2 cm apart on the gastric side of the GEJ. The usual target for placement of plications is 1 cm below the Z-line at three, six, and nine o'clock for the circumferential pattern, and at two o'clock 3, 2, and 1 cm below the z-line for the linear configuration. In the helical configuration, which can be applied to small hiatal hernias, a total of four to six plications are placed for a length of 3 to 4 cm below and up to the z-line.

In general, each placation requires passage of an endoscope seven to eight times (twice for suture placement, five times for the knotting process, and once to cut the knot). The need for repetitive knot tying has been eliminated by the development of the EndoCinch-2. Depending on anatomy and technical expertise, the procedure takes from 30 to 60 minutes to complete.

Clinical experience

To date, approximately 3000 procedures have been performed worldwide. Most of the available data are uncontrolled, with short follow-up, and are mostly available in abstract form. The EndoCinch system has been evaluated in two open-label prospective studies [6,7]. Mahmood and coworkers [7] recently published their experience with ELGP in 26 patients with 1-year follow-up using the EndoCinch-1 suturing system. They routinely use two plications. At endoscopy in 22 patients at 3 months, one of the placations had vanished in 3 patients and both placations had disappeared in 2 patients. In the remaining 17 patients (77%), both placations were intact. There was significant improvement in quality of life, heartburn symptom score, and regurgitation frequency at 1, 3, 6, and 12 months. Similarly, pH studies also demonstrated significant improvement at 3 months, but in only 48% of patients did the DeMeester score return to normal values. Manometric studies failed to demonstrate a significant difference in LES pressure and length. Thirty percent of the patients continued to require proton pump inhibitors (PPIs) therapy at follow-up ranging from 3 to 12 months after ELGP.

Filipi and associates [8] published the results of a multicenter trial in eight North American centers involving 64 patients. It should be noted that patients who have dysphagia, severe esophagitis, failure to improve with PPIs, morbid obesity (body mass index [BMI] > 40) and hiatal hernia greater than 2 cm were excluded. Treatment success was defined as a 50% decrease in the heartburn severity score and a reduction in the use of antisecretory medications to under four doses per month. Patients were randomized to a linear (52%) or circumferential (48%) plication configuration. The linear configuration consisted of plications stacked on the lesser curvature 1 cm apart, with the most proximal placation at or just below the squamocolumnar junction. For the circumferential group, placations were placed just below the squamocolumnar junction approximately 120° apart.

Mean time to complete the procedure was 68 minutes. Sixty nine percent of patients received conscious sedation, 14% monitored anesthesia, and 17% general anesthesia. There was significant improvement in heartburn severity score and in pH studies. Heartburn scores were decreased significantly at 3 and 6 months. The percent total time the pH was lower than 4, total number of reflux episodes, and percent upright time pH was lower than 4 were all significantly improved at 6 months follow-up, but none returned to the normal range. No significant change was found in LES resting pressure or length. There was no significant effect on mucosal healing, with 25% of patients having grade 2 esophagitis at baseline and 19% having it at 6-month follow-up. The configuration of the plication did not affect outcome. Success criteria were met in 58.8% of patients, and in 46.9% if it is assumed that the procedure was unsuccessful in the 10 patients that withdrew from the study. Improvement in symptoms did not always correlate with improvement of esophagitis or pH profiles. Repeat procedures for suboptimal results were performed on 11 patients between 49 and 405 days after the original attempt. Procedure failures were related to technical problems such as inappropriate plication positioning, complete or partial disruption of the plication, inadequate tissue inclusion, and poor knot tying resulting in an excessively loose plication. The intended suture location was accomplished for 81% of the plications. Adverse events included mucosal tears, gastric bleeding, and suture perforation. There was no mortality. Quality of life scores at 6 months postprocedure were significantly improved for social functioning and bodily pain.

In another recent study of 33 patients [9], heartburn severity score and frequency of regurgitation showed continued improvement at the 2 year follow-up compared with baseline; however, only 8 patients (25%) initially on antisecretory therapy with PPIs were completely off medications, 40% required full-dose medications, and 6% had undergone a laparoscopic fundoplication (LF) because of therapeutic failure.

Analysis of the available data shows that although initial success with ELGP is frequently achieved, with 75% to 85% of patients reporting symptom relief at 6 weeks, 30% to 75% of patients experience recurrent symptoms at 6 months and require resumption of antisecretory medications. Approximately 25% of patients treated by ELGP were off all PPIs, and slightly more than one quarter of patients were on less-than-baseline PPI therapy. Two-year follow-up studies are available from two centers [9,10]. In the report by Rothstein and coauthors [9], over 40% of patients were still on full-dose medications, whereas in the study by Haber et al [10], 7 of

23 patients (30.4%) eventually had an operative fundoplication. In a case-control study comparing ELGP and LF [11], 78% of patients undergoing ELGP were satisfied with their symptomatic outcome at 6 weeks, compared with 96% of patients undergoing LF. In a subsequent report [12], the same authors reported their experience with LF after failed ELGP. All patients who had typical symptoms benefited from LF.

A case-control study [13] compared the efficacy of the EndoCinch device in 18 patients with 16 age-matched patients who underwent LF. The mean duration of the procedure (52 versus 116 minutes) and hospital stay (0.05 versus 3.3 days) were shorter in those undergoing the endoscopic procedure. Symptom scores, need for PPIs, and quality of life were significantly improved in both groups; however, those undergoing LF showed greater control of esophageal acid exposure [13].

In addition to the EndoCinch, other suturing devices have been introduced by other companies and are being increasingly used in the hope of improving on the results from initial trials.

The full-thickness Endoscopic Plication System (NDO Surgical, Mansfield, Massachusetts) creates a single full-thickness placation near the GEJ with serosa-to-serosa apposition. The plication is formed with a pretied, suture-based implant delivered just below the GEJ with a gastroscope in a retroflexed manner. Direct visualization is accomplished using a 5.9 mm, outer-diameter, flexible pediatric gastroscope inserted through a dedicated channel in the instrument. A single pleat of full-thickness tissue with healing of serosa-to-serosa is accomplished.

Following a feasibility study in cadaveric human and pig stomachs, Chuttani and colleagues [14] used the Endoscopic Plication System in seven patients who had GERD. Plications were placed between the anterior wall and the fundus because it was deemed the safest area, avoiding major branches on the left and right gastric arteries and vagus nerves. Six of the seven patients were successfully plicated, with five being able to discontinue medications for GERD. Improvement in symptoms and pH exposure persisted at 6 months [15]. Pleskow et al [16] recently presented their experience with the Endoscopic Plication System in 64 patients who had mild-to-moderate GERD. Improvement in symptoms was seen in 75% of patients, normalization of pH in 30%, and 83% of patients were off antisecretory medications at 6 months of follow-up. No significant change in manometric studies was noted. Complications included chest pain, abdominal pain, pneumothorax, gastric perforation, gastric mucosal injury, and pneumoperitoneum.

The Wilson-Cook endoscopic suturing device (ESD, Wilson-Cook Medical, Winston-Salem, North Carolina) consists of several components: the flexible Sew-Right device, the flexible Ti-knot device, the external accessory channel to attach to any flexible upper endoscope, braided 2-0 polyester suture, and titanium knot clipping devices. No overtube is required. The Sew-Right and the Ti-knot devices are reloadable, and are passed through the accessory channel attached to the endoscope; therefore multiple placations can be created from only one initial intubation. The Sew-Right device contains two needles oriented in tandem and controlled by a toggle switch. A continuous single-suture loop is used to stitch two adjacent areas in the proximal stomach to form a placation. The device has a vacuum cap that slides over the distal end of the sewing device once it has been loaded with the suture. At this time, only limited clinical experience has been reported [17].

Radiofrequency energy

Radiofrequency energy (RFe) is commonly used in surgical and endoscopic procedures for cutting and coagulation of tissue. Cutting waveforms are purely sinusoidal and typically reside in the frequency range between 400 kHz and 1 MHz, whereas coagulation waveforms incorporate brief pauses in sinusoidal pattern to optimize tissue coagulation and hemostasis. The Stretta system (Curon Medical, Sunnyvale, California) consists of a radiofrequency (RF) generator and single-use RFe catheters [18]. The generator delivers pure sine-wave energy (465 kHz) and 2 to 5 W per channel. There are four RF channels, each powering a single needle electrode, a temperature feedback control system, and a peristaltic irrigation pump. The RF energy delivery catheter comprises a soft guidewire tip, a balloon-basket assembly, four electrode delivery sheaths positioned radially around the balloon, and suction and irrigation lines. When the catheter is positioned and the needles deployed into the circular muscle of the distal LES or cardia, RFe is delivered to each electrode to achieve a target temperature of 85°C in the muscle; the generator will discontinue power delivery to an individual electrode if tissue temperature exceeds 100°C, if mucosal temperature exceeds 50°C, or if tissue impedance exceeds 1000 Ohms. An integrated peristaltic pump delivers chilled plain water irrigation to the basket ports to maintain mucosal temperature at a safe level during RFe delivery. The result is a thermal lesion in the muscle coat, with intact overlying mucosa. This procedure is a promising new modality in the management of GERD [19]. It can be safely performed in one short session with endoscopy under conscious sedation.

Mechanism of action

The mechanism of action is believed to be twofold: (1) mechanical alteration of the GEJ, and (2) neural modulation of TLESR [20–22]. Whereas rapid heating of tissue results in desiccation, high impedance, and limitation of lesion propagation, thermocouple-controlled RFe delivery for GERD results in the propagation of a circumscribed area of thermal coagulative necrosis that targets the smooth muscle at or near the GEJ and cardia. This injury in the acute phase undergoes wound healing with influx of macrophages, polymorphonuclear leukocytes, and myofibroblasts. Over time, the wound volume is reduced as fibroblasts contract and collagen is deposited, resulting in tissue contraction and remodeling, leading to tightening and reduced compliance of the GEJ. Contraction of the collagen already present in the tissues occurs immediately on exposure to 65°C, resulting in tissue shrinkage. In a porcine model of botulinum-induced LES hypotension, RFe delivery substantially restored LES pressure within 8 weeks of treatment [22a]. Furthermore, RF treatment increased the GYP by 75% over controls. Augmentation of the GYP, similar to that occurring after fundoplication, indicates a more robust antireflux barrier.

In approximately 85% of patients who have GERD, TLESRs are the primary mechanisms of disease. RFe has been demonstrated to induce ablation of nerves that trigger TLESRs. TLESRs are triggered primarily by gastric distension and are mediated through vagal pathways; they are reduced by vagal blockade and the gamma-aminobutyric acid receptor agonist baclofen. Although the exact mechanism of action is still uncertain, RFe could interfere with triggering of TLESRs by several potential mechanisms. First, intramural lesions could interrupt neural signaling of distension, either by ablating mechanoreceptors at the gastric cardia or by interrupting the afferent nerve pathways that control relaxation of the LES. Interference with the efferent motor pathway seems less likely, because there is no effect on swallowing-induced LES relaxation. Second, it is known that RFe lesions heal by fibrosis and contraction, and can thereby alter the mechanics of the gastric cardia, resulting in less distension and therefore fewer stimuli to the mechanoreceptors, then resulting in reduction in nerve signaling and TLESRs.

Technique

The procedure is performed on an outpatient basis with conscious sedation. Twenty-five percent of patients experience mild discomfort during catheter passage, and 50% to 70% of patients have moderate discomfort during RFe delivery. Increased doses of midazolam and fentanyl usually are effective, but some patients require general anesthesia.

Unlike the EndoCinch method, the Stretta procedure is easy to learn and apply. It does not seem to be as operator-dependent as the Bard method. The average operative time is 45 ± 0.9 minutes.

Results

Wolfsen and Richards [23] recently published the registry results of the Stretta procedure for the treatment of GERD. Thirty-three institutions participated in this study, with a total of 558 patients suitable for analysis. At 6 months of follow-up, 91% of patients had experienced symptom control and 9% of patients had no improvement. At baseline, 50% of patients had symptom control while on drugs, compared with 90% at follow-up after Stretta ($P < 0.0001$). Satisfaction with symptom control on drugs at baseline was reported by 23% of patients, compared with an 87% satisfaction rate after Stretta ($P < 0.0001$). At baseline, 94% of patients required daily PPI therapy, compared with 49% after Stretta. Most patients (90%) would recommend Stretta to a friend.

Triadafilopoulos and coworkers [24] recently reported the 6- and 12-month results of an open label trial of Stretta in the treatment of patients who had GERD. This was a prospective multicenter trial involving 118 patients who had chronic heartburn or regurgitation, abnormal esophageal acid exposure, hiatal hernia less than 2 cm, and mild esophagitis (<grade 2). The procedure was successfully completed in all patients in 55 ± 13 minutes. At 12 months, 94 (79.6%) were available for follow-up. There was improvement in heartburn score, GERD score, and quality of life. Proton pump inhibitor requirement decreased from 88% to 30%, and esophageal acid exposure improved significantly, although it did not normalize in the majority of subjects. There was no significant improvement in the incidence and severity of esophagitis after treatment. There were 10 (8.6%) complications, all acute and self-limited.

In a more recent study, Tam and coauthors [25] found that RFe had significant effects on the function of the LES: the rate of TLESR was reduced by 24% and postprandial basal LES pressure increased significantly. These effects were associated with a reduction in reflux events and esophageal acid exposure, and improvement in quality of life. At 6 months, RFe treatment significantly reduced reflux episodes and esophageal acid exposure time; however, by 12 months, the effects on reflux episodes seemed to have been partially lost, because only the rate of recumbent reflux episodes remained statistically lower. Median total esophageal exposure time remained significantly reduced at 12 months. Clinical remission was present in 75% and 65% of patients at 6 and 12 months of follow-up, respectively. Two thirds (65%) of patients remained off acid suppression therapy at 1 year of follow-up.

Houston et al [26] also reported significant decrease in esophageal acid exposure time, DeMeester score, and use of antisecretory medications, and no change in LES pressure following RFe treatment; however, in this study, only 43% of patients returned at 6 months for follow-up manometric studies, limiting the interpretation of the results.

Richards and colleagues [27] prospectively evaluated 140 patients who had GERD and performed the Stretta procedure or laparoscopic fundoplication. The 65 patients undergoing the Stretta procedure had a small hiatal hernia (<2 cm), LES pressure equal to or greater than 8 mmHg, and absence of Barrett's esophagus. Seventy-five patients who had larger hernias, LES pressure less than 8 mmHg, or Barrett's underwent LF. There was significant and equal magnitude of improvement in GERD scores and quality of life in both groups after the procedures. Fifty-eight percent of Stretta patients were off PPIs, and 31% had reduced their dose significantly;

97% of LF patients were off PPIs. In the Stretta patients, there was a significant decrease in esophageal acid exposure time (8.2 ± 0.9% to 4.4 ± 0.5%, $P < 0.01$) and DeMeester score (39.4 ± 4.5 to 26.6 + 5.2, $P < 0.01$). There was no significant change in mean LES pressure (22.8 ± 2.4 to 23.5 ± 2.5, $P > 0.05$). Only eight of the 22 (36%) patients who underwent repeat pH testing had normalization of their acid exposure time. No manometric or pH studies are reported for the LF group. Both procedures resulted in improvements in asthma symptoms. Complete response, defined as no longer needing PPIs, was achieved in 58% of patients after Stretta and in 97% after LF. Partial (31%) or no response (11%) was observed in 42% of patients in the Stretta group and in 3% of the LF group. No cases of worsening dysphagia or new-onset dysphagia were identified in either group. Complications occurred in 1.5% of patients undergoing the Stretta procedure and in 11% of patients after LF. There was no mortality in either group.

Although the incidence of complications is decreased compared with LF, it should be noted that measures of success traditionally used to assess antireflux surgery were not achieved. At a relatively short follow-up, it appears that between 30% and 50% of patients still require PPI therapy after Stretta. Although improvement in 24-hour pH studies is reported, the DeMeester score rarely normalized in these studies.

Bulking techniques

The principle of this technique is to create a mechanical barrier in the GEJ to prevent gastroesophageal reflux. Three products have been used: (1) biopolymer augmentation (Enteryx); (2) Plexiglas implantation (PMMA) and (3) expandable hydrogel prosthesis (Gatekeeper). Currently only Enteryx has been approved by the FDA.

Enteryx

Enteryx (Enteric Medical Technologies, Foster City, California) is an injectable inert biocompatible solution containing 8% ethylene vinyl alcohol copolymer (EVOH) dissolved in demethyl sulfoxide (DMSO) [28]. Micronized tantalum powder (30% weight/volume) is suspended in the polymer/solvent mixture to provide contrast for visualization during fluoroscopy. Enteryx was recently approved for the treatment of GERD based on the results of a multicenter trial involving 85 patients [29].

Mechanism of action

The precise mechanism whereby Enteryx improves symptoms of GERD is still not determined. The liquid material comprised of EVOH has been used since 1996 in the embolization of arteriovenous malformations, cerebral aneurysms, and peripheral vascular abnormalities [30]. The viscosity of Enteryx before contact with tissue is extremely low, allowing injection through a 23- to 25-gauge needle. On injection through a selectively placed catheter into the deep layers of the esophagus, the solvent (DMSO) rapidly diffuses away, causing an in-situ precipitation of the polymer (EVOH) and formation of a spongy coherent polymeric mass. Complete solidification occurs in less than 1 minute, with no distal migration or fragmentation of the implant. Pathologic findings in a porcine model [31] demonstrated that initially its administration caused a marked acute inflammatory reaction with moderate cellular necrosis. Resolution of this acute reaction was followed by a chronic foreign-body granulomatous inflammatory process separated from the surrounding tissues by a fibrous capsule of varying thickness. By 3 months postimplantation, the process appeared to be very stable, with little or no active inflammation. Endoscopically, the implants appear as encapsulated, firm, smooth, and slightly mobile ovoid masses. These mechanical properties may impart an alteration in the compliance of the tissues, preventing sphincter shortening and improving the barrier function of the GEJ, as demonstrated by beneficial effects in esophageal acid exposure time and mild changes in LES pressure and TLESR.

The Enteryx procedure kit is commercially available from Boston Scientific (Natick, Massachusetts). As with other endoscopic therapies for GERD, the procedure is performed under conscious sedation in the endoscopy suite as an outpatient procedure. There have been no reports of serious adverse effects. The most common side effects seen are transient chest pain in 91% and dysphagia in 20% [31a]. The procedure is not recommended for patients who are unable to undergo endoscopy or who have esophageal varices.

Results

Johnson et al [32] conducted a prospective, multicenter, single-arm study to evaluate the safety and efficacy of Enteryx in 85 patients who had GERD. At 6 months of follow-up, PPI use was eliminated in 74% of patients and reduced by more than 50% in an additional 10% of subjects. Mean LES length increased from 2 cm at baseline to 3 cm after therapy ($P = 0.003$). Mean total esophageal acid exposure time (9.5% pretherapy to 6.7% post-therapy, $P < 0.001$) and quality of life improved significantly. This study, however, did not specify the proportion of patients in whom esophageal acid exposure time returned to normal levels.

Within the first 3 months of treatment, 22% of patients underwent repeat injections (the protocol prohibited repeat treatments after the first 3 months).

Lehman and associates [33] reported the results of a multicenter North American and European trial using Enteryx for GERD in 176 patients. As in the previous study, quality of life and esophageal acid exposure time improved significantly (13.8% to 9.6%), and up to 82% of patients were able to reduce or eliminate the need for antisecretory therapy with PPIs. Although many patients experienced improvement in their symptom score and medication requirements, there was evidence of persistent acid reflux in 61% of the patients and low grade esophagitis in 37% at 12 months of follow-up [34].

Other studies [35] have also demonstrated that, despite a significant symptomatic improvement and beneficial effects in quality of life and reflux episodes, normalization of esophageal acid exposure is achieved in only less than 50% of patients. In a recent imaging study [36], the average implant volume was approximately 80% of baseline at 3, 6, and 12 months. Conversely, among patients who had maintained or increased PPI use, the average implant volume was 40% of baseline, indicating that a higher residual implant volume is associated with a greater likelihood of successful clinical outcome. The decrease in implant volume between baseline and 3 months was attributable to sloughing resulting from superficial implantation of the Enteryx material. All patients who retained more than 5 cc of implant material eliminated or reduced PPI use by 50%, and the majority experienced significant improvement in quality of life scores.

Polymethylmethacrylates

Plexiglas microspheres, polymethylmethacrylates (PMMA), made of polymethyl methacrylate and marketed as PAMMA (Rolfs Medical International, Breda, Netherlands), are injected by needle under high pressure into the submucosal zone of the proximal GEJ, developing a bulklike barrier to augment LES pressure and decrease acid reflux [37].

Mechanism of action

PAMMA was first used in human applications in 1936 for dental prostheses, and is used extensively in plastic surgery to augment the diminished thickness of the chorium in cases of skin defects and wrinkles. Apart from its well-documented biocompatibility, PAMMA microspheres of 100 microns have a smooth, completely round surface that permits injection through a needle, hinders phagocytosis and migration from the implantation site, and evokes negligible foreign body reaction. The prepared implant is a 3:1 suspension of PAMMA in gelatin solution (3.5% spongious encephalitis-free gelatin solution). After implantation, the gelatin (75% of total volume) is phagocytized by macrophages within 3 months and replaced by fibroblasts and collagen fibers, a reaction stimulated by PAMMA spheres (25%). The spheres are encapsulated by connective tissue, which replaces at least 50% of the gelatin volume, allowing at least two thirds of the total volume of the implant to remain at the site of injection. These properties render it an attractive tissue bulking agent.

Results

Feretis and associates [38] recently reported their results in 10 patients. Over a period of 4 to 6 months of follow-up there was a significant improvement in symptom score (12.2 versus 7.7), medication use, and esophageal acid exposure time (24.5% versus 10.4%). Seven patients discontinued antisecretory therapy with PPIs. Although there was improvement in esophageal acid exposure, the DeMeester score values failed to normalize (74.6 versus 36.3) in 9 of the 10 patients.

Gatekeeper

This expandable hydrogel prosthesis is marketed commercially as the Gatekeeper Reflux Repair System (Medtronic, Minneapolis, Minnesota). The Gatekeeper system consists of a specially designed 16 mm overtube assembly, a 2.4 mm diameter prosthesis delivery system (1 mm diameter needle, dilator, and 2.4 mm diameter sheath), a pushrod assembly, and Gatekeeper prostheses [39]. With the help of the overtube, the hydrogel bioprostheses can be inserted in the submucosa of the distal esophagus. The prostheses are made from a biocompatible material similar to the substance used in contact lenses (polyacrylonitrile-based hydrogel [HYPAN]). HYPAN is one of the least reactive polymers when compared with silicone, polyethylene, and polytetrafluoroethylene. The overtube and endoscope contained within the lumen of the overtube are passed into the lower esophagus over a guide wire. Once in position, suction is applied via the endoscope, which pulls the esophageal wall into a shelf at the end of the overtube. Separate segments of the esophageal mucosa within the circumference of the GEJ are aspirated into the tip of the probe and dilated with saline injections, creating a tissue bleb or submucosal pocket. Subsequently, four to six expandable hydrogel prostheses are inserted through the mucosal slits into the submucosa under direct vision (Fig. 1). Although dry when inserted into the LES, the prostheses expand upon contact with moisture to about the size of a gelcap, creating a mechanical barrier against reflux. A pilot study in humans [40] showed that it is a safe technique, and that no prostheses migrated into the mediastinum. One of the definite advantages of this technique over other endoscopic treatments for GERD being developed is its reversibility. Multicenter studies have been initiated [41,42]. As with other therapies, beneficial effects have been reported in symptom score (21 versus 8), esophageal acid exposure time (8.6% versus 6.4%) and quality of life. Long-term results are still not available.

Discussion

Although there is currently immense interest in these new forms of endoscopic therapies for GERD, a few aspects should be kept in mind.

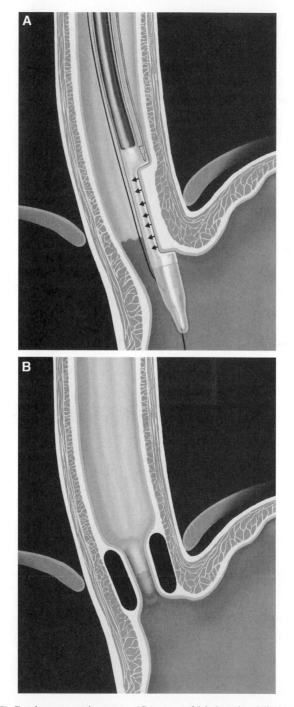

Fig. 1. (*A*,*B*) Gatekeeper repair system. (Courtesy of Medtronics, Minneapolis, MN.)

Available studies are small, open-label, with significant dropouts and lack of intention-to-treat analysis of data. Most studies include only patients who had mild-to-moderate disease, and who had adequately responded to antisecretory medications and had normal or near-normal manometric studies. Exclusion criteria generally include moderate to severe esophagitis, hiatal hernia greater than 2 cm, Barrett's esophagus, morbid obesity (BMI > 40), and systemic comorbidities. Although most studies demonstrate a decrease in the esophageal acid exposure time, symptoms, and medication use, and improvements in quality of life, most have failed to demonstrate normalization of esophageal acid exposure or to reliably heal esophagitis. Only 30% to 50% of patients achieve normalization of esophageal acid exposure when studied by pH-metry after therapy. Although half to two thirds of patients initially discontinued or reduced significantly the use of PPIs, resumption of medication occurred in up to 50% of patients by 6 to 12 months of follow-up. These results are inferior to those reported after open or LF, which normalize esophageal acid exposure in 90% of the patients and heal esophagitis in excess of 90% of patients. Additionally, patients undergoing antireflux surgery usually have more severe forms of GERD, compared with the patient populations that have undergone studies with ET. Despite the success of laparoscopic fundoplication, operative morbidity and the small risk for mortality remain issues. For this reason, ET will continue to be introduced into clinical practice, and will probably become the procedure of choice for selected groups of patients. Issues that need to be resolved include optimizing patient selection, defining long-term outcomes, and doing comparative studies between the different approaches used. In the meantime, potential patients must be made aware that the efficacy demonstrated to date is modest, and that long-term outcome is still uncertain. For the patient who has severe GERD, LF should remain the procedure of choice.

References

[1] Swain CP, Mills TN. An endoscopic sewing machine. Gastrointest Endosc 1986;32:36.

[2] Swain CP, Brown GJ, Mills TN. An endoscopic stapling device: the development of a new flexible endoscopically controlled devise for placing multiple transmural staples in gastrointestinal tissue. Gastrointest Endosc 1989;35:338.

[3] Tam W, Holloway R, Dent J, et al. Impact of endoscopic suturing of the gastroesophageal junction on lower esophageal sphincter function and gastroesophageal reflux in patients with reflux disease. Gastroenterology 2002;122:390–8.

[4] Kadirkamanathan SS, Evans DF, Gong F, et al. Antireflux operations at flexible endoscopy using endoluminal stitching techniques: an experimental study. Gastrointest Endosc 1996;44:133–43.

[5] Kadirkamanathan SS, Yazaki E, Evans DF, et al. An ambulatory porcine model of acid reflux to evaluate endoscopic gastroplasty. Gut 1999;44:782–8.

[6] Endoscopic suturing for gastroesophageal reflux disease: clinical outcome with the Bard EndoCinch. Gastrointest Endosc Clin N Am 2003;13:89–101.

 [7] Mahmood Z, McMahon BP, Arfin Q, et al. Endocinch therapy for gastro-oesophageal reflux disease: a one year prospective follow up. Gut 2003;52:34–9.

 [8] Filipi CJ, Lehman GA, Rothstein RI, et al. Transoral, flexible endoscopic suturing for treatment of GERD: a multicenter trial. Gastrointest Endosc 2001;53:416–22.

 [9] Rothstein RI, Pohl H, Grove M, et al. Endoscopic gastric plication for the treatment of GERD: two year results [abstract]. Am J Gastroenterol 2001;96:S53.

[10] Haber GB, Marcon NE, Kortan P, et al. A 2-year follow-up of 25 patients undergoing endoluminal gastric plication (ELGP) for gastroesophageal reflux disease (GERD) [abstract]. Gastrointest Endosc 2000;53:116.

[11] Velanovich V, Ben-Menachem T, Goel S. Case-control comparison of endoscopic gastroplication with laparoscopic fundoplication in the management of gastroesophageal reflux disease. Surg Laparosc Endosc 2002;12:219–33.

[12] Velanovich V, Ben Menachem T. Laparoscopic Nissen fundoplication after failed endoscopic gastroplication. J Laparoendosc Adv Surg Tech A 2002;12:305–8.

[13] Mahmood Z, Byrne PJ, McCullough J, et al. A comparison of BARD EndoCinch transesophageal endoscopic placation (BETEP) with laparoscopic fundoplication (LNF) for the treatment of gastroesophageal reflux disease (GORD) [abstract]. Gastrointest Endosc 2002;55:AB90.

[14] Chuttani R, Sud R, Sachdev G, et al. Endoscopic full-thickness plication for GERD: final results of human pilot study [abstract]. Gastrointest Endosc 2002;55:AB258.

[15] Chuttani R. Endoscopic full-thickness placation: the device, technique, pre-clinical and early clinical experience. Gastrointest Endosc Clin N Am 2003;13:109–16.

[16] Pleskow D, Rothstein R, Kozarek R, et al. Endoscipic full-thickness plication for GERD: a multi-center study [abstract]. Gastroenterology 2003;(Suppl): abstract ID 103782.

[17] Rosen M, Ponsky J. Wilson-Cook sewing device: the device, technique, and preclinical studies. Gastrointest Endosc Clin North Am 2003;13:103–8.

[18] Utley DS. The Stretta procedure: device, technique, and preclinical study data. Gastrointest Endosc Clin N Am 2003;13:135–45.

[19] Triadafilopoulos G. Clinical experience with the Stretta procedure. Gastrointest Endosc Clin N Am 2003;13:147–55.

[20] DiBaise JK, Brand RE, Quigley EM. Endoluminal delivery of radiofrequency energy to the gastroesophageal junction in uncomplicated GERD: efficacy and potential mechanism of action. Am J Gastroenterol 2002;97:833–42.

[21] Triadafilopoulos G, Utley DS. Temperature-controlled energy delivery for gastroesophageal reflux disease: the Stretta procedure. J Laparoendosc Adv Surg Tech A 2001;11: 333–9.

[22] Triadafilopoulos G, Dibaise JK, Nostrant TT, et al. Radiofrequency energy delivery to the gastroesophageal junction for the treatment of GERD. Gastrointest Endosc 2001;53: 407–15.

[22a] Utley DS, Kim M, Vierra MA, et al. Augmentation of lower esophageal sphincter pressure and gastric yield pressure after radiofrequency energy delivery to the gastroesophageal junction: a porcine model. Gastrointest Endosc 2000;52:81–6.

[23] Wolfsen HC, Richards WO. The Stretta procedure for the treatment of GERD: a registry of 558 patients. J Laparoendosc Adv Surg Tech A 2002;12:395–402.

[24] Triadafilopoulos G, Dibaise JK, Nostrant TT, et al. The Stretta procedure for the treatment of GERD: 6 and 12 month follow-up of the US open label trial. Gastrointest Endosc 2002; 55:149–56.

[25] Tam WC, Schoeman MN, Zhang Q, et al. Delivery of radiofrequency energy to the lower oesophageal sphincter and gastric cardia inhibits transient lower oesophageal sphincter relaxations and gastro-oesophageal reflux in patients with reflux disease. Gut 2003;52: 479–85.

[26] Houston H, Khaitan L, Holzman M, et al. First year experience of patients undergoing the Stretta procedure. Surg Endosc 2003;17:401–4.

[27] Richards WO, Houston HL, Torquati A, et al. Paradigm shift in the management of gastroesophageal reflux disease. Ann Surg 2003;237:638–49.

[28] Louis H, Deviere J. Endoscipic implantation of Enteryx for the treatment of gastroesophageal reflux disease: technique, pre-clinical and clinical experience. Gastrointest Endosc Clin N Am 2003;13:191–200.

[29] Johnson DA, Ganz R, Aisenberg J, et al. Endoscopic deep mural implantation of Enteryx for the treatment of GERD: 6-month follow-up of a multicenter trial. Am J Gastroenterol 2003;98:250–8.

[30] Nishi S, Taki W, Nakahara I, et al. Embolization of cerebral aneurysms with a liquid embolus, EVAL mixture: report of three cases. Acta Neurochir (Wien) 1996;138:294–300.

[31] Mason RJ, Hughes M, Lehman GA, et al. Endoscopic augmentation of the cardia with a biocompatible injectable polymer (Enteryx) in a porcine model. Surg Endosc 2002;16: 386–91.

[31a] Johnson DA, Ganz R, Aisenberg J, et al. Endoscopic implantation of enteryx for treatment of GERD: 12 month results of a prospective multi-center trial. Am Journal of Gastroenterology 2003;98:1921–30.

[32] Johnson DA, Ganz R, Aisenberg J, et al. Endoscopic deep mural implantation of Enteryx for the treatment of GERD: 6 month follow-up of a multicenter trial. Am J Gastroenterol 2003;98:250–8.

[33] Lehman GA, Hieston KJ, Aisenberg J, et al. Enteryx solution, a minimally invasive injectable treatment for GERD: current world-wide multicenter human trial results [abstract]. Gastrointest Endosc 2003;57(Suppl):AB96.

[34] Lehman GA, Hieston KJ, Johnson D, et al. Enteryx solution, a minimally invasive injectable treatment for GERD: analysis of pH-metry and manometry findings over 12 months. Digestive Disorders Week May 19, 2003, abstract 100910.

[35] Neuhaus H, Schumacher B, Preiss C, et al. Enteryx solution, a minimally invasive injectable treatment for GERD: German multicenter experience. Digestive Disorders Week May 19, 2003, abstract 100951.

[36] Johnson DA, Aisenberg J, Deviere J, et al. Enteryx solution, a minimally invasive injectable treatment for GERD: analysis of X-ray findings over 12 months. Digestive Disorders Week 2003, abstract 107493.

[37] Feretis C, Benakis P, Dimopoulos C, et al. Plexiglas (polymethylmethacrylate) implantation: technique, pre-clinical and clinical experience. Gastrointest Endosc Clin N Am 2003;13:167–78.

[38] Feretis C, Benakis P, Dimopoulos C, et al. Endoscopic implantation of Plexiglas (PAMMA) microspheres for the treatment of GERD. Gastrointest Endosc 2001;53;423–6.

[39] Fockens P. Gatekeeper reflux repair system: technique, pre-clinical and clinical experience. Gastrointest Endosc Clin N Am 2003;13:179–89.

[40] Fockens P, Bruno MJ, Hirsch DP, et al. Endoscopic augmentation of the lower esophageal sphincter. Pilot study of the Gatekeeper reflux repair system in patients with GERD. Gastrointest Endosc 2002;55:AB257.

[41] Lehman G, Watkins JL, Hieston K, et al. Endoscopic gastroesophageal reflux disease (GERD) therapy with Gatekeeper system. Initiation of a multicenter prospective randomized trial. Gastrointest Endosc 2002;55:AB261.

[42] Fockens P, Costamagna G, Gabbrielli A, et al. Endoscopic augmentation of the lower esophageal sphincter (LES) for the treatment of GERD: multicenter study of the Gatekeeper reflux repair system. Gastrointest Endosc 2002;55:AB90.

ELSEVIER
SAUNDERS

Surg Clin N Am 85 (2005) 483–493

SURGICAL
CLINICS OF
NORTH AMERICA

Achalasia

Todd A. Woltman, MD, PhD, Carlos A. Pellegrini, MD,
Brant K. Oelschlager, MD*

*Department of Surgery, University of Washington, 1959 NE Pacific Street, Box 356410,
Seattle, WA 98195-6410, USA*

Achalasia is a primary esophageal motor disorder of unknown etiology. It is an uncommon ailment, with a reported incidence of 0.5 to 1 per 100,000 in the United States. Achalasia affects both sexes equally, typically presenting between the ages of 20 and 50, though it can occur at all ages. Ineffective relaxation of the lower esophageal sphincter (LES) combined with loss of esophageal peristalsis leads to impaired emptying and gradual esophageal dilation. Dysphagia is the cardinal feature of achalasia, accompanied by varying degrees of aspiration, weight loss, and pain. The anatomic defect appears to be a decrease or loss of inhibitory nonadrenergic, noncholinergic ganglion cells in the esophageal myenteric plexus. Histological analysis of esophagi resected from patients who had end-stage achalasia demonstrates myenteric inflammation and progressive depletion of ganglion cells and subsequent neural fibrosis [1]. There is also a significant reduction in the synthesis of nitric oxide and Vasoactive Intestinal Polypeptide (VIP), the most important mediators of relaxation in the lower esophageal sphincter. Macroscopically, there may often be thickening of the circular layer of the distal esophagus. Achalasia also carries a slightly increased risk of cancer, squamous cell carcinoma in particular.

Patient presentation

Most patients who have achalasia present with progressive dysphagia to solids and liquids, although symptoms may be subtle and nonspecific early in its course. The mean duration of symptoms before presentation is 2 years, and the diagnosis often takes much longer because the symptoms are often attributed to gastroesopahageal reflux disease (GERD) or other disorders.

---

* Corresponding author.
E-mail address: brant@u.washington.edu (B.K. Oelschlager).

0039-6109/05/$ - see front matter © 2005 Elsevier Inc. All rights reserved.
doi:10.1016/j.suc.2005.01.002   *surgical.theclinics.com*

Initially, the patient may complain of the sensation of a retrosternal "sticking" of foodstuffs. Stress or cold liquids may exacerbate dysphagia. Patients may regurgitate undigested food, especially after meals or when lying supine. Patients may stand after eating or raise their arms over their head to enlist gravity and to increase the intrathoracic pressure in an attempt to aid esophageal emptying. If unable to force food into the stomach by the ingestion of liquids or other means, spontaneous or forced regurgitation are often employed to evacuate the esophagus. Occasionally, physicians even confuse the disease with an eating disorder. As a result of regurgitation, aspiration of esophageal contents may lead to pulmonary disease. In fact, up to 10% of patients who have achalasia experience significant bronchopulmonary complications [2].

Many patients express a sensation of heartburn, explaining why many are initially diagnosed with GERD. Though patients who have achalasia may experience gastroesophageal (GE) reflux [3], more often heartburn is secondary to fermentation of retained undigested food in the esophagus. Chest pain, clearly distinguishable from heartburn, occurs in 30% to 50% of patients. The etiology of this pain is unclear, and is unpredictably relieved by esophageal myotomy and other treatments. Weight loss is variable and tends to be insidious. The magnitude of weight loss tends to correlate with the severity of the underlying disease. Rapid onset of symptoms (≤ 6 months), advanced age (>50 years), or significant weight loss (>15 lbs) should raise suspicion for pseudoachalasia, usually secondary to malignancy or extaluminal obstruction. In these cases, a thorough work-up with a CT scan or endoscopic ultrasound must be performed before further therapy is considered.

Evaluation

A barium esophagram is typically the first imaging study used in the evaluation of dysphagia. The scout film may demonstrate an air-fluid level in the esophagus with a paucity of gastric air. The classical appearance of achalasia on a barium study is the "bird's beak" tapering of the distal esophagus, with a column of contrast in the esophageal lumen (Fig. 1A , B). Variable esophageal dilation is seen, ranging from mild in the early stages to the massive sigmoid-shaped esophagus of end-stage achalasia. Fluoroscopic evaluation may also reveal nonpropulsive, tertiary contractions of the esophageal body, with failure to clear the barium bolus from the esophagus.

Manometry is the gold standard for confirming the diagnosis of achalasia. The resting LES pressure may be elevated, but is usually normal, and fails to relax completely with swallowing. Complete absence of peristalsis is the sine qua non of achalasia. The waveforms are usually simultaneous and of low amplitude (Fig. 2). When present, they are simultaneous and nonpropulsive in nature. A subset of patients who have "vigorous" achalasia are found to have high-amplitude contractions. In patients who have a dilated and

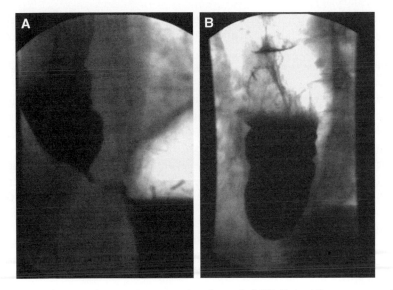

Fig. 1. (*A*) Barium esophagram demonstrating the typical "bird's beak" appearance of the distal esophagus in a patient with achalasia. (*B*) Esophagram showing a significantly dilated csophagus with an air-fluid level.

tortuous esophagus, the LES may be difficult to intubate, requiring fluoroscopic guidance for manometry catheter placement. In the patient who will not tolerate esophageal manometry, nuclear scintigraphy can be used to cvaluate esophageal transit.

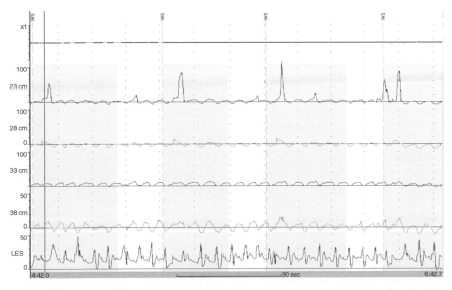

Fig. 2. Manometry tracing from a patient with achalasia. Note the absence of peristalsis throughout the esophageal body and the lack of LES relaxation.

Twenty-four-hour pH monitoring is neither required nor usually helpful. Although patients who have achalasia may experience some element of GE reflux, it is not clinically relevant. Further, acidification of esophageal contents secondary to fermentation of retained food may lead to a false positive study [4].

Endoscopic evaluation is used to rule out other processes that may mimic achalasia. The characteristic appearance is an atonic, dilated esophagus with a tightly closed LES that does not open with insufflation. With gentle pressure, the scope is admitted through the LES with a "pop," in contrast with a peptic stricture or a malignancy, which do not yield. TheGE junction, including a retroflexed view of the gastric cardia, should be carefully inspected. Biopsies of any mucosal abnormality should be obtained. If pseudoachalasia cannot be ruled out, endoscopic ultrasound or a CT scan may prove informative.

Treatment

Any treatment of achalasia is directed at the palliation of symptoms and cannot change the underlying pathology. The neuromuscular defect is not corrected. The goal of all therapeutic options is to relieve the functional obstruction of the distal esophagus, thus improving esophageal emptying.

Pharmacotherapy

The use of drugs to treat achalasia would seem to be attractive because of its noninvasive nature. Several agents relax smooth muscle, and thus theoretically decrease LES pressure. Unpredictable and incomplete absorption of oral formulations secondary to poor esophageal emptying is one limitation; thus sublingual administration is the most efficacious route. Nitrates and calcium-channel blockers are the most commonly used medications. They are more effective in patients who have mild symptoms without severe esophageal dilation. Side effects such as headaches and peripheral edema are common, limiting their adoption. Relief from these agents is inconsistent and generally short-lived, with most patients showing continued progression of their disease [5–7]. Their usefulness is limited to temporizing symptoms until more effective therapy is attempted, or in those patients deemed too frail to undergo a more invasive treatment.

Botulinum toxin

Botulinum toxin A (Botox, Allergan, Irvine, California) is a neurotoxin produced by Clostridium botulinum that binds to cholinergic nerves and irreversibly inhibits acetylcholine release. This effect is eventually overcome by regeneration of new synapses. Botox is injected into the LES through the working port of a flexible endoscope, with minimal incidence of immediate complications. Early enthusiasm has waned because results have not proven to be durable. Botox injection is initially effective in 60% to 85% of patients, but 50% develop recurrent symptoms within 6 months [8]. Repeat administration is possible, but efficacy is diminished with subsequent injections. Because Botox is a relatively expensive therapy, the need for repeat treatment limits both its convenience and cost-effectiveness. Another problem with this therapy is that Botox injection can cause an intense inflammatory reaction of the GE junction, with subsequent fibrosis. This may impact future surgical therapy, because most patients have continued or progressive symptoms. The authors' experience during esophageal myotomy is that there is more difficulty in finding the submucosal plane in patients who have had prior Botox therapy than in untreated patients (53% versus 7%). Although there does not appear to be a difference in the ultimate relief of dysphagia, we did experience an increased rate of perforation (7% versus 2%) in patients who have had prior Botox therapy [9]. Although this is not well understood, Botox appears to be more effective in older patients and in those who have vigorous achalasia. Botox should be reserved for patients unwilling or deemed unfit to undergo an invasive procedure. Also, in patients who have atypical presentations, Botox may be considered as a diagnostic procedure. By simulating the effect of esophageal myotomy, it can identify patients who are likely to have relief with an operation.

Pneumatic dilatation

The oldest treatment of achalasia is forceful dilatation of the LES, originally accomplished by the passage of a piece of whalebone with a sponge affixed to the end [10]. This therapy has become more effective with the development of graded polyethylene balloons. Under fluoroscopic guidance, balloons (at least 30 mm in diameter) are passed through the LES and inflated, disrupting the fibers of the LES. The balloon is kept inflated from 1 to 3 minutes and then deflated. This is followed by an esophagram with water-soluble contrast to evaluate the LES diameter and to evaluate for perforation. If no extravasation is seen, the patient is observed for 6 hours and then discharged to home. The "graded" approach refers to the use of serially larger balloons (up to 40 mm) with subsequent dilatations for initial nonresponders. Only a single dilatation is performed per session. Response rates of 60% to 90% can be achieved, with approximately 70% of patients obtaining substantial relief of dysphagia after 1 year [11]. Repeat dilatation is often used, but its efficacy is diminished after two sessions. Patients who have a poor result after initial dilatation or early return of their symptoms are predictably less likely to respond with subsequent dilations. Most patients are able to tolerate pneumatic dilatation. Interestingly, younger patients do not respond as well as older patients [12]. This is thought to be due to their tissues being more compliant, and simply stretching during dilatation rather that tearing. The presence of a hiatal hernia, significantly dilated esophagus (>7 cm), or an epiphrenic diverticulum increases the risk of perforation and these are relative contraindications. Although the likelihood of improving dysphagia increases with increasing balloon diameter, so does the likelihood of perforation. Overall, the incidence of perforation is about 2% per dilation attempt [13]. Whether to treat achalasia initially with pneumatic dilatation depends on physician and surgeon expertise, patient age and comorbidities, and patient preference. If dilation fails, a myotomy can usually be performed without additional difficulties.

Surgical therapy

Ernest Heller first described cardiomyotomy for achalasia in 1914. His original description was of two myotomies, one anterior and one posterior, along the GE junction. This has been modified, and now only an anterior myotomy is performed. Excellent results with cardiomyotomy can be achieved in 90% to 95% of patients. Extramucosal cardiomyotomy provides more reliable relief of dysphagia than pneumatic dilation, because it allows accurate division of LES muscle fibers rather than blind disruption. Traditionally, this was accomplished either by a transthoracic or a transabdominal approach. Each approach is associated with an obvious incision and postoperative stays of 7 to 10 days. For this reason, despite superior long-term results from surgical myotomy [11], most patients were treated by less invasive therapies, such as pneumatic dilatation. Recent developments in minimally invasive techniques now allow performance of cardiomyotomy by either a thoracoscopic [14] or a laparoscopic [15] approach. Reduction in postoperative pain and morbidity, as well as improved cosmesis, has made the surgical option more attractive. Some feel that a megaesophagus (>8 cm) is a contraindication to a myotomy because of poor relief of dysphagia. The authors feel that with laparoscopy that there is little to lose by attempting a myotomy and reserving an esophagectomy for failures. Using this approach, the majority of patients obtain relief and avoid subsequent esophagectomy.

The first approach using minimally invasive techniques was thoracoscopy [14]. Through a left thoracoscopic approach, a long myotomy could be performed, extending approximately 0.5 cm across the GE junction (similar to the open approach). The thought was that this would provide relief of dysphagia without rendering the cardia completely incompetent and resulting in significant reflux. Initial results were promising, with 89% of patients experiencing relief of dysphagia [16]; however, over time several patients (9/35) in the authors' series required myotomy extension or postmyotomy dilation to relieve dysphagia [17]. Furthermore, over 60% had abnormal reflux when 24-hour pH monitoring was performed. Thus it became clear that successful relief of dysphagia often depends on extending the myotomy well onto the stomach, which can only be done from an abdominal approach. Also, even a limited gastric myotomy and hiatal dissection, such as is performed with a thoracoscopic myotomy, results in a high incidence of reflux.

For these reasons, the authors and most esophageal surgeons perform a Heller myotomy via a laparoscopic approach. The advantages include excellent visualization of the distal esophagus and the stomach, so that an extended gastric myotomy and an antireflux procedure may be performed. Moreover, it avoids the anesthetic complexity of single-lung ventilation required for thoracoscopy. The authors have substantial experience with both approaches, and have found that laparoscopy is more effective in relieving dysphagia (93% versus 85%) with a shorter hospital stay (48 versus 72 hours) and less postoperative reflux (17% versus 60%) [17].

There are two main controversies surrounding Heller myotomy. One is the extent of the esophageal myotomy; the other is whether an antireflux procedure should be performed, and if so, which one. Although there is agreement that the proximal extent of the myotomy should reach 6 to 7 cm above the GE junction, this distal extent of the myotomy is controversial. Some consider that the goal in performing a myotomy is to adequately relieve dysphagia without unnecessarily disrupting the antireflux barrier. The authors have found that there is no length of esophageal myotomy that maximally relieves dysphagia and minimizes the occurrence of reflux. This is emphasized by the thoracoscopic approach that, despite a limited distal extension of the myotomy, produced GERD in most patients. We recently compared a more traditional approach (a 1.5–2 cm gastric myotomy) with an extended gastric myotomy (at least 3 cm). We found that the longer myotomy resulted in less dysphagia (1.2 versus 2.1 on a 5-point frequency scale) and fewer interventions for recurrent dysphagia (3% versus 17%) [18]. Because we advocate an extended gastric myotomy, we feel that an antireflux procedure is prudent in most cases. Those who advocate not performing an antireflux procedure cite good clinical results and low incidence of heartburn [19,20]; however, few groups perform postmyotomy 24-hour pH monitoring to evaluate for the true incidence of GE reflux without a fundoplication. Moreover, this practice results intervention rates for dysphagia as high as 14% [20], which we think is likely the result of a limited gastric myotomy.

Most surgeons find that performing an antireflux procedure in conjunction with laparoscopic myotomy does not add significant time or morbidity to the operation, and is not associated with increased postoperative dysphagia. Certainly, a partial fundoplication (Dor or Toupet) is the best option. A total fundoplication (eg, Nissen fundoplication) may cause a functional obstruction for a nonpropulsive esophagus, resulting in a high incidence of dysphagia [21]. An anterior (Dor) fundoplication requires less posterior dissection, and thus is easier and theoretically preserves more of the antireflux barrier. Also, because the wrap is brought anterior the myotomy, it potentially covers any undetected mucosal injuries. A posterior (Toupet) fundoplication is the preferred partial fundoplication when indicated for GERD; however, its superiority in preventing reflux after myotomy has not been demonstrated. Because it holds the edges of the myotomy open, a Toupet may provide protection against recurrent dysphagia. For these reasons, it is the procedure of choice for the author's group. Although each of these antireflux techniques has its own theoretical benefits and champions, there is no strong evidence supporting one over the other.

Laparoscopic Heller myotomy—operative technique

The setup is the same as that for a Nissen fundoplication (Fig. 3). The patient is placed in a modified lithotomy position, with a standard five-port placement. In the authors' group, we routinely mobilize the gastric fundus and short gastric vessels to minimize tension on the subsequent fundoplication. An extensive anterior and lateral hiatal and mediastinal esophageal dissection is performed to maximize the length of the myotomy. It is important to identify the left (anterior) vagus and separate it from the esophagus to enable the performance of a continuous esophagogastric myotomy.

A lighted 52 Fr bougie is passed into the body of the stomach. The bougie illuminates the esophagus, which helps with identification and stability when performing the myotomy. The fat pad overlying the cardioesophageal

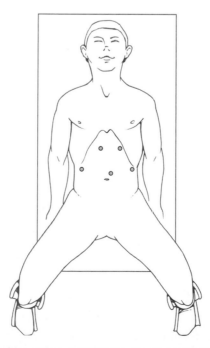

Fig. 3. Patient position and port-site location for laparoscopic Heller myotomy.

junction is excised, a step critical to accurately identifying the GE junction. A Babcock clamp opened over the bougie just distal to the GE junction provides exposure of the distal esophagus. We perform the myotomy with an L-shaped hook electrocautery device, although minimal energy is used so as to minimize mucosal injury. The appropriate plane may be more difficult to identify in patients who have previously undergone treatment with Botox or pneumatic dilatation The longitudinal muscle fibers are divided first, exposing the inner circular muscle, which is then separated from the mucosa. For this reason most submucosal bleeding should be controlled with pressure and time. The myotomy should be carried as proximal as safely as possible (usually 6–8 cm) and 2 to 3 cm onto the stomach. As discussed previously, we routinely perform a 3-cm distal myotomy. The distal dissection is the most difficult, because the muscular layers are poorly defined and the mucosa is thinner. Mucosal perforations should be repaired with fine (4-0 or 5-0) absorbable suture, and rarely require other intervention. Endoscopy may be used to check the completeness of the myotomy and for unrecognized mucosal injury.

As we perform an extended distal myotomy, we routinely perform an antireflux procedure. We prefer a standard Toupet fundoplication, securing both edges of the fundus to each side of the myotomy as well as to the diaphragm (Fig. 4). Nausea is aggressively treated with antiemetics, and patients are generally start liquids the night of their procedure. Average length of stay is 1 to 2 days, and resumption of normal diet and activities occurs within 2 to 3 weeks.

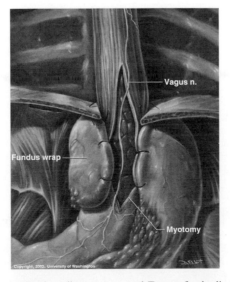

Fig. 4. Drawing of a completed cardiomyotomy and Toupet fundoplication. (Courtesy of the University of Washington, Seattle, WA.)

Summary

Surgical therapy (Heller myotomy) is the most effective treatment to relieve dysphagia associated with achalasia. The advent of minimally invasive techniques, specifically the laparoscopic approach, significantly reduced the morbidity of surgical therapy, making it the procedure of choice for most patients who have achalasia. Pneumatic dilatation is a viable alternative, though is associated with inferior results and a higher risk of esophageal perforation than surgical therapy. Pharmacotherapy and Botox provide inferior results and should be reserved for temporizing therapy, or for patients who are deemed too frail for surgical intervention. For best results, a laparoscopic myotomy should be carried at least 3 cm onto the stomach, and a partial fundoplication should be performed to reduce the incidence of postoperative GE reflux.

References

[1] Goldblum JR, Rice TW, Richter JE. Histopathological features in esophagomyotomy specimens from patients with achalasia. Gastronenterol 1996;111:648–54.
[2] Howard PJ, Maher L, Pryde A, et al. Five year prospective study of the incidence, clinical features, and diagnosis of achalasia in Edinburgh. Gut 1992;33:1011–5.
[3] Shoenut JP, Trenholm BG, Micflickier AB, et al. Reflux patterns in patients with achalasia without operation. Ann Thorac Surg 1988;45:303–5.
[4] Smart HL, Foster PN, Evans DF, et al. Twenty four hour oesophageal acidity in achalasia before and after pneumatic dilatation. Gut 1987;28:883–7.
[5] Gelfond M, Rozen P, Keren S, et al. Effect of nitrates on LOS pressure in achalasia: a potential therapeutic aid. Gut 1981;22:312–8.
[6] Traube M, Dubovik S, Lange RC, et al. The role of nifedipine therapy in achalasia: results of a randomized, double-blind, placebo-controlled study. Am J Gastroenterol 1989;84: 1259–62.
[7] Gelfond M, Rozen P, Gilat T. Isosorbide dinitrate and nifedipine treatment of achalasia: a clinical, manometric and radionuclide evaluation. Gastroenterology 1982;83:963–9.
[8] Vaezi MF, Richter JE. Current therapies for achalasia: comparison and efficacy. J Clin Gastroenterol 1998;27(1):21–5.
[9] Horgan S, Hudda K, Eubanks T, et al. Does botulinum toxin injection make esophagomyotomy a more difficult operation? Surg Endosc 1999;13:576–9.
[10] Willis T. In: Hagae Comitis. Pharmaceutice rationalis sive diatribe de medicamentorum operationibus in human corpore. London: 1674. [in Latin].
[11] Csendes A, Braghett I, Hernriquea A, et al. Late results of a prospective randomized study comparing forceful dilatation and oesphagomyotomy in patients with achalasia. Gut 1989; 30:299–304.
[12] Clouse RE, Abramson BK, Todorczuk JR. Achalasia in the elderly: effects of aging on clinical presentation and outcome. Dig Dis Sci 1991;36:225.
[13] Reynolds JC, Parkman HP. Achalasia. Gastroenterol Clin North Am 1989;18:223–55.
[14] Pellegrini C, Wetter LA, Patti M, et al. Thoracoscopic esophagomyotomy: initial experience with a new approach for the treatment of achalasia. Ann Surg 1992;216:291–9.
[15] Cuschieri A, Shimi S, Nathanson LK. Laparoscopic cardiomyotomy for achalasia. J R Coll Surg Edinb 1991;36:152–4.
[16] Pelligrini CA, Leichter R, Patti M, et al. Thoracoscopic esophageal myotomy in the treatment of achalasia. Ann Thorac Surg 1993;56:680–2.

[17] Patti MG, Pellegrini CA, Horgan S, et al. Minimally invasive surgery for achalasia: an 8-year experience with 168 patients. Ann Surg 1999;230(4):587–94.

[18] Oelschlager BK, Chang L, Pellegrini CA. Improved outcome after extended gastric myotomy for achalasia. Arch Surg 2003;138:490–7.

[19] Sharp KW, Khaitan L, Scholz S, et al. 100 consecutive minimally invasive Heller myotomies: lessons learned. Ann Surg 2002;235:631–9.

[20] Richards WO, Clements RH, Wand PC, et al. Prevalence of gastroesophageal reflux after laparoscopic Heller myotomy. Surg Endosc 1999;13:1010–4.

[21] Wills VL, Hunt DR. Functional outcome after Heller myotomy and fundoplication for achalasia. J Gastrointest Surg 2001;5:408–13

ELSEVIER
SAUNDERS

SURGICAL
CLINICS OF
NORTH AMERICA

Surg Clin N Am 85 (2005) 495–503

Diverticula of the Esophagus

Stephen D. Cassivi, MD, Claude Deschamps, MD*,
Francis C. Nichols III, MD, Mark S. Allen, MD,
Peter C. Pairolero, MD

*Division of General Thoracic Surgery, Mayo Clinic College of Medicine,
200 First Street SW, Rochester, MN 55905, USA*

Most esophageal diverticula are acquired and occur mostly in adults. They can be divided into two categories: pseudodiverticula and true diverticula. Pulsion or pseudodiverticula result from transmural pressure gradients that develop from within the esophagus, resulting in herniation of the mucosa through a weak point of the muscle layer. Two types are recognized: pharyngoesophageal (Zenker's) diverticulum and epiphrenic diverticulum. Traction or true diverticula result from inflammation in neighboring lymph nodes, and are composed of all layers of the esophageal wall.

Pharyngoesophageal (Zenker's) diverticulum

Pharyngoesophageal (Zenker's) diverticulum is the most common diverticulum of the esophagus, and is situated posteriorly just proximal to the cricopharyngeus muscle [1–4]. It is most prevalent in the fifth to eighth decades. The diverticulum may be asymptomatic, but most patients develop symptoms early in the course of the disease. Once the condition is established, it progresses in size, and in frequency and severity of symptoms and complications. Symptoms include oropharyngeal dysphagia, and spontaneous regurgitation of bland, undigested food and saliva. Swallowing may be noisy, and patients often complain of halitosis. Eating and drinking may be interrupted by episodes of regurgitation and aspiration, with or without coughing or choking. Respiratory complications include hoarseness,

---

* Corresponding author.
E-mail address: deschamps.claude@mayo.edu (C. Deschamps).

0039-6109/05/$ - see front matter © 2005 Elsevier Inc. All rights reserved.
doi:10.1016/j.suc.2005.01.016   *surgical.theclinics.com*

bronchospasm, pneumonia, and even lung abscess. Carcinoma arising in a pharyngoesophageal diverticulum is extremely uncommon.

Diagnosis is confirmed by barium swallow, which will demonstrate the sac. Manometry and endoscopy are of little clinical value in this setting. If an endoscopy is indicated for other reasons, the endoscopist should be warned of the possibility of a pharyngoesophageal diverticulum, because of the risk of instrumental perforation. There is no medical therapy for this condition, and all patients who have such a diverticulum should be considered candidates for surgical treatment. Nutritional or chronic respiratory complications are not contraindications to the surgery. To the contrary, operation in such patients should be performed promptly, because recurrent hypoxic episodes of aspiration are poorly tolerated in this elderly population, as emphasized by Payne [4]. Advanced age is also not a contraindication to surgical treatment. A review by Crescenzo and coauthors [5] from the Mayo Clinic of patients 75 years or older who underwent surgical treatment of a Zenker's diverticulum demonstrated an improvement in 94%, with no operative deaths. Treatment is best done on an elective basis while the pouch is of small or moderate size, and before complications have occurred. When nutritional or respiratory complications are present or when neoplasia is suspected, surgical intervention becomes more urgent. Diverticular perforation is a surgical emergency.

General endotracheal anesthesia is used, and the patient is placed in the supine position, with the neck extended and the head turned toward the right. The authors favor diverticulectomy and cricopharyngeal myotomy for diverticula 2 cm and larger, and myotomy alone for smaller ones (Figs. 1–4). The incision is oblique, along the anterior border of the left sternocleidomastoid muscle. The sternocleidomastoid muscle and carotid sheath are

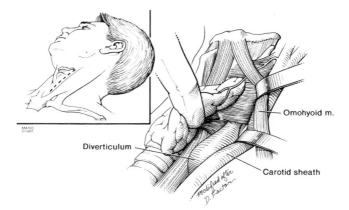

Fig. 1. Oblique left cervical incision along the anterior border of the left sternocleidomastoid muscle (*inset*). The thyroid and trachea are retracted medially and the carotid sheath laterally to expose the diverticulum. Note: the finger is used to retract the thyroid to avoid recurrent nerve injury. (Courtesy of the Mayo Clinic Foundation, Rochester, MN; with permission.)

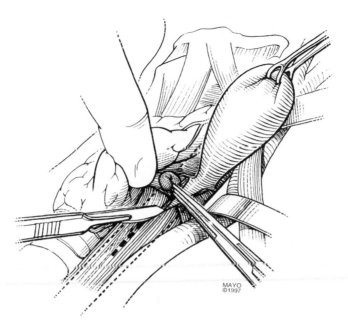

Fig. 2. The myotomy is initiated immediately at the neck of the diverticulum and is extended caudally for 4 cm. A peanut dissector is used to retract the divided muscle laterally. A 36-Fr bougie has been introduced in the esophagus. (Courtesy of the Mayo Clinic Foundation, Rochester, MN; with permission.)

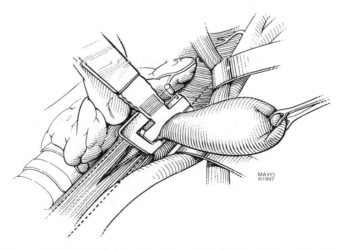

Fig. 3. A TA stapling device is used to close the neck of the diverticulum. The device is placed parallel to the long axis of the esophagus. (Courtesy of the Mayo Clinic Foundation, Rochester, MN; with permission.)

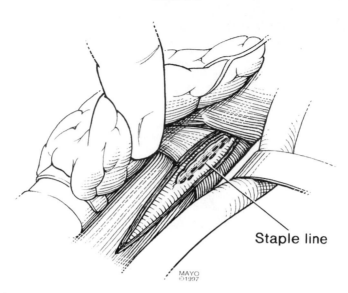

Staple line

MAYO
©1997

Fig. 4. The staple line is left uncovered. Note: the myotomy includes the cricopharyngeal muscle and 4 cm of cervical esophageal muscle. (Courtesy of the Mayo Clinic Foundation, Rochester, MN; with permission.)

retracted laterally, and the thyroid gland and trachea retracted medially with a finger to avoid injury to the recurrent laryngeal nerve, which runs in the tracheoesophageal groove. The neck of the diverticulum is located between the inferior constrictor of the pharynx above and the cricopharyngeal muscle below. The omohyoid muscle crosses over the area and serves as a convenient landmark. Once the diverticulum is identified, it is mobilized and elevated with a Babcock clamp. At this point, a 36-Fr Maloney bougie may be introduced in the esophagus to facilitate the dissection. The area of the neck is freed from surrounding fibrofatty tissue. The myotomy is performed with a #15 blade with the dilator in place. It is initiated at the neck of the diverticulum, and is extended inferiorly for about 4 cm. Simultaneously, the surgeon uses a small peanut dissector to retract the divided muscle layer laterally. The myotomy is placed so that it is oriented roughly at 135° laterally from the anterior aspect of the esophagus. Most sacs smaller than 2 cm simply disappear after the myotomy. For diverticula between 2 and 4 cm, the diverticulum may be transected by the cut-and-sew technique, and the mucosal defect closed with interrupted 4-0 silk. Larger diverticula should be removed using a stapling device, which improves the speed and accuracy of closure. To avoid stricture, the bougie is left in place while the stapler device is applied and fired. The bougie is removed, the mucosal closure is left uncovered, and a small suction drain (Jackson-Pratt) is placed in the retropharyngeal space. The neck incision is closed, and the patient is sent to the regular ward after the recovery room. A radiographic examination of the esophagus using contrast study is done the following day, and if satisfactory, diet is resumed. The drain is removed 2 days after the operation, and the patient is discharged home on the third postoperative day.

Cricopharyngeal myotomy with or without diverticulectomy carries a very low morbidity. The Mayo Clinic reported a mortality rate of 1.2% in a series of 888 consecutive patients [6]. Vocal cord paralysis, mostly transient, occurred in 3.1% of patients, and esophagocutaneous fistula occured in 1.8%. Long-term follow-up revealed that 93% of patients had excellent or good functional result. Recurrence rate was 3.6%. Reoperation for recurrent or persistent pharyngoesophageal diverticulum can be a technical challenge. Although late results are satisfactory after reoperation, surgical morbidity is increased, with a higher incidence of fistula and recurrent nerve paralysis.

Other approaches have also been used successfully. Dohlman and Mattsson [7] first described peroral endoscopic diathermic division of the septum or common wall between the diverticulum and the esophagus. Van Overbeek [8] has further described the use of a carbon dioxide laser to divide the common wall. Collard and coworkers [9] and Peracchia and associates [10] have used an endoluminal stapler to effect an endoscopic cricopharyngeal myotomy. Collard's experience over 16 years was recently published (Gutschow et al [11]). It showed that open techniques, including diverticulectomy, diverticulectomy with cricopharyngeal myotomy, and myotomy alone, provide improved symptomatic relief over endoscopic techniques. This was especially true with smaller diverticula.

Epiphrenic diverticulum

Diverticulum of the lower esophagus, or epiphrenic diverticulum, is rare [12–14]. It is more common in the sixth decade, and may arise anywhere within the thoracic esophagus, but most often in the lower 10 cm. An associated esophageal motility disorder is often present; the causative relationship with the diverticulum, however, is unclear. The clinical manifestations of epiphrenic diverticulum are variable and unpredictable. Many patients are asymptomatic and others have only mild dysphagia. Other symptoms include regurgitation, repetitive episodes of aspiration, chest pain, and pyrosis. No correlation exists between the size of the diverticulum and the severity of symptoms. Likewise, distinguishing between symptoms caused by the diverticulum and those caused by an underlying motility disorder is difficult.

All patients who have suspected epiphrenic diverticulum should have barium upper-gastrointestinal roentgenographic examination. Barium swallow provides proof of diagnosis; serves as a baseline if the patient is asymptomatic; provides clues to any associated motility disorder; and may detect other lesions, such as cancer or stricture, that are causing symptoms.

Those patients who have incapacitating symptoms should have further evaluation with both esophagoscopy and esophageal manometry. Esophagoscopy allows careful evaluation of the esophageal mucosa for esophagitis and the rare presence of cancer. It may also be of value in removing retained debris from the sac before operation in patients who have severe retention and regurgitation. Manometry is mandatory to define associated motility disorders. These manometric findings may help determine the length of esophagomyotomy required to relieve functional obstruction; however, manometry may underestimate the extent of abnormal motility, because of the difficulty in passing the probe into the stomach. If gastroesophageal reflux is suspected, a 24-hour pH study can also be performed to confirm reflux before proceeding with an antireflux procedure on clinical findings alone. If not confirmed, the symptoms thought to be related to reflux may be caused by other conditions, such as abnormal motility or regurgitation of diverticular contents. The decision to proceed with surgical repair can be difficult. The surgeon must balance the risk of the procedure against the potential benefit when selecting surgical candidates. Thus the authors believe that patients who have minimal or no symptoms should be managed conservatively, because progression of symptoms is unlikely. If symptoms are incapacitating, an operation should be advised.

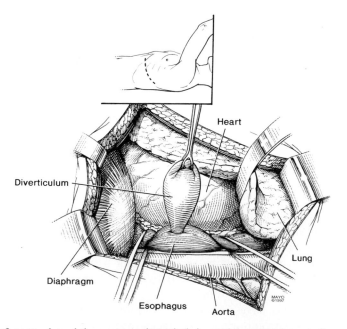

Fig. 5. Left posterolateral thoracotomy through the seventh intercostal space allows adequate access to the thoracic esophagus and hiatus (*inset*). The esophagus is rotated to bring the diverticulum into the view. (Courtesy of the Mayo Clinic Foundation, Rochester, MN; with permission.)

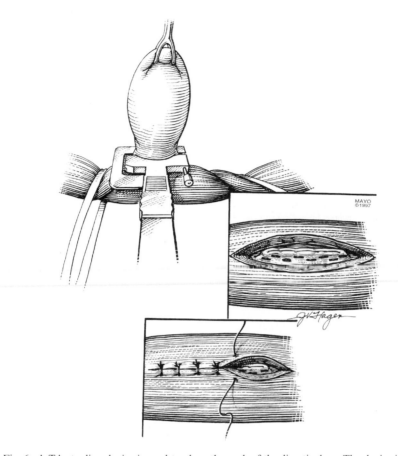

Fig. 6. A TA stapling device is used to close the neck of the diverticulum. The device is placed parallel to the long axis of the esophagus. The muscular wall is closed over the stump with interrupted 3-0 silk sutures (*inset*). (Courtesy of the Mayo Clinic Foundation, Rochester, MN; with permission.)

The authors' current treatment of choice is diverticulectomy combined with a long esophagomyotomy (Figs. 5–7). A left posterolateral thoracotomy through the seventh interspace provides adequate exposure. The esophagus is circled with tapes, and is rotated to bring the diverticulum into view. The sac is mobilized and dissected to its neck, and the diverticulectomy performed longitudinally over a 50F dilator. We prefer to use a TA stapling device, and to close the muscular wall to cover the stump. The esophagomyotomy should be performed opposite the site of the diverticulectomy, and should be carried onto the stomach for a few millimeters and extended cephalad through all regions of the esophagus documented to have abnormal motility. If motility is normal, the esophagomyotomy should be carried to a level above the diverticulum, which is usually between the inferior pulmonary vein and the arch of the aorta. The frequently thickened

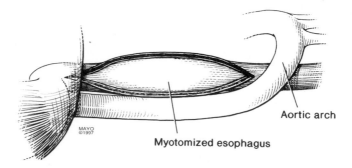

Aortic arch

Myotomized esophagus

Fig. 7. The myotomy is performed opposite the site of the diverticulectomy. The long myotomy begins from the esophagogastric junction and extends up to the aortic arch. The thickened muscle layer is retracted laterally to uncover approximately 50% of esophageal circumference. (Courtesy of the Mayo Clinic Foundation, Rochester, MN; with permission.)

muscle layer is retracted laterally to uncover approximately 50% of esophageal circumference.

The authors do not routinely add an antireflux procedure in the absence of preoperative gastroesophageal reflux or hiatal hernia. If either is present, a less obstructive antireflux procedure, such as Belsey Mark IV, should be performed. A radiographic contrast study is done on the fifth postoperative day, and if normal, diet is resumed. Leaks are usually contained and are best treated with parenteral nutrition until resolution. The risk of surgery is significant, and portends the difficulties in performing multiple concomitant procedures on the esophagus.

The Mayo Clinic reported a series of 112 patients who had epiphrenic diverticulum, 33 of whom underwent operation [13]. There were 3 deaths (9.1%), all occurring in patients who had abnormal manometry. Clinically significant leak rate was 6%. Long-term results were excellent or good in 66% of patients. There was no recurrence. Despite substantial operative risks, most patients will have long-term symptomatic palliation after operation. More recently, a laparoscopic approach has been performed successfully in selected patients.

Traction diverticulum

A traction diverticulum usually sits in the midesophageal area, and is secondary to a granulomatous inflammatory reaction (often histoplasmosis or tuberculosis) in the adjacent lymph nodes [2]. Midesophageal traction diverticula are usually small and asymptomatic, and do not require surgery. Rare complications such as fistulization to the tracheobronchial tree or great vessels require thoracotomy, excision of the inflammatory mass, and primary closure of the esophagus and the airway or vessel. Recurrence is minimized by the interposition of viable tissue such as pleura or muscle.

References

[1] Allen MS. Pharyngoesophageal diverticulum: technique of repair. Chest Surg Clin N Am 1995;5:449–58.

[2] Deschamps C, Trastek VF. Esophageal diverticula. In: Shields TW, LoCicero J III, Ponn RB, editors. General thoracic surgery, vol. 1. Fifth edition. Philadelphia: Lippincott Williams & Wilkins; 2000. p. 1839–50.

[3] Payne WS, King RM. Pharyngoesophageal (Zenker's) diverticulum. Surg Clin North Am 1983;63:815–24.

[4] Payne WS. The treatment of pharyngoesophageal diverticulum: the simple and complex. Hepato-Gastroenterol 1992;39:109–14.

[5] Crescenzo DG, Trastek VF, Allen MS, et al. Zenker's diverticulum in the elderly: is operation justified? Ann Thorac Surg 1998;66:347–50.

[6] Rocco G, Deschamps C, Martel E, et al. Results of reoperation on the upper esophageal sphincter. J Thorac Cardiovasc Surg 1999;117(1):28–31.

[7] Dohlman G, Mattsson O. The role of the cricopharyngeal muscle in cases of hypopharyngeal diverticula: a cineroentgenographic study. AJR Am J Roentgenol 1959;81:561.

[8] van Overbeek JJM. Microendoscopic CO2 laser surgery of the hypopharyngeal (Zenker's) diverticulum. Adv Otorhinolaryngol 1995;49:140.

[9] Collard JM, Otte JB, Kestens PJ. Endoscopic stapling technique of esophagodiverticulostomy for Zenker's diverticulum. Ann Thorac Surg 1993;56:573.

[10] Peracchia A, Bonavina L, Narne S, et al. Minimally invasive surgery for Zenker diverticulum: analysis of results in 95 consecutive patients. Arch Surg 1998;133:695–700.

[11] Gutschow CA, Hamoir M, Rombaux P, et al. Management of pharyngoesophageal (Zenker's) diverticulum: which technique? Ann Thorac Surg 2002;74:1677.

[12] Tirnaksiz MB, Deschamps C. Diverticula of the esophagus. In: Cameron JL, editor. Current surgical therapy. 6th edition. St. Louis: Mosby; 1998. p. 29–33.

[13] Benacci JC, Deschamps C, Trastek VF, et al. Epiphrenic diverticulum: results of surgical treatment. Ann Thorac Surg 1993;55:1109–14.

[14] Klaus A, Hinder RA, Swain J, et al. Management of epiphrenic diverticula. J Gastrointest Surg 2003;7(7):906–11.

ELSEVIER
SAUNDERS

SURGICAL
CLINICS OF
NORTH AMERICA

Surg Clin N Am 85 (2005) 505–514

Indications and Technique of Colon and Jejunal Interpositions for Esophageal Disease

Mary S. Maish, MD[a], Steven R. DeMeester, MD[b],*

[a]Department of Surgery, Keck School of Medicine, University of Southern California,
1510 San Pablo Street, Suite 514, Los Angeles, CA 90033, USA
[b]Department of Cardiothoracic Surgery, Keck School of Medicine, University of Southern
California, 1510 San Pablo Street, Suite 514, Los Angeles, CA 90033, USA

Esophageal reconstruction is often the most challenging component of an esophagectomy, and is certainly the aspect most noted and evaluated by the patient. Unfortunately, there is no replacement organ that is able to mimic the function of a healthy esophagus. Instead, all suffer from a lack of effective peristalsis and the absence of a physiologic barrier to reflux. Despite these shortcomings, available esophageal replacement organs permit most patients to eat very satisfactorily, and in patients who undergo esophagectomy for large tumors or severe strictures, swallowing is often significantly improved.

The most common esophageal substitute is the stomach. Advantages of a gastric pull-up include the relative speed and ease with which the stomach can be mobilized, the need for only one anastomosis, and the generally reliable blood supply through the right gastroepiploic arcade along the greater curvature. Disadvantages of a gastric pull-up include the fact that there is often relative ischemia at the tip of the fundus, and the leak and stricture rate of a cervical esophago-gastric anastomosis can be as high as 30%. In addition, the long-term presence of acid-secreting gastric mucosa juxtaposed to acid-sensitive squamous esophageal mucosa with no intervening barrier can lead to complications of reflux, including Barrett's esophagus and adenocarcinoma [1]. Finally, in patients who have large tumors near the gastroesophageal junction, use of the stomach may compromise the oncologic resection, because the gastric staple line along the lesser curve is likely to be within a few centimeters of the neoplasm.

---

* Corresponding author.
E-mail address: sdemeester@surgery.usc.edu (S.R. DeMeester).

0039-6109/05/$ - see front matter © 2005 Elsevier Inc. All rights reserved.
doi:10.1016/j.suc.2005.01.014   *surgical.theclinics.com*

In contrast, use of the colon to replace the esophagus allows an excellent oncologic resection of tumors near the gastroesophageal junction. The colon is acid-resistant, and by virtue of its long length, it prevents exposure of esophageal mucosa to refluxed gastric juice, thereby decreasing the risk of Barrett's developing in the residual esophagus. Typically, the transverse colon graft has an excellent blood supply via the left colic and marginal artery, and because the tip of the colon graft is well-perfused, the esophago-colo anastomosis heals reliably in most patients. The authors have found that compared with an esophago-gastric anastomosis, the stricture rate of an esophago-colo anastomosis is significantly decreased (University of Southern California data, [2]). In addition, because the colon is outside the field of radiation for distal esophageal cancers, a colon interposition in patients who have had neoadjuvant chemoradiotherapy allows healthy, nonradiated tissue to be used for the esophageal anastomosis. Another benefit of the colon graft is that length is seldom an issue, even if the reconstruction is at the level of the pharynx; however, compared with a gastric pull-up, a colon interposition is more difficult to mobilize, entails three anastomoses rather than one, and takes longer in the operating room. Further, meticulous attention to operative detail is required when using the colon in order to ensure both short- and long-term success with the graft.

Although both the stomach and colon are acceptable replacement organs for the entire esophagus, jejunal grafts are more suitable for limited esophageal replacement. Long Roux-en-Y limbs are useful to reconstruct the alimentary tract following gastrectomy and distal esophagectomy, whereas free grafts are used to bridge gaps either between the esophagus itself, or between the esophagus and another conduit such as the stomach or colon. Although not impossible, complete replacement of the esophagus by small intestine is difficult, given the curvature induced by the mesenteric vessels.

Step one: planning the operation

There are several decisions that need to be made when planning esophageal reconstruction. First, a decision needs to be made as to whether the patient will be reconstructed at the time of the esophagectomy or in a delayed fashion. Delayed reconstruction is generally reserved for emergency resections and complex redo operations. This possibility should be discussed preoperatively with patients as a possible "bailout" during any esophagectomy, in the event that the patient becomes unstable or is having a problem of some sort during the resection phase of the procedure. Second, the type of conduit needs to be chosen: stomach, colon, jejunum, or a composite graft. Third, the position of the conduit is determined, generally either in the posterior mediastinum or in a substernal location.

In most circumstances, the esophageal replacement organ should be selected before the esophagectomy. This is necessary for scheduling purposes, but more importantly, to ensure that the replacement organ has been suitably evaluated and prepared. In some cases, the patient's history alone will suggest the likely replacement organ. For example, patients who have had a prior fundoplication or gastric resection are likely to need a colon interposition, whereas those who have had a prior colectomy will typically require either a gastric pull-up or a jejunal graft.

All patients who have esophageal malignancy should have an upper endoscopy to evaluate the location and size of the tumor, so that a judgment can be made about the oncologic suitability of the stomach for esophageal replacement. Preferably, this should be done by the surgeon planning the resection. If a gastric pull-up is decided upon, no other conduit-specific evaluation is generally necessary; however, if a colon graft is chosen or considered as a backup because of concern regarding suitability of the stomach, then additional evaluation is required. Likewise, if a jejunal graft will be used, then additional preoperative planning and scheduling may be necessary, although no other testing is generally required.

Choosing the graft

Given its reliability and simplicity, the stomach is most commonly used as the replacement organ for the esophagus; however, there are several circumstances in which alternatives should be sought. These include: (1) situations in which the stomach is involved by the primary disease process, such as caustic injury or tumors at the gastroesophageal junction extending into the lesser curve; (2) altered gastric anatomy or blood supply secondary to previous interventions such as antireflux or gastric surgery; (3) situations in which there is concern about the length of the stomach, such as when a pharyngeal anastomosis will be necessary; and (4) in young patients who have a benign disease process and who will live a long time with the graft in place, particularly when a vagal-sparing procedure with total gastric preservation is appropriate. In these circumstances, a colon interposition should be strongly considered, and if the colon is unavailable or unsuitable, then a free jejunal or composite graft may be necessary.

Preoperative evaluation and scheduling for colon or jejunal grafts

Before use of the colon for an esophageal substitute, a colonoscopy or dual-contrast barium enema should be obtained to assess the graft for polyps or other lesions that should either be addressed before the use of the colon for esophageal replacement, or that would preclude use of the colon for this purpose. In addition, the authors often obtain a visceral arteriogram to assess patency of the inferior mesenteric artery; completeness of the marginal artery; and presence of aberrant anatomy, including early branching or separate middle colic arterial take-offs from the aorta. A standard colon graft is unlikely to be feasible after repair of an abdominal aortic aneurysm, because the inferior mesenteric artery is often ligated during this procedure. Other conditions that discourage use of the colon include ulcerative colitis, extensive diverticulosis, prior diverticulitis, Hirschsprung's disease as an infant, or previous colonic resection. Although no specific evaluation is necessary for planned small-bowel grafts, it is important to schedule the use of an operating microscope in the operating room, and the procedure should be scheduled in conjunction with a surgeon familiar with microvascular procedures (usually a plastic surgeon) if the esophageal surgeon is uncomfortable with microvascular anastomoses.

Operative technique: general

Although important with any esophageal replacement graft, anesthetic management is critical when using colon or jejunal free grafts. In particular, intravascular volume needs to be adequately maintained, and additional fluids given in anticipation of the greater third-spacing that accompanies a larger dissection, especially with use of the colon. It is also essential that no pressors or vasoconstrictive agents be given, because the small mesenteric vessels of the colon and jejunum are exquisitely sensitive to these drugs, and spasm or constriction can lead to thrombosis of these small vessels, with loss of the graft. Likewise, maintenance of a normal pH and acid-base balance is vital throughout these procedures.

Operative technique: colon interposition

The left, right, and transverse colon can be used as interposition grafts. Regardless of the planned graft, the ascending and descending portions of the colon and the hepatic and splenic flexures are mobilized. It is helpful to pack the small bowel into a bag to keep it out of the way during mobilization of the colon and dissection of the mesentery. Typically, the colon graft is prepared at the start of the operation, so that the viability of the graft, especially the anticipated area of anastomosis, can be evaluated some hours later. Most commonly, the transverse colon is used in an isoperistaltic fashion and the graft is based on the inferior mesenteric artery, the ascending branch of the left colic artery, the marginal artery of Drummond, and communication between the left and right branches of the middle colic artery. It is critical to maintain communication between branches of the middle colic artery, because the proximal extent of the graft is almost always to the right of the middle colic trunk.

The necessary length of colon is determined by measuring from the left ear to the xiphoid with an umbilical tape. The tape is cut to this distance.

Next, the splenic flexure/descending colon is brought up to the hiatus, being careful to minimize tension on the left colic vessels, and a 3-0 silk stitch is placed in a tinea as a mark. The umbilical tape is then laid out on the colon, starting from the marking stitch and going proximally. Typically, the umbilical tape ends near the hepatic flexure or in the distal ascending colon. A second 3-0 silk marking stitch is placed here, and the colon is remeasured to be certain of the stitch placement sites.

The mesenteric dissection commences along the inferior edge of the pancreas, at the root of the transverse mesocolon in the lesser sac. Often the middle colic vein can be visibly traced downward into this vicinity, and with careful dissection the superior mesenteric vein (SMV) and the junction with the middle colic vein are identified. In some cases, an accessory middle colic vein is present, with a separate entrance into the SMV. An important variant to recognize is one in which the gastroepiploic vein joins either the middle colic vein, or more commonly, the accessory middle colic vein before joining the SMV. It is critical to preserve the gastroepiploic vein, because this will be the primary drainage of the residual antrum if the colon is used, and is essential if a gastric pull-up is necessary. Next, the middle colic artery is identified and dissected to its origin from the superior mesenteric artery (SMA). It is often easiest to do this dissection by holding the transverse colon up in a cephalad direction while working at the root of the mesentery medial to the ligament of Treitz. The SMA is identified just lateral to the SMV. It is important to identify the middle colic artery at its origin from the SMA in order to be certain there is not an early bifurcation that would be compromised by dividing the vessel distally. At this point the anatomy is identified, but no vessels are ligated or divided.

Next, the mesentery at the site of the proximal stitch in the colon is dissected, and the colon wall is cleaned in preparation for division. Deeper in the mesentery, the arcade vessels joining the middle colic circulation with the right colic vessels are encountered. A bulldog clamp is placed on this arcade, and the mesentery is divided centrally below these vessels and carried toward the middle colic vessels. Generally, this portion of the mesentery is avascular, but occasionally a small arterial or venous branch is encountered. Arterial branches are clamped with fine bulldog or microvascular clamps. The dissection is continued beyond the middle colic vessels toward the ligament of Treitz, and here again, the mesentery should be largely avascular. Any small arteries identified should be clamped with a microvascular or bulldog clamp. Care is taken to prevent injury to the inferior mesenteric vein as the splenic flexure region is approached.

Once the distal colon stitch is reached, the mesenteric dissection is finished. Now the portion of transverse colon between the stitches is receiving arterial supply only from the ascending branch of the left colic and the middle colic arteries. The pulse in the middle colic artery should be palpated, and then a bulldog clamp should be placed proximally on the middle colic artery at its origin, and the pulse rechecked. At this point, the graft is perfused only by the ascending branch of the left colic artery. Doppler signals should be ascertained, and the colon should be inspected for evidence of ischemia. Commonly, the distal portion of the graft (the area near the proximal stitch) will spasm initially, but over time it should dilate, and in a good colon, the small mesenteric vessels adjacent to the bowel wall will be visibly pulsatile after several minutes with the clamps in place. Once the surgeon is satisfied with the vascularity of the graft, the clamped arteries are ligated and divided, as are the corresponding veins. Ideally, only a single middle colic artery and vein are ligated, but often an accessory small vein or artery is present and needs to be divided.

Finally, the colon itself is divided at the site of the proximal stitch with a linear stapler, and the graft is held straight up in the air. If the mesentery restricts straightening the graft, then it is incised, often tangentially, using transillumination to avoid any vessels. This will usually allow the graft to be nearly straight. The graft can then be tucked into the pelvis while the esophageal resection is performed.

The colon graft can be placed in either the posterior mediastinal or a substernal position. The graft is pulled through the designated space, while carefully wrapped in a camera bag to minimize trauma and maintain anatomic alignment. Once the graft is passed up to the neck, an end-to-end, esophago-colo anastomosis is performed with a single layer of full-thickness 4-0 monofilament absorbable sutures. Size discrepancy must be taken into account, although with dilatation of the esophagus secondary to distal obstruction the size match is often close. After completing the proximal anastomosis the graft is pulled firmly down into the abdomen. This is facilitated by removal of the camera bag used to pull the graft up to the neck. An important next step is to suture the colon graft to the left crus of the diaphragm at the hiatus with several permanent sutures. This will help prevent intrathoracic redundancy of the graft, and also prevents herniation of other abdominal organs into the posterior mediastinum. Failure to secure the colon graft to the left crus of the diaphragm likely contributed to the relatively high reoperation rates for redundancy reported by some centers [3].

When used substernally, it is recommended that the thoracic inlet be opened by removing the left half of the manubrium, clavicular head, and the medial portion of the left first rib, in order to accommodate the graft and prevent compression as it transitions from the posterior neck to a substernal location. Similarly, the exit from the substernal tunnel should be inspected. It is advisable to separate the diaphragm from the undersurface of the sternum and medial portions of the thorax anteriorly in order to create space for the graft. If the left lateral segment of the liver is large, it may be necessary to excise it in order to prevent interference with the course of the graft as it descends to join the gastric remnant. Further, in some patients the pericardium acts as a shelf and leads to acute angulation of the graft as it descends to join the gastric remnant. If necessary, this angle can be softened by opening the pericardium in an anterior-posterior direction, and then closing it transversely. The colon should be sutured to the left portion of the diaphragm, again to prevent redundancy and herniation of abdominal viscera into the substernal space.

The distal colon graft is then divided with a linear stapler, preserving about 10 cm of intra-abdominal colon below the haitus. Excess intra-abdominal colon can lead to stasis and regurgitation, and must be avoided. Great caution is used when dividing the colon, in order to prevent injury to the underlying mesenteric vessels supplying the graft. Unless the vagus nerves are spared, the stomach is divided, leaving only the antrum, and a pyloroplasty is performed. The colo-gastric anastomosis is completed using two layers of 3-0 silk sutures. When the vagus nerves are preserved only the gastroesophageal junction is excised, and no pylorpolasty is necessary. In this circumstance, the proximal short gastric vessels are divided to allow passage of the colon graft from the hiatus to the posterior aspect of the stomach, and a stapled colo-gastric anastomosis is performed to the posterior gastric body.

The final step is the colo-colostomy. When using the transverse colon this anastomosis ends up in the left upper quadrant near the colo-gastric anastomosis. It sometimes is necessary to mobilize the distal colon a few centimeters to facilitate performance of this anastomosis, but again, caution is necessary to avoid injury to the mesenteric vessels supplying the graft, and to prevent ischemia of the mobilized end of the colon. A nasogastric tube is carefully passed into the stomach, the mesenteric defect is closed, and a feeding jejunostomy is placed.

What if ... ?

Numerous aberrances are possible in the circulation to the transverse colon, and some are commonly encountered. One is the joining of the right gastroepiploic vein to either the middle colic vein or an accessory vein before joining the SMV. This vein must be preserved. Another not uncommon problem is proximal bifurcation of the middle colic artery into left and right branches. The communication between these vessels must be maintained; thus ligation of the middle colic artery needs to be proximal to the bifurcation. In some cases, a side-biting clamp must be applied to the SMA to divide the middle colic vessel and preserve the communication between left and right branches. In some patients, however, there are two completely separate origins of the middle colic artery from the SMA. In these patients, either a different portion of colon is used, and the graft is based on the middle colic vessels, or one of the divided middle colic arteries is anastomosed to the internal mammary artery or a neck vessel to supercharge the graft. The authors' experience has been that when two separate middle colic arteries are present, the graft is at high risk for ischemia, and it would be unwise to use it without supercharging. Two veins are relatively common, and provided one is small and there is visible collateral communication between the veins, this seldom poses a problem for the graft. Three veins or no clear communication between two major vein branches should be cause for significant concern, however. In this circumstance, consideration should be given to either abandoning the colon graft or to performing a microvascular anastomosis between one of the middle colic veins and the innominate vein, with the colon in a substernal location. Regardless of the arterial and venous anatomy, the absence of a Doppler signal at the proximal end of the graft is also an indication to supercharge the graft; perform an esophagostomy and reinspect the colon at about 48 hours; or to abandon the transverse colon and use an alternate conduit.

Alternate colon grafts

If the transverse colon is not available or suitable for use, the right or left colon can be used as an interposition graft. Compared with the left colon, the right colon is thin-walled and bulky. It can be used in an isoperistaltic fashion based on the middle colic vessels, and is a reasonable choice if colon is required and there are two independent middle colic arteries arising from the SMA. The right colon, including the cecum, will usually reach to the neck, but if not, a portion of terminal ileum can be left attached to the cecum. The ascending colon graft relies on an intact arcade between the right branch of the middle colic and the right colic artery.

The left colon is also a suitable conduit, and the wall thickness and caliber of the lumen of the left colon make it more suitable for esophageal replacement than the right colon. The drawback to use of the left colon is the requirement that it be used in a retroperistaltic fashion based on the middle colic vessels, and the greater propensity for the descending colon to be involved with diverticulosis.

Jejunal grafts: operative technique

Selection of an appropriate jejunal free graft begins with transilluminating the mesentery. The length of jejunum necessary as a free graft is measured with an umbilical tape, and marked with stitches on the jejunum. A different stitch is used to mark the proximal bowel, in order to prevent inadvertent placement in an antiperistaltic fashion. Before vascular isolation, the insertion site of the free graft is prepared. There are several suitable cervical vessels for anastomosis to the jejunal free graft, including the transverse cervical artery, but in most circumstances, the authors' preference has been the internal thoracic (mammary) artery. With adequate mobilization this artery easily reaches to the neck, and it provides reliable arterial inflow. The mammary vein, though, is flimsy and quite small, and our preference is to use a large-caliber vein such as the innominate or a jugular vein.

To make room for the graft as it courses from the neck to a substernal location, it is best to remove the left half of the manubrium, left clavicular head, and the medial end of the first rib. This exposure also allows mobilization of the left mammory artery. If long lengths of mammory artery are necessary the entire sternum may need to be divided and the mammory mobilized, similar to when it is used for coronary grafting.

Once the site and recipient vessels are prepared, the jejunal graft is harvested. It is important to dissect the mesenteric vessels as proximally as possible, so as to ensure an adequate caliber for the anastomosis. Only the proximal ends of the vessels are ligated, and this is done as the last step, after transection of the bowel with a GIA stapler and division of the mesentery to the area where the vessels are going to be ligated and divided. After division of the vessels, the authors flush the graft with iced saline containing 1000 units of heparin, and wrap the jejunum in a slush-ice filled lap pad to keep it cool. Warm ischemic time for the jejunum can extend to 3 hours, but cooling the bowel reduces the edema of the reperfused graft in our experience [4].

The graft is then brought into the prepared neck site, and under the operating microscope the vessels are dissected to remove adjacent fat and flimsy tissue that could get caught in the anastomosis and lead to thrombosis. The authors tend to do the arterial anastomosis first, although the order is not important. Plenty of redundancy should be left in the artery to accommodate movement and positioning of the graft. This does not predispose to kinking or thrombosis, particularly with the mammory artery. The venous anastomosis should be as straight as possible, however, with a minimum of kinking. It is critical to avoid any twisting of either anastomosis. Each anastomosis is completed using interrupted fine (8-0 or 9-0) monofilament micovascular sutures, and generally only 6 to 8 sutures are necessary for each. The arterial anastomosis is performed end-to-end, and the authors typically align the sides with a corner stitch, and place two or three stitches between each corner on the anterior and posterior wall. All knots must be on the outside of the vessel, and tiny bites are taken to prevent stenosis and thrombosis. The venous anastomosis is generally end-to-side into the innominate vein, which has been occluded with vessel loops. The vessels are flushed with heparinized saline, and papaverine is used to prevent spasm as necessary, particularly for the mammory artery. The venous clamps are released first to de-air and flush the graft, followed by the arterial clamps. Unless an obvious technical problem with suture placement is present, the authors prefer to loosely wrap each anastomosis with oxidized cellulose (Surgicel) for a few minutes, and then inspect for hemostasis. The jejunum should turn pink immediately with reperfusion and begin peristalsing. The vessels are checked with a Doppler, and the graft is positioned to prevent kinking or twisting of the vessels. The graft should be trimmed to minimize redundant length, and then the esophago-jejunal anastomosis is performed, followed by the distal anastomosis. Commonly, the free graft produces an exuberant amount of mucous and secretions after reperfusion. Other than a daily aspirin started postoperatively, and subcutaneous heparin for prophylaxis against deep vein thrombosis, the authors do not routinely use any blood-thinning agents for the free graft. In the absence of technical errors, vascular patency rates for jejunal free grafts are excellent, particularly when the venous anastomosis is performed to a large vein.

Over time, jejunal grafts, particularly long ones, have a propensity to become redundant and require trimming. Generally, this is accomplished with segmental resection of a portion of the graft and primary anastomosis. Grafts that have been in place for several years are typically very hardy and tolerate trimming well; however, disruption of the mesenteric vessels will lead to loss of the graft, so patients should be warned that before undergoing any surgery in the area of the graft, they must make sure that the surgeon is aware of the altered anatomy and the consequences of injury to the mesenteric vessels supplying the graft. This is less of a problem with a jejunal free graft in the neck, but it is extremely important for patients who have a colon interposition, because the graft relies on its native abdominal vessels for perfusion.

Summary

Esophageal replacement is a significant undertaking for both surgeon and patient. Because eating and drinking are some of life's great pleasures, the outcome of this undertaking has a direct impact on a patient's quality of life. The primary esophageal replacement organs are the stomach and colon, and each has advantages and disadvantages. As such, the choice of the graft should be tailored to the patient and the disease process in order to maximize the likelihood that the disease will be effectively treated, and that the patient's ability to enjoy a meal with family and friends will be restored.

References

[1] Oberg S, Johansson J, Wenner J, et al. Metaplastic columnar mucosa in the cervical esophagus after esophagectomy. Ann Surg 2002;235:338–45.

[2] Briel IW, Tamhankar AP, Hagen JA, et al. Prevalence and risk factors for ischemia, leak, and stricture of esophageal anastomosis: gastric pull-up versus colon interposition [see comment]. J Am Coll Surg 2004;198(4):536–41; discussion 541–2.

[3] DeMeester SR. Colon interposition following esophagectomy. Dis Esophagus 2001;14(3–4): 169–72.

[4] Hikida S, Takeuchi M, Hata H, et al. Free jejunal graft autotransplantation should be revascularized within 3 hours. Transplant Proc 1998;30(7):3446–8.

ELSEVIER
SAUNDERS

Surg Clin N Am 85 (2005) 515–524

SURGICAL
CLINICS OF
NORTH AMERICA

Boerhaave's Syndrome: Diagnosis and Treatment

Conrad M. Vial, MD, Richard I. Whyte, MD*

Department of Cardiothoracic Surgery, Stanford University School of Medicine, CVRB 205, 300 Pasteur Drive, Stanford, CA 94305-0344, USA

Boerhaave's syndrome, or postemetic rupture of the esophagus, first described in 1724, represents a special instance of barogenic trauma to the esophagus, leading to a challenging clinical syndrome that still bears its describer's name [1]. Perforation of the esophagus may result from a variety of iatrogenic or otherwise acquired conditions. In modern medical contexts, instrumentation of the esophagus for diagnostic or therapeutic purposes represents the most common etiology; however, other forms of traumatic insult to the esophagus secondary to penetrating, blunt force, or corrosive injury—accidental or intentional—remain important causes of esophageal disruption. Indeed, to the extent that noniatrogenic esophageal injury occurs in a medically unsupervised setting, the clinical sequelae may be more grievous, particularly when one considers the prognostic significance of the time course to recognition and treatment. The local inflammation and systemic sepsis that result from the expulsion of both gastric and oral secretions into the mediastinum and pleural cavities in such cases can be particularly severe, with mortality rates approaching 30%, in comparison with rates of 10% documented in thoracic units managing iatrogenic injuries [2,3]. The factors underlying this disparity in outcomes illustrate less about any peculiarities in the causes and consequences of Boerhaave's syndrome per se than they do about the significance of prompt recognition and early, aggressive intervention in all cases of esophageal disruption. In this light, the following overview construes an episode of forceful vomiting as one of several clinical scenarios that may incite a common pathophysiologic response, and that mandate the same meticulous diagnostic and therapeutic approach.

* Corresponding author.
E-mail address: riwhyte@stanford.edu (R.I. Whyte).

0039-6109/05/$ - see front matter © 2005 Elsevier Inc. All rights reserved.
doi:10.1016/j.suc.2005.01.010

Clinical presentation and pathophysiology

Regardless of the cause of esophageal perforation, a fulminant mediastinal inflammatory response may result from extrusion of bacteria and enzyme rich salivary, gastric, and biliary secretions. Circulation of these noxious stimuli throughout the mediastinum and pleural spaces may be exacerbated by the negative intrathoracic pressure that results from the mechanics of ventilation. Fluid transit across excoriated mediastinal and pleural surfaces can lead to systemic hypovolemia, hypoperfusion, systemic inflammation, sepsis, and multisystem organ dysfunction, typically affecting the respiratory apparatus first. Left untreated, this injury has a mortality approaching 100%. Although the final common pathophysiologic pathway is possible if not probable in most cases of untreated esophageal rupture, certain factors can modulate the presentation and outcome of a given patient. These are: (1) the location of the tear or laceration, (2) the cause of injury as it relates to the extent of damage or the presence of intrinsic disease of the esophagus, and (3) the time elapsed from insult to intervention.

Disruptions of the cervical esophagus are commonly associated with neck or upper chest pain, whereas those of the middle and lower esophagus may lead to interscapular or epigastric discomfort, respectively. The physical examination may be unremarkable, although it may demonstrate subcutaneous emphysema, dullness to percussion (secondary to a pleural effusion), Hamon's sign (a crunchlike noise due to movement of mediastinal air), or other more ominous signs such as tachycardia, tachypnea, and hypotension. Patients who have upper esophageal injuries may present with chest radiographs that demonstrate either pneumomediastinum alone or a right-sided pleural effusion, whereas those who have distal esophageal perforations (as is most often the case in Boerhaave's syndrome) more commonly exhibit a left-sided effusion.

The cause of injury may serve as a marker of the extent of damage or the likelihood and severity of concomitant intrinsic disease of the esophagus, and this may bear significantly upon the management strategy indicated. For example, although discrete intramural dissections of the cervical esophagus created during the course of pneumatic dilatation of a benign, "soft" stricture may often be treated conservatively, attempted dilatation of a "hard" stricture in the setting of carcinoma or overzealous pneumatic dilatation for achalasia may cause injury that requires operative intervention to address not only the esophageal tear in and of itself, but also the associated obstructive lesion. By the same token, a high-velocity gunshot wound involving the esophagus may be attended by such a degree of tissue devitalization that the esophagus is rendered unsalvageable. In the case of postemetic esophageal rupture, the syndrome's frequent association with antecedent alcohol and food intake, along with the distal location of the tear (generally the left lateral wall of the esophagus just above the diaphragm), often portend a more aggressive inflammatory response because of the forced extrusion of voluminous gastric contents into the mediastinum [3].

Finally, the aggravated clinical course often attributed to Boerhaave's syndrome may illustrate the significance of time in the prognosis of patients who have esophageal disruptions. To the extent that the so-called "classic triad" of vomiting, lower chest pain, and subcutaneous emphysema is either not always manifest or not recognized in cases of postemetic esophageal perforation, a number of these patients present late (ie, longer than 24 hours postinjury) [3]. It stands to reason that the longer the course of undetected mediastinal soilage, the worse the patient's condition is likely to be at the time of clinical evaluation. Indeed, delayed diagnosis and therapy have been associated with poorer outcomes historically, and, as will be discussed, this has been used in the past as the basis for recommendations for supposedly more conservative modes of therapy in such patients [4,5]. Suffice it to say at this point that late-presenting patients do exhibit higher complication rates, but in recent series, such morbidity is more accurately attributed to the patients' clinical status at presentation, rather than being used as the impetus for less than definitive interventional strategies [6].

Diagnosis

The essential attribute of the diagnostic approach to esophageal rupture is the maintenance of a high index of suspicion. Any patient who presents with pain or fever following forceful vomiting, esophageal instrumentation, or chest trauma should be aggressively evaluated, with the aim of ruling out perforation of the esophagus. Notwithstanding the aforementioned comments regarding plain chest radiograph findings in such settings, a negative or normal chest roentgenogram does not suffice. Contrast esophagography—using a water-soluble agent initially, followed by a barium study if the initial result is negative—represents the most reliable test for demonstrating the presence and location of a perforation, and as such, is mandatory for a complete evaluation (Fig. 1). Contrast-enhanced CT of the chest may, on rare occasions, be a useful test in the event of a persistent clinical suspicion after a normal barium esophagram, or when contrast esophagography is impractical, as in the case of an intubated/sedated patient [7]. Likewise, esophagoscopy has little role in the evaluation of suspected Boerhaave's syndrome, except to the extent that a normal-appearing distal esophagus reliably rules out the presence of a distal esophageal perforation.

Treatment

In all cases in which an esophageal disruption has been demonstrated, the goals of the initial phase of therapy are the same: resuscitation of the patient; establishment of appropriate physiologic monitoring capabilities;

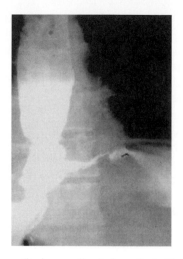

Fig. 1. Contrast esophagogram (barium swallow) of a patient with Boerhaave's syndrome. The study shows extravasation of barium from the distal esophagus.

and limiting the extent of ongoing mediastinal contamination through cessation of oral intake, broad-spectrum antibiotic therapy, and nasogastric tube decompression. The approach to subsequent phases of treatment depends on several of the factors already reviewed, including the time course, location, cause, and extent of injury, as well as the presence of intrinsic disease of the esophagus.

As has already been alluded, nonoperative management of esophageal perforations is advisable only in a minority of cases, and is exceedingly rare in the setting of Boerhaave's syndrome. Nevertheless, some patients are well-served by such an approach, the criteria for which have been fairly clearly delineated: a contained rupture with evidence of reflux of extravasated barium back into the esophagus and no associated pleural contamination, combined with minimal symptoms and no evidence of systemic infection [8]. Almost by definition, these features are most reliably established in patients who present late, because enough time for true containment to be discernible has to have elapsed in order for a given patient to be appropriately risk-stratified. Thus, the potentially high cost of not intervening in early presenters is that of "sitting on," a septic process that remains in a state of uncontrolled evolution. Those who truly declare themselves candidates for the most conservative of management strategies tend to have small cervical tears following esophago-scopy or traumatic endotracheal intubation, well-circumscribed intramural dissections following pneumatic dilatation for achalasia (in 4%–6% of such patients), or small anastamotic disruptions detected on routine barium swallow following esophageal surgery [2,9]. These patients are generally well-managed by maintenance of oral hygiene, cessation of oral intake, antibiotics, and nutritional support delivered parenterally or enterally distal to the site of injury.

In the overwhelming majority of patients who have esophageal rupture, however, some type of operative intervention is required. Treatment may take the form of exploration and drainage, esophageal exclusion/diversion, primary repair with or without autogenous tissue reinforcement, or esophagectomy with immediate versus delayed reconstruction/replacement. With particular emphasis on more complex injuries such as are likely to occur in Boerhaave's syndrome, the essential elements of these surgical techniques will be outlined before undertaking a critical assessment of the role played by each in current management of esophageal perforation.

Cervical esophageal perforations (including those of the upper thoracic esophagus) are often amenable to drainage alone, provided extruded oral secretions have not drained dependently to such an extent that the lower mediastinum or either pleural space has become significantly contaminated. A skin incision is made along the anterior border of the left sternocleido-mastoid (SCM) from the level of the cricoid cartilage to the sternal notch. Underlying tissues are mobilized so as to permit retraction of the SCM and carotid sheath laterally while the trachea and thyroid are displaced medially. Care is taken to avoid injury to the recurrent laryngeal nerves as a blunt, finger-dissection technique is employed to gain access to the prevertebral space and to develop a plane along the posterolateral aspect of the esophagus. The abscess contained therein is evacuated and irrigated; drains are placed within the area and brought out via the skin incision. In the event of more extensive contamination and erosion beyond the upper mediastinum, some form of additional transthoracic drainage may be required.

Intrathoracic esophageal disruptions require generally aggressive mediastinal and pleural drainage. This is accomplished via posterolateral thoracotomy on the side, and at the intercostal level appropriate for the location of the tear (ie, right side, fourth or fifth interspace for upper-third and midesophageal injuries; left side, sixth or seventh interspace for distal-third ruptures). The mediastinal-pleural interface is widely incised, and both the mediastinum and pleural space are debrided, irrigated, and then drained by large-caliber thoracostomy tubes. Although these elements represent the fundamental point of departure for all surgical approaches to esophageal rupture, the literature has characterized a number of different end points of operative intervention.

The technique of esophageal exclusion/diversion was described many decades ago as involving division and closure of the esophagus proximal and distal to the site of injury, with creation of an end-cervical esophagostomy. This approach has evolved to one that preserves esophageal continuity by the placement of either a staple line or removable ligature distally (with or without t-tube drainage), and creation of a side cervical esophagostomy proximally for diversion of oral secretions [10]. The ongoing presence of the original septic focus within the thorax, in combination with the often suboptimal control of ongoing mediastinal soilage and difficulties with eventual esophageal reconstruction, have limited the technical application of this strategy in either its original or modified form, particularly as methods of repair or replacement of the perforated esophagus have been refined and the outcomes analyzed. In fact, as will become apparent below, the exclusion/diversion paradigm is instead most often employed either in the setting of an extensively devitalized or otherwise dysfunctional esophagus, wherein segmental resection actually represents the least radical treatment alternative for esophageal rupture, or when the patient is too unstable to tolerate definitive repair or resection.

Fundamental elements of primary repair of esophageal perforations have been well-described [11–13]. Of paramount significance is the full exposure of the mucosal defect (Fig. 2A), the extent of which can be obscured by the more limited muscular disruption, requiring that a longitudinal esophago-myotomy be performed proximally and distally. Necrotic tissue along the perimeter of injury is debrided, and healthy mucosal and submucosal edges are placed under gentle traction, so as to permit their mobilization away from the overlying rim of investing muscular tissue. A 40F to 46F bougie is then placed into the esophagus, and the mucosal/submucosal edges burgeoning through the muscular defect are reapproximated in a tension-free, stapled (Fig. 2B) or interrupted, handsewn fashion. Muscular tissue is then closed over this first layer, using a running or interrupted absorbable suture technique. This two-layer closure may then be reinforced with a variety

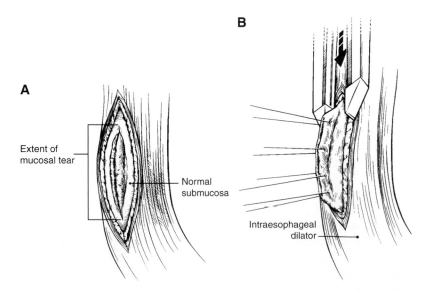

Fig. 2. Primary repair of esophageal perforation. (*A*) exposure of the entire mucosal injury (which often extends beyond the muscular tear). (*B*) Reapproximation of the mucosal and submocsal edges using a surgical stapler. *Data from* Iannettoni MD, Whyte RI, Orringer, MB. Catastrophic complications of the cervical esophagogastric anastomosis. J Thorac Cardiovasc Surg 1995;110(5):1493–500; discussion 1500–1.

of vascularized autogenous tissues, including intercostal muscle on its pedicle, omentum, pericardial fat pad, or thickened pleura. Most advocates of reinforcement suggest an onlay patch rather than wrap technique, in order to minimize the possibility of inducing stricture at the repair site. The essential corollary to any approach to primary repair, however, is the elimination or amelioration of any obstruction distal to the site of repair. Such lesions commonly take the form of reflux strictures or achalasia, requiring intraoperative esophageal dilatation combined with full fundoplication or esophagomyotomy with partial fundoplication, respectively. Failure to relieve a source of obstruction places any proximal esophageal repair at high risk for breakdown. Multiple zones of obstruction or lesions not amenable to correction constitute an indication for esophagectomy.

Segmental resection of the esophagus as a therapy for perforation is undertaken as a prelude to either immediate or delayed reconstruction/replacement using transposed stomach, colon or, rarely, small bowel [14]. Preparation of a gastric pull-up concomitant with esophagectomy and mobilization of the same through the native esophageal bed to a cervical esophagogastric anastamosis is preferable to using an unprepared colon interposition; however, success with the latter has been reported. If delayed reconstruction is deemed necessary, the entire intrathoracic esophagus is mobilized, and the damaged segment is excised, taking care to preserve as much healthy proximal esophagus as is possible so that it may be tunneled subcutaneously for construction of a left-sided cervical or anterior thoracic end esophagostomy [15]. (Stomal appliances are easier to apply and care for on the chest wall.) In these circumstances, the gastric inlet is oversewn, and the esophago-diaphragmatic hiatus is closed to prevent herniation of peritoneal contents into the thorax. After the patient's septic insult has been overcome and his or her metabolic condition fortified, alimentary continuity can be established via retrosternal esophageal replacement using stomach or colon.

In settings both of primary repair and esophagectomy, creation of a feeding jejunostomy with or without a decompressing gastrostomy is prudent [3,12,14]. The need to provide for enteral nutrition in the case of delayed esophageal reconstruction is obvious, but the high incidence of foregut dysfunction and the possibility of even straightforward anastamotic or repair site complications when intestinal continuity is restored from the outset renders these precautions advisable in most other cases. Interrogation of a repair or anastamosis by barium swallow is undertaken several days following operation. Once the integrity of the native esophagus or its replacement has been confirmed, the patient may be started on an oral diet. If a subclinical disruption is documented on the esophagram, the patient is supported nutritionally and kept nulla per os (NPO) until repeat examination indicates healing. In the context of postoperative esophago-pleurocutaneous fistula development, reoperation is generally warranted, although healing may occur, provided that the chest is well-drained, the patient is well-supported metabolically, and there is no distal obstruction or foreign body.

The final destination targeted by all surgical approaches to esophageal perforation is therefore the same: drainage of the infected mediastinum and elimination of ongoing soilage—what varies is the pathway to achieve these goals. Because esophageal disruptions such as those generally associated with Boerhaave's syndrome are both relatively uncommon and highly morbid, surgical management guidelines have been historically divergent and controversial. The wisdom of undertaking operative repair of a per-forated esophagus more than 24 hours after injury was frequently called into question in the past [4,10]. Reluctance to intervene aggressively in these circumstances was prompted by apparently high mortality rates in this subpopulation, and perceived technical challenges in handling fragile esophageal tissues. More recent series [11–13] support meticulous primary repair of nonmalignant, intrathoracic disruptions, even in the setting of delayed presentation or diagnosis. Important caveats to this strategy include the recognition of any intrinsic esophageal disease or complicating factors that would unduly imperil the repair, or that render the esophagus unworthy of salvage. Herein lie the chief sources of challenge and controversy in the current management of esophageal rupture.

A series examining the outcome of primary repair for postemetic perforation of the esophagus [3] documented an overall mortality rate of 14.3%; over half the patients presented more than 24 hours after rupture, and 81% of the cohort underwent unreinforced operative repair combined with aggressive mediastinal toilet and gastrostomy. This compares favorably with the mortality rates and prevalence of delayed referral/diagnosis quoted by Port et al [6] in a review of their and others' experience with esophageal disruptions of multiple etiologies. Although there are authors who strongly favor reinforcement of primary repairs due to some evidence indicating improved postoperative clinical leak rates [11,12], outcome differences in this regard are inconsistently documented, suggesting that individualized patient management with respect to the technique of repair is perhaps the most compelling strategy. Indeed, the same thesis may be put forth regarding the decision to reject primary repair in favor of esophagectomy in these patients. Several series have indicated that in certain clinical settings, greater morbidity is incurred with conservative procedures and even attempts at primary repair than with esophageal resection [14,16,17]. As has already been mentioned, the circumstances favoring esophagectomy as therapy for esophageal disruption include unreconstructable tissue defects and incorrigible intrinsic disease of the esophagus. These criteria may be realized in the setting of Boerhaave's syndrome, if not due to the magnitude of the initial insult, then because of the frequent delay in presentation/ diagnosis, leading to advanced mediastinal sepsis. It is important to note that in addition to frankly devastating esophageal injuries, more subtle, antecedent functional deficiencies in a patient's native esophagus may represent an important consideration. A report by Iannettoni and colleagues [18] that reviewed intermediate-term outcomes following surgical treatment of intrathoracic esophageal perforation revealed that substantial fraction of patients who survived primary repair required some additional form of significant endoscopic or surgical intervention for dysphagia. By contrast, no further operative therapy was needed in those patients in whom esophagectomy was performed.

In the final analysis, effective management of esophageal rupture requires an aggressive approach to diagnosis and treatment, tempered by an understanding of the individual patient's background and status at presentation. Although a patient recently instrumented with an endoscopic balloon may be managed nonoperatively without adverse outcome, one with a self-inflicted corrosive injury may well require esophageal resection, cervical esophagostomy, and delayed reconstruction with a substernal colonic interposition graft in order for success to be achieved. Boerhaave's syndrome encompasses a good deal of the spectrum of complexity and diversity that characterizes patients who have esophageal disruptions. Although it often occurs in otherwise relatively healthy patients, postemetic perforation of the esophagus can result in a devastating injury exacerbated by delayed diagnosis, and therefore requires one to be versed in all potentially applicable therapies.

References

[1] Derbes VJ, Mitchell RE Jr. Hermann Boerhaave's Atrocis, nec Descripti Prius, Morbi Historia, the first translation of the classic case report of rupture of the esophagus, with annotations. Bull Med Libr Assoc 1955;43:217.

[2] Lawrence DR, Ohri SK, Moxon RE, et al. Iatrogenic oesophageal perforations: a clinical review. Ann R Coll Surg Engl 1998;80:115–8.

[3] Lawrence DR, Ohri SK, Moxon RE, et al. Primary esophageal repair for Boerhaave's syndrome. Ann Thorac Surg 1999;67:818–20.

[4] Skinner DB, Little AG, DeMeester TR. Management of esophageal perforation. Am J Surg 1980;139:760–4.

[5] Jones WG, Ginsberg RJ. Esophageal perforation: a continuing challenge. Ann Thorac Surg 1992;53:534–43.

[6] Port JL, Kent MS, Korst RJ, et al. Thoracic esophageal perforations: a decade of experience. Ann Thorac Surg 2003;75:1071–4.

[7] White CS, Templeton PA, Attar S. Esophageal perforation: CT findings. AJR Am J Roentgenol 1993;160:767–70.

[8] Cameron JL, Kieffer RH, Hendrix TR, et al. Selective nonoperative management of contained intrathoracic esophageal disruptions. Ann Thorac Surg 1979;27:404–8.

[9] Lo AY, Surick B, Ghazi A. Nonoperative management of esophageal perforation secondary to balloon dilatation. Surg Endosc 1993;7:529–32.

[10] Fell SC. Esophageal perforation. In: Pearson FG, Cooper JD, Deslauriers J, et al, editors. Esophageal surgery. New York: Churchill Livingstone; 2002. p. 615–36.

[11] Gouge T, Depan H, Spencer F. Experience with the Grillo pleural wrap procedure in 18 patients with perforation of the thoracic esophagus. Ann Surg 1989;209:612–7.

[12] Wright CD, Mathisen DJ, Wain JC, et al. Reinforced primary repair of thoracic esophageal perforation. Ann Thorac Surg 1995;60:245–8.

[13] Whyte RI, Iannetoni MD, Orringer MB. Intrathoracic esophageal perforation—the merit of primary repair. J Thorac Cardiovasc Surg 1995;109:140–4.

[14] Orringer MB, Stirling MB. Esophagectomy for esophageal disruption. Ann Thorac Surg 1990;49:35–42.

[15] Orringer MB. Complications of esophageal surgery and trauma. In: Greenfield LJ, editor. Complications in surgery and trauma. Philadelphia: JB Lippincott Co; 1990. p. 302–5.

[16] Altorjay A, Kiss J, Voros A. The role of esophagectomy in the management of esophageal perforations. Ann Thorac Surg 1998;65:1433–6.

[17] Salo JA, Isolauri JO, Heikkila LJ, et al. Management of delayed esophageal perforation with mediastinal sepsis; esophagectomy or primary repair? J Thorac Cardiovasc Surg 1993;106: 1088–91.

[18] Iannettoni MD, Vlessis AA, Whyte RI, et al. Functional outcome after surgical treatment of esophageal perforation. Ann Thorac Surg 1997;64:1606–9.

ELSEVIER
SAUNDERS

SURGICAL
CLINICS OF
NORTH AMERICA

Surg Clin N Am 85 (2005) 525–538

Functional Problems Following Esophageal Surgery

Pavlos Papasavas, MD*

Temple University School of Medicine at the Western Pennsylvania Hospital Clinical Campus, 4800 Friendship Avenue, Pittsburgh, Pennsylvania 15224, USA

Antireflux surgery is performed to address functional esophageal symptoms such as heartburn, regurgitation, dysphagia, and chest pain. The occurrence of postoperative functional problems such as dysphagia and gas bloat has inspired criticism of laparoscopic fundoplication, which has maintained that patients trade gastroesophageal reflux disease (GERD) symptoms for new functional problems.

Persistent and recurrent gastroesophageal reflux disease symptoms

The two main reasons for a dissatisfied patient following fundoplication are poor patient selection and operative technical errors. It is important to differentiate between persistent and recurrent symptoms. A successful fundoplication should have a dramatic and immediate effect on preoperative GERD symptoms. Several studies have linked the success of fundoplication with the presence of typical GERD symptoms and objective documentation of GERD. In patients who have heartburn that does not improve postoperatively, the appropriateness and indications for surgical treatment should be questioned. These patients may have been suffering from other diseases, and may have been erroneously labeled as GERD patients. Lack of objective preoperative evidence of GERD, such as abnormal 24-hour pH study and endoscopic presence of significant esophagitis, should initiate investigation for other diseases such as esophageal or gastric dysmotility, gallbladder disease, irritable bowel syndrome, and heart disease.

* Department of Surgery, The Western Pennsylvania Hospital, N4600, 4800 Friendship Avenue, Pittsburgh, PA 15224.

E-mail address: ppapasav@wpahs.org

0039-6109/05/$ - see front matter © 2005 Elsevier Inc. All rights reserved.
doi:10.1016/j.suc.2005.01.007   *surgical.theclinics.com*

The majority of patients who have persistent postoperative symptoms do not require a reoperation to take down the fundoplication, providing that a structural wrap problem is not present. These patients are treated with antisecretory agents according to the severity of their symptoms. Proof of the adequacy of the fundoplication to eliminate acid reflux can be easily provided with a 24-hour pH study. When symptoms persist following what is considered an adequate repair, then other esophageal disorders must be ruled out. Patients who have functional heartburn have esophageal hypersensitivity to physiologic esophageal acid exposure or esophageal mechanosensitivity [1,2]. Psychological factors may also play a role. In such patients, treatment with a low-dose tricyclic antidepressant may be successful [3].

In patients who initially experience improvement in their GERD symptoms and who subsequently complain of recurrent symptoms or development of new symptoms, a thorough evaluation should be undertaken to exclude an anatomic deformity of the fundic wrap. The work-up should include a barium esophagram and esophagogastroduodenscopy (EGD). EGD is complementary to barium esophagram, and can detect 10% to 50% of abnormalities missed by esophagram [4,5]. With the aforementioned evaluation, anatomic failures such as herniation of the wrap, a slipped or misplaced wrap, a disrupted fundoplication, or a tight fundoplication may be diagnosed in the majority of patients.

In the era of laparoscopic surgery, the most common pattern of anatomic wrap failure is the herniation of the wrap across the diaphragm (Figs. 1, 2) [4,6–8]. Acute wrap herniation may occur in patients who have early postoperative retching and straining. Diagnosis is made by barium esophagram, and a laparoscopic repair may be successful if the patient is treated

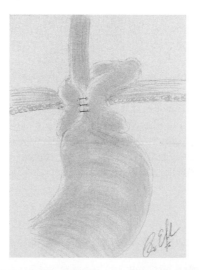

Fig. 1. Transdiaphragmatic herniation of fundic wrap. (Courtesy of Ramy Eskander, MD, with permission).

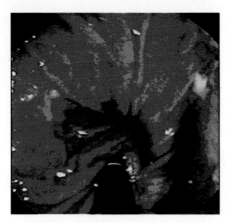

Fig. 2. Endoscopic view of center of herniated fundoplication. (*From* Hunter JG, Smith CD, Branum GD, et al. Laparoscopic fundoplication failures: patterns of failure and response to fundoplication revision. Ann Surg 1999;230:525–36; with permission.)

within the first 48 hours following diagnosis [4]. To prevent acute wrap herniation, postoperative nausea should be aggressively treated pharmacologically. Transdiaphragmatic wrap herniation that occurs later in the postoperative period may be associated with short esophagus, inadequate closure, or breakdown of the diaphragmatic crura closure and inadequate intrathoracic esophageal mobilization. The laparoscopic technique is associated with less inflammatory reaction and adhesion formation, and possibly weaker fixation of the fundoplication to the subdiaphragmatic area compared with the open technique [6,8]. Multivariate analysis in one study [6] revealed that surgical technique (routine closure of the crura and short gastric transection), hiatal hernia size, early postoperative vomiting, and diaphragmatic stressors (chronic coughing, sneezing, vomiting, weight lifting, motor vehicle accidents) are associated with a higher incidence of anatomic wrap failure. In another study [9], obesity was associated with a higher failure rate. A foreshortened esophagus is suspected preoperatively if the endoscopic distance between the gastroesophageal junction and the diaphragmatic impression is greater than 5 cm, or intraoperatively if an intra-abdominal length of 2 to 3 cm of adequately mobilized esophagus cannot be secured. In these patients, a Collis gastroplasty should be considered to create 3 cm of neoesophagus [10–12]; however, the actual existence of short esophagus is questioned by a number of surgeons [13,14]. In addition, extensive mediastinal esophageal dissection may eliminate the need for a gastroplasty [8,15].

Another reason for recurrent symptoms is a slipped or misplaced wrap (Fig. 3). Whether the stomach slips through the wrap or the wrap is misplaced around the stomach instead of the esophagus is not clear; however the consequences are the same: heartburn, regurgitation, and dysphagia. EGD reveals gastric folds above the fundic wrap. Proper intraoperative mobilization of the fundus and anchoring of the wrap to the esophagus

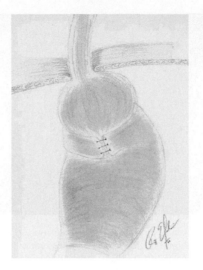

Fig. 3. Slipped or misplaced fundoplication. (Courtesy of Ramy Eskander, MD, with permission).

prevents either misplacement or slippage. Occasionally, a disrupted fundoplication is found. In this case, EGD reveals a patulous wrap that does not hug the scope.

Before embarking on a reoperation for a failed fundoplication, a full preoperative work-up must include barium esophagram and EGD in every patient, 24-hour pH study in selected patients who have a suspicion of a disrupted or loose fundoplication, and esophageal manometry in those patients presenting with dysphagia and esophageal emptying complaints. In addition, patients presenting with delayed gastric emptying should undergo a nuclear gastric emptying study. A laparoscopic approach for the reoperation may be attempted by an experienced surgeon, with an expected conversion rate of 0% to 33% [4,6,8,16–19]. The primary reasons for conversion are usually dense perihiatal adhesions and intraoperative injury to the esophagus or the stomach. The mortality of laparoscopic reoperation for failed fundoplication ranges from 0% to 1%, and the postoperative morbidity ranges from 4% to 32% [4,6,8,16,18,19]. Intraoperative morbidity can be as high as 35%, underlying the technical difficulties of the reoperation [19]. The success of fundoplication declines following each reoperation; from an initial 90% to 95%, down to 80% to 90% after a second surgery, and 50% to 65% after a third surgery [4,20]. These patients become "esophageal cripples," and they can end up undergoing an esophageal resection [21].

Dysphagia

Dysphagia is a common and often debilitating post-fundoplication symptom. The incidence of dysphagia following an antireflux procedure is variable. This is partially due to different definitions of dysphagia and various methods of assessment. Early post-fundoplication dysphagia is probably due to transient edema of the esophagus at the site of the fundoplication, or to temporary esophageal hypomotility [22,23]. It occurs in 4% to 100% of patients, and in the vast majority of patients it improves within the first 6 weeks [24–30]. Patients are instructed to follow a liquid diet for 2 weeks, and to progressively introduce solid foods over a period of 4 to 6 weeks. Reassurance and dietary guidance should be offered to all patients who have mild early postoperative dysphagia, in order to avoid bolus obstruction [31]. A small percentage of patients (0%–36%) develop severe or persistent dysphagia [27–29,32–36]. The causes of chronic dysphagia include poor patient selection for total fundoplication, incomplete preoperative work-up, and problems related to the surgical technique. The routine use of preoperative manometric and endoscopic esophageal evaluation identifies patients who have achalasia, diffuse esophageal spasm, scleroderma, strictures, and short esophagus, and enables the surgeon to differentiate these various esophageal disorders and tailor the appropriate operation as indicated.

Many studies have investigated the impact of the operative technique on the development of postoperative dysphagia. Randomized studies failed to identify any difference in chronic postoperative dysphagia between open and laparoscopic fundoplication [37–40]. In the era of open fundoplication, the introduction of a short, floppy fundoplication by DeMeester et al [41] and Donahue and colleagues [42] decreased significantly the occurrence of postoperative dysphagia, to the point that those modifications became the standard of care. Most surgeons perform a short 1 to 2 cm fundoplication over a 48 to 60 Fr Bougie. A number of surgeons tailor the fundoplication technique by performing a partial wrap in patients who have impaired esophageal motility [25,34,43]. The rationale for performing a partial wrap is to decrease the resistance of the bolus transfer that is seen following a Nissen fundoplication [31]. Several studies [33,44–49], however, have shown that preoperative manometric evidence of abnormal esophageal peristalsis does not predict development of postoperative dysphagia. Abnormal esophageal peristalsis often improves after fundoplication [34,46,47,50]. Studies comparing full with partial fundoplication [35,51] indicate that there is a smaller incidence of early dysphagia after a partial fundoplication, but that there is no difference regarding chronic dysphagia between the two techniques.

It is controversial whether or not complete mobilization of the gastric fundus by division of the short gastric vessels is associated with less early and late postoperative dysphagia [24,30,49]. Double-blinded, randomized studies failed to show a relationship between division of the short gastric vessels and development of dysphagia [30]; however, Rosetti-Nissen fundoplication has been associated with two distinct anatomic fundoplication deformities: the twisted fundoplication and the two-compartment stomach [24]. The use of the anterior wall of the stomach to create the fundic wrap places tension at the gastroesophageal junction, and a spiral deformity of the distal esophagus as this is seen endoscopically (Fig. 4). The two-compartment stomach is created by the use of the greater curvature distal to the unmobilized fundus to create the fundoplication (Fig. 5).

The majority of studies that examined whether preoperative dysphagia is a risk factor for the development of chronic postoperative dysphagia revealed no correlation [32,35,49,52]. Patients who have a normal lower esophageal sphincter (LES) or high mean LES pressures are at increased risk for developing postoperative dysphagia compared with patients who have abnormal LES [53]. Other risk factors such as age, diabetes, and degree of esophagitis have been investigated and found to have no correlation with postoperative dysphagia [49,54,55].

Dysphagia may be secondary to a structural cause, such as tight fundoplication, slipped fundoplication, twisted fundoplication, or a paraesophageal hernia. Anatomic deformity of the wrap occurs in 1% to 9% of cases [4,6,8,56,57]. Nonclosure or incomplete closure of the diaphragmatic crura can lead to paraesophageal hernia and dysphagia [58]. Manometric evaluation of the patients who develop postoperative dysphagia demonstrates higher mean LES basal and nadir pressures, suggesting that tightness of the wrap or failure of the wrap to relax may play a role in chronic postoperative dysphagia [33]. Other manometric parameters, such as the ramp pressure and the residual relaxation pressure, have been studied [30,44,59]; however, the clinical importance of these findings is not clear [59].

Lastly, patient personality and, more specifically, the degree of control patients feel they have over their outcome "health locus of control" seem to play a role in the development of postoperative dysphagia. Patients who

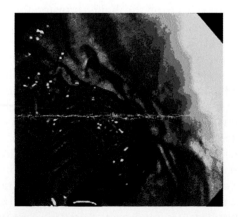

Fig. 4. A twisted valve seen after Rossetti fundoplication. (*From* Hunter JG, Smith CD, Branum GD, et al. Laparoscopic fundoplication failures: patterns of failure and response to fundoplication revision. Ann Surg 1999;230:525–36; with permission.)

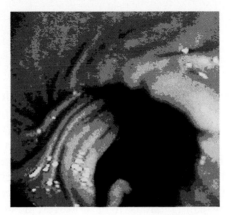

Fig. 5. A two-compartment stomach is an extreme variant of the twisted valve. The proximal pouch (fundus) is seen as the dark cavity in the center for the photo. (*From* Hunter JG, Smith CD, Branum GD, et al. Laparoscopic fundoplication failures: patterns of failure and response to fundoplication revision. Ann Surg 1999;230:525–36; with permission.)

have low expectations for their own abilities experience more postoperative dysphagia compared with patients who have higher expectations [26].

Postoperatively, patients unable to tolerate a liquid diet after 2 weeks or a solid diet after 6 weeks should be further evaluated to rule out an anatomic deformity of the fundoplication. The first recommended study to investigate persistent postoperative dysphagia is a barium swallow. It depicts the location of the fundic wrap in relation to the gastroesophageal junction, and identifies any anatomic deformities of the wrap. If a 12.5-mm barium pill can pass though the gastroesophageal junction, then severe dysphagia can be excluded and other causes of dysphagia, such as psychogenic causes, should be sought. In such patients, manometric esophageal evaluation is performed to exclude subtle esophageal dysmotility disorders. Endoscopy is complementary to barium swallow by identifying fundic wrap disruptions that are missed with barium swallow [5]. Surgical correction of the anatomic deformity of the fundoplication results in resolution of dysphagia in the majority of patients [4,8]. Patients who do not have any anatomic abnormalities following investigation with radiographic contrast studies and endoscopy are managed with pneumatic dilatation with a 30 to 40 mm balloon, with a 50% success rate [60,61]. Pneumatic dilation is less successful in patients with more than one prior fundoplication, abnormal esophageal peristalsis, and a slipped wrap [60,61]. If patients fail the aforementioned treatment, they are considered for a surgical revision of the fundoplication, converting a full wrap to a partial wrap [62]. The decision to reoperate in patients who have chronic postoperative dysphagia is based on the severity of their symptoms. Patients unable to tolerate solid diet or in whom the amount of tolerated diet is causing weight loss should be offered early reoperative treatment; however, patients who have milder symptoms and stable weight can be observed, because dysphagia may improve with time.

Gas bloat

Inability to belch, hyperflatulence, and abdominal bloating are a constellation of symptoms that have emerged as common functional problems following fundoplication. The occurrence of gas bloat has allowed the part of the medical community that criticizes laparoscopic fundoplication to maintain that patients trade GERD symptoms for gas bloat symptoms. The majority of patients who experience gas bloat and hyperflatulence in the early postoperative period improve with time as they adjust to their new eating habits [63]; however, a small percentage of patients develop chronic debilitating symptoms that cause weight loss and limit social life and overall quality of life [57,63–65]. The etiology of gas bloat is unclear, although a number of factors have been proposed to explain the mechanism of postoperative gas bloat: aerophagia, vagus nerve injury, gastroparesis, inability to belch, and altered perception of gastric filling by the patient [66–70].

A large percentage of patients who have GERD swallow saliva frequently to mitigate the acidic environment in their esophagi [71]. Along with saliva swallowing, these patients develop a habit of aerophagia. Postoperatively, the majority of patients who have successful control of GERD lose the stimulus for aerophagia, and eventually unlearn this habit. Vagal injury has been described as a complication of fundoplication [67]. Even injury to vagal branches, such as the nerve of McRae that innervates the pylorus, can cause postoperative pyloric dysfunction and gastroparesis [72]. Undiagnosed pre-existent gastroparesis or new development of postoperative gastroparesis may explain persistent gas bloat symptoms in a small number of patients [68,73]. Patients who have GERD symptoms and complaints of vomiting should undergo preoperative work-up to rule out gastroparesis. Diagnosis is made with a nuclear gastric emptying study and endoscopy that shows significant amount of old food in the stomach. To be able to belch following a fundoplication, the intragastric pressure needs to overcome the valve resistance at the fundic wrap. Following Nissen fundoplication, there is a dramatic increase in the valve resistance that can explain the inability of some patients to belch [74]. Altered perception of gastric distension may also play a role in the reporting of gas bloat symptoms postoperatively. Patients who have functional dyspepsia have altered perception of gastric distension, and can be distinguished from those who have organic dyspepsia [69].

Postprandial gas bloat has been reported in up to 73% of GERD patients undergoing fundoplication [70,75]. The majority of patients who have preoperative gas bloat symptoms improve following laparoscopic Nissen fundoplication; however, patients who have minimal or absent preoperative gas bloat have a one-in-three chance of experiencing worsening of their gas bloat postoperatively. Development of gas bloat appears to bear no correlation with the lower esophageal sphincter manometric profile [70]. In another study [75], patients who had minimal preoperative gas bloat and a supine pattern of GERD were more prone to developing gas bloat postoperatively compared with patients who had an upright or mixed GERD pattern. Preoperative abnormal gastric emptying appears to be predictive for the development of postoperative gas bloat [73]. Patients who have an established preoperative mechanism of aerophagia may demonstrate less postoperative symptomatic relief from GERD symptoms [76].

The pharmacologic treatment of gas bloat consists of prokinetic agents and antigas medications such as simethicone and charcoal caps. It is crucial that patients receive dietary guidelines to ameliorate the symptoms, such as advice to avoid drinking with a straw and to avoid carbonated beverages. Consultation with a speech pathologist to educate patients on how to unlearn the habit of aerophagia can also be helpful. In case of recalcitrant gas bloat, a nuclear gastric emptying study should be performed to rule out gastroparesis. Invasive therapeutic modalities with variable results include pneumatic dilation of the wrap, revision of a full to a partial fundoplication, laparoscopic pyloroplasty, and subtotal gastrectomy with Roux-en-Y gastrojejunostomy.

Minimizing the risk of postoperative recalcitrant gas bloat syndrome can be achieved by careful identification and preservation of the vagal nerves intraoperatively, and by identification of patients who have gastroparetic symptoms preoperatively.

Diarrhea

Post-fundoplication diarrhea may occur in up to 26% of patients [63,77,78]. The diarrhea usually presents postprandially, and resembles dumping syndrome. The mechanism of post-fundoplication diarrhea involves vagal nerve injury, either permanent or traction injury. Injury to the celiac branch of the posterior vagal trunk, which normally innervates the pancreas and the small and large intestine, may cause diarrhea by decreasing pancreatic secretions and fat absorption. It is difficult to establish the diagnosis of solitary vagal branch injury, because tests such as pentagastrin stimulation, sham feeding, and nuclear gastric emptying studies may be normal. Another mechanism of post-fundoplication diarrhea is the increase in gastric emptying that is observed following a fundoplication [79,80]. Patients who have irritable bowel syndrome have a higher incidence of gas bloat and diarrhea both pre- and postoperatively; therefore it is important to question the patient about the existence of preoperative symptoms [63,81].

The majority of patients who have post-fundoplication diarrhea improve with time. Reassurance and antidiarrheal medications are usually the only necessary measures. In case of persistent symptoms, other causes of diarrhea should be ruled out, such as pseudomembranous colitis, gastrinoma, food allergy, and VIPoma (pancreatic endocrine tumor, vasoactive intestinal peptide-producing tumor).

Is antireflux surgery worth these functional problems?

Despite the aforementioned shortcomings of surgical management of GERD, several studies have documented a dramatic improvement in GERD symptoms and quality of life following fundoplication. The author and his associates [82] have previously reported on 297 patients who had recalcitrant GERD and who underwent laparoscopic fundoplication. At 2-year follow-up, the average symptom scores (scale from 0 to 10) decreased significantly in comparison with the preoperative values: heartburn from 8.4 to 1.7, regurgitation from 7.2 to 0.7, and dysphagia from 3.7 to 1.0. Only 10% of patients were on proton pump inhibitors (PPI) for typical GERD symptoms at 2 years after surgery. Fernando and coworkers [83] compared 51 patients on medical treatment for GERD with 120 patients who underwent laparoscopic fundoplication. Quality of life was evaluated with two validated questionnaires. The number of dissatisfied patients was significantly lower in the surgical group (5.9%) compared with the medical group (21.6%). In a meta-analysis by Van Den Boom and coauthors [84], cost effectiveness of medical treatment with omeprazole was compared with open and laparoscopic fundoplication. Long-term therapy with omeprazole was less cost-effective after 4 years compared with open fundoplication, and after only 1.4 years compared with laparoscopic fundoplication.

Summary

Functional problems following esophageal surgery for GERD are not infrequent. The majority of patients improve with time. Careful patient selection and attention to surgical technique are key factors in preventing such functional disorders. When anatomic abnormalities related to the fundoplication are identified, reoperation may offer symptom relief. Before embarking on re-fundoplication, a thorough preoperative evaluation of the esophageal physiology is recommended.

References

[1] Tack J, Janssens J. Functional heartburn. Curr Treat Options Gastroenterol 2002;5:251–8.
[2] Fass R, Tougas G. Functional heartburn: the stimulus, the pain, and the brain. Gut 2002;51: 885–92.
[3] Clouse RE. Antidepressants for functional gastrointestinal syndromes. Dig Dis Sci 1994;39: 2352–63.

[4] Hunter JG, Smith CD, Branum GD, et al. Laparoscopic fundoplication failures: patterns of failure and response to fundoplication revision. Ann Surg 1999;230:595–604 [discussion: 604–6].

[5] Jailwala J, Massey B, Staff D, et al. Post-fundoplication symptoms: the role for endoscopic assessment of fundoplication integrity. Gastrointest Endosc 2001;54:351–6.

[6] Soper NJ, Dunnegan D. Anatomic fundoplication failure after laparoscopic antireflux surgery. Ann Surg 1999;229:669–76 [discussion: 676–7].

[7] Dallemagne B, Weerts JM, Jehaes C, et al. Causes of failures of laparoscopic antireflux operations. Surg Endosc 1996;10:305–10.

[8] Horgan S, Pohl D, Bogetti D, et al. Failed antireflux surgery: what have we learned from reoperations? Arch Surg 1999;134:809–15 [discussion: 815–7].

[9] Perez AR, Moncure AC, Rattner DW. Obesity adversely affects the outcome of antireflux operations. Surg Endosc 2001;15:986–9.

[10] Johnson AB, Oddsdottir M, Hunter JG. Laparoscopic Collis gastroplasty and Nissen fundoplication. A new technique for the management of esophageal foreshortening. Surg Endosc 1998;12:1055–60.

[11] Jobe BA, Horvath KD, Swanstrom LL. Postoperative function following laparoscopic collis gastroplasty for shortened esophagus. Arch Surg 1998;133:867–74.

[12] Demeester SR, Demeester TR. Editorial comment: the short esophagus: going, going, gone? Surgery 2003;133:364–7.

[13] Gastal OL, Hagen JA, Peters JH, et al. Short esophagus: analysis of predictors and clinical implications. Arch Surg 1999;134:633–6 [discussion: 637–8].

[14] Korn O, Csendes A, Burdiles P, et al. Length of the esophagus in patients with gastroesophageal reflux disease and Barrett's esophagus compared to controls. Surgery 2003;133:358–63.

[15] O'Rourke RW, Khajanchee YS, Urbach DR, et al. Extended transmediastinal dissection: an alternative to gastroplasty for short esophagus. Arch Surg 2003;138:735–40.

[16] Watson DI, Jamieson GG, Game PA, et al. Laparoscopic reoperation following failed antireflux surgery. Br J Surg 1999;86:98–101.

[17] Szwerc MF, Wiechmann RJ, Maley RH, et al. Reoperative laparoscopic antireflux surgery. Surgery 1999;126:723–8 [discussion: 728–9].

[18] Curet MJ, Josloff RK, Schoeb O, et al. Laparoscopic reoperation for failed antireflux procedures. Arch Surg 1999;134:559–63.

[19] Floch NR, Hinder RA, Klingler PJ, et al. Is laparoscopic reoperation for failed antireflux surgery feasible? Arch Surg 1999;134:733–7.

[20] Gadenstatter M, Hagen JA, DeMeester TR, et al. Esophagectomy for unsuccessful antireflux operations. J Thorac Cardiovasc Surg 1998;115:296–300.

[21] Watson TJ, DeMeester TR, Kauer WK, et al. Esophageal replacement for end-stage benign esophageal disease. J Thorac Cardiovasc Surg 1998;115:1241–7 [discussion: 1247–9].

[22] Polk HC Jr. Fundoplication for reflux esophagitis: misadventures with the operation of choice. Ann Surg 1976;183:645–52.

[23] Low DE. Management of the problem patient after antireflux surgery. Gastroenterol Clin North Am 1994;23:371–89.

[24] Hunter JG, Swanstrom L, Waring JP. Dysphagia after laparoscopic antireflux surgery. The impact of operative technique. Ann Surg 1996;224:51–7.

[25] DeMeester TR, Stein HJ. Minimizing the side effects of antireflux surgery. World J Surg 1992;16:335–6.

[26] Kamolz T, Bammer T, Pointner R. Predictability of dysphagia after laparoscopic nissen fundoplication. Am J Gastroenterol 2000;95:408–14.

[27] Perdikis G, Hinder RA, Lund RJ, et al. Laparoscopic Nissen fundoplication: where do we stand? Surg Laparosc Endosc 1997;7:17–21.

[28] Dallemagne B, Weerts JM, Jeahes C, et al. Results of laparoscopic Nissen fundoplication. Hepatogastroenterology 1998;45:1338–43.

[29] O'Reilly MJ, Mullins SG, Saye WB, et al. Laparoscopic posterior partial fundoplication: analysis of 100 consecutive cases. J Laparoendosc Surg 1996;6:141–50.

[30] Watson DI, Pike GK, Baigrie RJ, et al. Prospective double-blind randomized trial of laparoscopic Nissen fundoplication with division and without division of short gastric vessels. Ann Surg 1997;226:642–52.

[31] Wills VL, Hunt DR. Dysphagia after antireflux surgery. Br J Surg 2001;88:486–99.

[32] Herron DM, Swanstrom LL, Ramzi N, et al. Factors predictive of dysphagia after laparoscopic Nissen fundoplication. Surg Endosc 1999;13:1180–3.

[33] Anvari M, Allen C. Esophageal and lower esophageal sphincter pressure profiles 6 and 24 months after laparoscopic fundoplication and their association with postoperative dysphagia. Surg Endosc 1998;12:421–6.

[34] Patti MG, De Pinto M, de Bellis M, et al. Comparison of laparoscopic total and partial fundoplication for gastroesophageal reflux. J Gastrointest Surg 1997;1:309–15.

[35] Rydberg L, Ruth M, Abrahamsson H, et al. Tailoring antireflux surgery: a randomized clinical trial. World J Surg 1999;23:612–8.

[36] Gotley DC, Smithers BM, Rhodes M, et al. Laparoscopic Nissen fundoplication—200 consecutive cases. Gut 1996;38:487–91.

[37] Luostarinen M, Virtanen J, Koskinen M, et al. Dysphagia and oesophageal clearance after laparoscopic versus open Nissen fundoplication. A randomized, prospective trial. Scand J Gastroenterol 2001;36:565–71.

[38] Chrysos E, Tsiaoussis J, Athanasakis E, et al. Laparoscopic vs open approach for Nissen fundoplication. A comparative study. Surg Endosc 2002;16:1679–84.

[39] Heikkinen TJ, Haukipuro K, Bringman S, et al. Comparison of laparoscopic and open Nissen fundoplication 2 years after operation. A prospective randomized trial. Surg Endosc 2000;14:1019–23.

[40] Laine S, Rantala A, Gullichsen R, et al. Laparoscopic vs conventional Nissen fundoplication. A prospective randomized study. Surg Endosc 1997;11:441–4.

[41] DeMeester TR, Bonavina L, Albertucci M. Nissen fundoplication for gastroesophageal reflux disease. Evaluation of primary repair in 100 consecutive patients. Ann Surg 1986;204:9–20.

[42] Donahue PE, Samelson S, Nyhus LM, et al. The floppy Nissen fundoplication. Effective long-term control of pathologic reflux. Arch Surg 1985;120:663–8.

[43] Hunter JG, Trus TL, Branum GD, et al. A physiologic approach to laparoscopic fundoplication for gastroesophageal reflux disease. Ann Surg 1996;223:673–85 [discussion: 685–7].

[44] Mathew G, Watson DI, Myers JC, et al. Oesophageal motility before and after laparoscopic Nissen fundoplication. Br J Surg 1997;84:1465–9.

[45] Fibbe C, Layer P, Keller J, et al. Esophageal motility in reflux disease before and after fundoplication: a prospective, randomized, clinical, and manometric study. Gastroenterology 2001;121:5–14.

[46] Beckingham IJ, Cariem AK, Bornman PC, et al. Oesophageal dysmotility is not associated with poor outcome after laparoscopic Nissen fundoplication. Br J Surg 1998;85:1290–3.

[47] Baigrie RJ, Watson DI, Myers JC, et al. Outcome of laparoscopic Nissen fundoplication in patients with disordered preoperative peristalsis. Gut 1997;40:381–5.

[48] Bessell JR, Finch R, Gotley DC, et al. Chronic dysphagia following laparoscopic fundoplication. Br J Surg 2000;87:1341–5.

[49] Gotley DC, Smithers BM, Menzies B, et al. Laparoscopic Nissen fundoplication and postoperative dysphagia—can it be predicted? Ann Acad Med Singapore 1996;25:646–9.

[50] Gill RC, Bowes KL, Murphy PD, et al. Esophageal motor abnormalities in gastroesophageal reflux and the effects of fundoplication. Gastroenterology 1986;91:364–9.

[51] Lundell L, Abrahamsson H, Ruth M, et al. Long-term results of a prospective randomized comparison of total fundic wrap (Nissen-Rossetti) or semifundoplication (Toupet) for gastro-oesophageal reflux. Br J Surg 1996;83:830–5.

[52] Patti MG, Feo CV, De Pinto M, et al. Results of laparoscopic antireflux surgery for dysphagia and gastroesophageal reflux disease. Am J Surg 1998;176:564–8.

[53] Blom D, Peters JH, DeMeester TR, et al. Physiologic mechanism and preoperative prediction of new-onset dysphagia after laparoscopic Nissen fundoplication. J Gastrointest Surg 2002;6:22–7 [discussion: 27–8].

[54] Trus TL, Laycock WS, Wo JM, et al. Laparoscopic antireflux surgery in the elderly. Am J Gastroenterol 1998;93:351–3.

[55] Watson DI, Foreman D, Devitt PG, et al. Preoperative endoscopic grading of esophagitis versus outcome after laparoscopic Nissen fundoplication. Am J Gastroenterol 1997;92: 222–5.

[56] Watson DI, Baigrie RJ, Jamieson GG. A learning curve for laparoscopic fundoplication. Definable, avoidable, or a waste of time? Ann Surg 1996;224:198–203.

[57] Low DE, Mercer CD, James EC, et al. Post Nissen syndrome. Surg Gynecol Obstet 1988; 167:1–5.

[58] Watson DI, Jamieson GG, Devitt PG, et al. Paraoesophageal hiatus hernia: an important complication of laparoscopic Nissen fundoplication. Br J Surg 1995;82:521–3.

[59] Bais JE, Wijnhoven BP, Masclee AA, et al. Analysis and surgical treatment of persistent dysphagia after Nissen fundoplication. Br J Surg 2001;88:569–76.

[60] Wo JM, Trus TL, Richardson WS, et al. Evaluation and management of postfundoplication dysphagia. Am J Gastroenterol 1996;91:2318–22.

[61] Gaudric M, Sabate JM, Artru P, et al. Results of pneumatic dilatation in patients with dysphagia after antireflux surgery. Br J Surg 1999;86:1088–91.

[62] Skinner DB. Surgical management after failed antireflux operations. World J Surg 1992;16: 359–63.

[63] Swanstrom L, Wayne R. Spectrum of gastrointestinal symptoms after laparoscopic fundoplication. Am J Surg 1994;167:538–41.

[64] Hinder RA, Filipi CJ, Wetscher G, et al. Laparoscopic Nissen fundoplication is an effective treatment for gastroesophageal reflux disease. Ann Surg 1994;220:472–81 [discussion: 481–3].

[65] Anvari M. Complications of laparoscopic Nissen fundoplication. Semin Laparosc Surg 1997;4:154–61.

[66] Ferguson MK. Pitfalls and complications of antireflux surgery. Nissen and Collis-Nissen techniques. Chest Surg Clin N Am 1997;7:489–509 [discussion: 510–1].

[67] Kozarek RA, Low DE, Raltz SL. Complications associated with laparoscopic anti-reflux surgery: one multispecialty clinic's experience. Gastrointest Endosc 1997;46:527–31.

[68] Hunter RJ, Metz DC, Morris JB, et al. Gastroparesis: a potential pitfall of laparoscopic Nissen fundoplication. Am J Gastroenterol 1996;91:2617–8.

[69] Mertz H, Fullerton S, Naliboff B, et al. Symptoms and visceral perception in severe functional and organic dyspepsia. Gut 1998;42:814–22.

[70] Anvari M, Allen C. Postprandial bloating after laparoscopic Nissen fundoplication. Can J Surg 2001;44:440–4.

[71] Hinder RA, Klingler PJ, Perdikis G, et al. Management of the failed antireflux operation. Surg Clin North Am 1997;77:1083–98.

[72] Anvari M, Jamieson GG. Surgical applications of the function of the pylorus. Surg Annu 1992;24:181–94.

[73] Lundell LR, Myers JC, Jamieson GG. Delayed gastric emptying and its relationship to symptoms of "gas float" after antireflux surgery. Eur J Surg 1994;160:161–6.

[74] O'Sullivan GC, DeMeester TR, Joelsson BE, et al. Interaction of lower esophageal sphincter pressure and length of sphincter in the abdomen as determinants of gastroesophageal competence. Am J Surg 1982;143:40–7.

[75] Papasavas PK, Keenan RJ, Yeaney WW, et al. Prediction of postoperative gas bloating after laparoscopic antireflux procedures based on 24-h pH acid reflux pattern. Surg Endosc 2003; 17:381–5.

[76] Kamolz T, Bammer T, Granderath FA, et al. Comorbidity of aerophagia in GERD patients: outcome of laparoscopic antireflux surgery. Scand J Gastroenterol 2002;37:138–43.

[77] Beldi G, Glattli A. Long-term gastrointestinal symptoms after laparoscopic nissen fundoplication. Surg Laparosc Endosc Percutan Tech 2002;12:316–9.

[78] Bammer T, Hinder RA, Klaus A, et al. Five- to eight-year outcome of the first laparoscopic Nissen fundoplications. J Gastrointest Surg 2001;5:42–8.

[79] Farrell TM, Richardson WS, Halkar R, et al. Nissen fundoplication improves gastric motility in patients with delayed gastric emptying. Surg Endosc 2001;15:271–4.

[80] Jamieson GG, Maddern GJ, Myers JC. Gastric emptying after fundoplication with and without proximal gastric vagotomy. Arch Surg 1991;126:1414–7.

[81] Raftopoulos Y, Papasavas P, Hayetian F, et al. Clinical outcome of laparoscopic antireflux surgery in patients with irritable bowel syndrome. Surg Endosc 2004;18:655–9.

[82] Papasavas PK, Keenan RJ, Yeaney WW, et al. Effectiveness of laparoscopic fundoplication in relieving the symptoms of gastroesophageal reflux disease (GERD) and eliminating antireflux medical therapy. Surg Endosc 2003;17:1200–5.

[83] Fernando HC, Schauer PR, Rosenblatt M, et al. Quality of life after antireflux surgery compared with nonoperative management for severe gastroesophageal reflux disease. J Am Coll Surg 2002;194:23–7.

[84] Van Den Boom G, Go PM, Hameeteman W, et al. Cost effectiveness of medical versus surgical treatment in patients with severe or refractory gastroesophageal reflux disease in the Netherlands. Scand J Gastroenterol 1996;31:1–9.

ELSEVIER
SAUNDERS

SURGICAL
CLINICS OF
NORTH AMERICA

Surg Clin N Am 85 (2005) 539–553

Molecular Biology of Esophageal Cancer in the Genomics Era

King F. Kwong, MD, FCCP

Division of Thoracic Surgery, Greenebaum Cancer Center, University of Maryland School of Medicine, 22 South Greene Street, Room N4E35, Baltimore, MD 21201, USA

Esophageal cancers are highly lethal malignancies. Overall 5-year survival from esophageal cancer is 13% [1]. Even early-stage esophageal cancer carries a sobering survival rate at 27% [2]. Unfortunately, the incidence of esophageal cancer is rising in the United States and other Western countries.

Esophageal cancer is composed of two main histological types and should not be viewed as one homogeneous entity. Histologically, adenocarcinoma and squamous cell carcinoma of the esophagus account for over 95% of all primary esophageal cancers. The incidence, prevalence, and biologic behavior between these two histological types are uniquely different from each other. Given such differences, future therapy options may be different for each type of esophageal cancer.

Despite better understanding of the risk factors and cellular derangements associated with esophageal cancer, the clinical treatment of esophageal cancer has changed surprisingly little, and long-term survival from esophageal cancer remains poor. In contrast, our general understanding about carcinogenesis from a cellular level has never been greater than at present. Advances in molecular biology techniques and the ability to detect precise genetic alterations in the cancer cell have added greatly to our understanding of tumorigenesis in all malignancies. Because of these advances, there is now great opportunity to identify key molecular mechanisms leading to the development and progression of esophageal cancers, and to tailor new therapies targeting specific molecular pathways.

Epidemiology of esophageal cancer

The epidemiology of esophageal adenocarcinoma (EAC) is strikingly different from that of esophageal squamous cell carcinoma (SCC).

E-mail address: kkwong@smail.umaryland.edu

0039-6109/05/$ - see front matter © 2005 Elsevier Inc. All rights reserved.
doi:10.1016/j.suc.2005.01.004   *surgical.theclinics.com*

Important clues to potential differences in the biologic behavior of esophageal cancers may be gleaned from understanding their epidemiologic differences.

In the United States and other Western countries (ie, Scotland, England, Wales, Sweden, Denmark, Norway, Australia, and New Zealand) the incidence of EAC has been rising since the late 1970s [3–8]. By 1994, for the first time since 1959, the incidence of EAC exceeded that of SCC [9]. Before 1978 in the United States, adenocarcinoma of the esophagus was found only rarely compared with squamous cell carcinoma [10].

Recent analyses based on the incidence and survival trends of esophageal cancer in the United States reveal several very interesting disparities. The 1973 to 1998 data from the US National Cancer Institute's (NCI) Surveillance, Epidemiology, and End Results (SEER) program shows that the incidence of adenocarcinoma is still rising at 7.8% per year for white males [11]. The incidence of EAC in black males and females has remained insignificantly low. In black males, SCC represents the predominant esophageal cancer type; however, the incidence of SCC has been steadily declining in white males and females and black females since 1973. Also, SCC has declined in black males starting in 1992 (down 8.5% per year) [11]. Paralleling the US experience, during this same time period other Western countries saw a dramatic increase in EAC incidence among white males [12–13].

Conversely, the epidemiology of esophageal cancer in China is quite the opposite of the Western experience. China has historically reported some of the highest mortality rates related to esophageal cancer in the world [14]. Five geographical regions in mid-Northern China (Linxian of Henan province, Yang City of Shanxi, Huaian of Jiangsu, Yanting of Sichuan, and Shenxian of Hebei) and one region in Southern China (Nanao area of Guangdong province) have some of the highest risk for esophageal cancer in the world. In sharp contrast to the rising incidence of EAC in Western countries, a contemporary analysis of 1970 to 1990 data from population-based registries in these high-risk regions shows surprising decreases in esophageal cancer incidence [15]. Moreover, the predominant histology seen in China has been and remains SCC. The incidence of EAC in China and other Asian countries remains fairly low, and none of these countries have seen increases in EAC such as those seen in the West during this same time period [16,17]). Given increased Westernization of their diets and lifestyles, and increased incidence of gastroesophageal reflux among their populations it is quite remarkable that more EAC is not seen in these Asian countries, [16].

The etiology of this sharp rise in EAC in the United States and other Western countries is unclear. Many clinicians speculate that EAC is related to the increased incidence of gastroesophageal reflux, leading to Barrett's esophagus, dysplasia, and ultimately carcinoma [18]; however, more recent population-based studies examining the prevalence of Barrett's esophagus cast serious doubts on the notion that gastroesophageal reflux-induced

Barrett's can account for the rise in EAC found in the last three decades [19–27]. These contemporary epidemiologic studies show that the true frequency of Barrett's esophagus in the general population may have been previously grossly underestimated [22–24]; if the Barrett's metaplasia-dysplasia-carcinoma hypothesis were true, then an even higher EAC incidence would be predicted. Moreover, as suggested by meta-analysis, the actual number of EAC cases arising from Barrett's may have been reported vigorously in the literature due to publication bias [28]. This means that far fewer Barrett's actually becomes EAC. Recent studies also reveal that the overall mortality rate in patients who have Barrett's esophagus is fairly similar to that of the non-Barrett's population [20], and that few patients who are diagnosed and treated for EAC also had Barrett's dysplasia predating their cancers [25–26]. The results of these recent studies also raise concerns regarding the cost-effectiveness of endoscopic surveillance in patients who have asymptomatic Barrett's, and possibly even in patients who have Barrett's with low-grade dysplasia [22,23,27].

Interestingly, even though the use of antiacid medications such as histamine receptor antagonists and proton-pump inhibitors has become widespread in the last decade, recent studies do not show that these medications are associated with an increased risk for esophageal cancer [29–32]. Although these and other studies highlight risk factors for esophageal cancer and suggest significant differences between EAC and SCC, the molecular mechanisms underlying esophageal carcinogenesis remain incompletely understood.

Tumor cell biology

The cell cycle

Normal noncancerous cells abide by an intricately regulated cell cycle (Fig. 1). The nonreplicating quiescent cell, in the G_0 phase, represents the overwhelming majority of the cell population in any given tissue. When prompted by appropriate external stimuli, such as hormones, growth factors, and cytokines, the G_0 cell enters into the first gap phase (G_1). G_1 is characterized by the activation of genes and synthesis of housekeeping proteins needed for the subsequent S phase, where DNA synthesis occurs. At the completion of S phase, the cell has doubled its DNA content and assumes a transient tetraploid state. Next, the second gap phase (G_2), is highlighted by heightened translational activity and abundant production of structural proteins. This cell is now primed to undergo mitosis, in which DNA segregates as discrete chromosomes and culminates with nuclear division. Cytokinesis, or cellular cytoplasmic division, marks the completion of the cell cycle—thus, forming two diploid cells. At this point, the cell can rejoin the G_0 cell pool or proceed to repeat the cell cycle if intra-cellular signals favor continued proliferation.

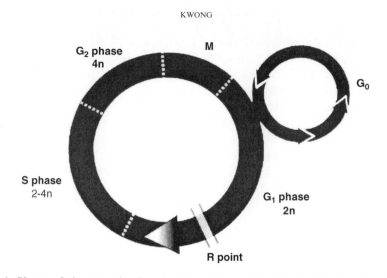

Fig. 1. Phases of the normal cell cycle. (*From* Souza RF, Morales CP, Spechler SJ. A conceptual approach to understanding the molecular mechanisms of cancer development in Barrett's esophagus. Ailiment Pharmacol Ther 2001;15(8):1088; with permission.)

Tumorigenesis

Cellular processes integral to the regulation of the cell cycle include those responsible for controlling the passage of the replicating cell through each phase of the cell cycle. These cell cycle checkpoints act negatively to prevent unregulated cellular replication. The restriction point (R-point) is a critical gate-keeping mechanism at the $G_1 \rightarrow S$ transition. Wild-type retinoblastoma (*RB*) gene protein is normally unphosphorylated, and serves to block cell progression through the R-point; however, hyperphosphorylation inactivates Rb and releases transcriptional factor E2F, which leads to activation of genes favoring cell replication (Fig. 2). Irreparable errors in the molecular pathways of cell cycle regulation may lead either to cell death or to transformation of the somatic cell into an immortalized cell—the cancer cell.

Other modulators of the cell cycle include oncogenes, tumor suppressor genes, and transcriptional factors. Oncogenes occur normally in the cell's DNA. Genetic mutations in oncogenes, such as *ras* and *c-myc*, produce gene products that override normal functioning of checkpoint processes, thus promoting cellular replication. Conversely, mutations in tumor suppressor genes, such as *p53* and *RB*, can lead to defective or absent gene products and remove important negative regulators of the cell cycle. Transcriptional factors are proteins that translocate into the nucleus and activate translation of its target gene.

Hanahan and Weinberg [33] recently summarized that the cancer cell exhibits six distinguishing phenotypic features. They are: exhibits autonomous growth, ignores antiproliferative signals, averts apoptosis, replicates unregulated, promotes angiogenesis, and invades locally and disseminates.

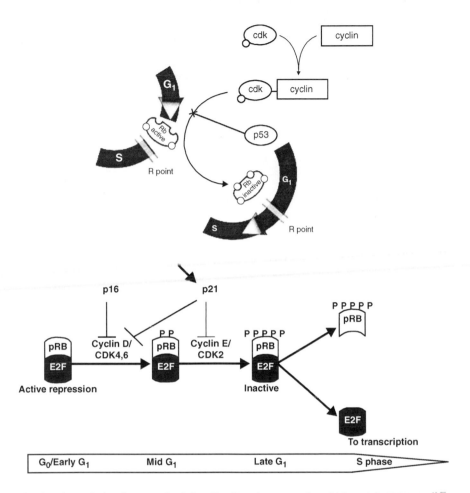

Fig. 2. *Rb* regulation in control of G₁→S cell cycle progression. (*Adapted from* Souza RF, Morales CP, Spechler SJ. A conceptual approach to understanding the molecular mechanisms of cancer development in Barrett's esophagus. Ailiment Pharmacol Ther 2001;15(8):1089; with permission.)

These quintessential features of the cancer cell have been the subject of many investigations attempting to elucidate the molecular mechanisms of esophageal cancer (Tables 1 and 2).

Autonomous growth

Growth signals such as hormones, growth factors, and cytokines are required exogenous stimuli that propel the quiescent G₀ cell into the cell cycle. These molecules bind to cell surface receptors and initiate a complex set of cell signaling pathways mediated by a class of molecules known as cyclins. In the

Table 1
Recent molecular studies: esophageal adenocarcinoma

Study	Tumorigenic molecule	Target type	Alteration	Host	Tissue type
[34]	Mcm2 (minichromosome maintenance protein)	sustained DNA replication	mutation	Hu	EAC
[35]	Chromosome 17p	TSG	deletion	Hu	EAC
[36]	Glutathione Peroxidase	detoxification	downreg.	Hu	Barrett's
[37]	nm23 protein	TSG	mutation	Hu	EAC
[38]	*Cdx2* intestinal homeobox	oncogene	mutation	Mo	eso. Cancer
[39]	TNF-α, β-catenin, *c-myc*	oncogene	activation	Hu	EAC, Barrett's
[40]	VEGF	angiogenesis	upreg.	Hu	Barrett's
[41]	Cyclo-oxygenase-2 (COX-2)	anti-apoptosis	upreg.	Rat	Barrett's
[42]	*p73* gene	TSG	LOH, AT/GC polymorphism	Hu	EAC, SCC
[43]	Chromosomes 4q, 14q, 12p, 17q, 5q, 8p, 2q, 6p, 12q	TSG, oncogenes	mut., deletet., alter. DNA copies	Hu	Barrett's
[44]	NF-κB	anti-apoptosis	upreg.	Rat	Barrett's
[45]	*c-myb*	oncogene	activation	Hu	EAC, Barrett's
[46]	p53 protein	TSG	mutation	Hu	Barrett's
[47]	Cyclo-oxygenase-2 (COX-2)	anti-apoptosis	upreg.	Hu	Barrett's
[48]	*RB, CDK4* genes	TSG	LOH, allelic imbalance, amplification	Hu	EAC
[49]	*APC, RB, p53* genes	TSG	LOH, micro-satellite instability	Hu	Barrett's
[50]	Chromosome 17 (*p53*)	TSG	LOH	Hu	EAC
[51]	*p53, p21*	TSG	mutation	Hu	EAC, Barrett's
[52]	K-*ras* gene	oncogene	point mutation	Hu	EAC, Barrett's
[53]	*DCC, APC, p53* genes	TSG	LOH	Hu	EAC
[54]	GST -α, -π	detoxification	downreg.	Hu	EAC, SCC
[55]	*p53* gene	TSG	mutation	Mo	EAC
[56]	Hsp27 protein	cytotoxic stress prot.	downreg.	Hu	Barrett's EAC
[57]	GST *P1* gene	detoxification	polymorphism	Hu	EAC, Barrett's
[58]	Telomerase	DNA replication	upreg.	Hu	EAC, Barrett's
[59]	*FHIT, FRA3B*	TSG	LOH, deletion	Hu	EAC, Barrett's
[60]	*CDKN2/p16*	cyclin, cell signal	LOH	Hu	Barrett's
[61]	p53 protein	TSG	mutations	Hu	Barrett's
[62]	*c-src* gene	oncogene	activation	Hu	Barrett's
[63]	*CDKN2/p16*	cyclin, cell signal	mutation	Hu	EAC, Barrett's
[64]	*p53*	TSG	allelic loss	Hu	Barrett's
[65]	*p53*	TSG	polymorphism	Hu	EAC, Barrett's
[66]	*p53*	TSG	mutation, single base substitution	Hu	EAC
[67]	c-erbB-2	growth factor receptor	upreg.	Hu	EAC, Barrett's

Abbreviations: EAC, esophageal adenocarcinoma; Hu, human; LOH, loss of heterozygosity; Mo, mouse; SCC, esophageal squamous cell carcinoma; TSG, tumor suppressor gene.

Table 2
Recent molecular studies: esophageal squamous cell carcinoma

Ref.	Tumorigenic molecule	Target type	Alteration	Host	Tissue type
[68]	Annexin I	signal transduction	nuclear translocation	Hu	SCC
[69]	*ETS2* (erythroblastosis virus oncogene)	oncogene	activation	Hu	SCC
[70]	$p16^{INK4a}$, $p14^{ARF}$ genes	TSG	hypermethyl.	Hu	SCC
[71]	*NMES1* (chromosome 15q)	novel gene, ?fxn	downreg.	Hu	SCC
[72]	*p53, MDM2, cyclinD1, p21, p16, RB*	TSG	mutation	Hu	SCC
[73]	*Reelin* gene (chromo. 7q)	?oncogene	activation	Hu	SCC
[74]	*TGIF* gene (chromo. 18p)	anti-apoptosis	amplification	Hu	SCC
[75]	*FHIT* gene (chromo. 3p)	TSG	mutation	Hu	SCC
[76]	Annexin I protein	cell cycle regulator	downreg.	Hu	SCC
[77]	$p21^{waf1/cip1}$ gene (chrom. 6p)	DNA replication	polymorphism	Hu	SCC
[78]	*MDM2* gene (binds p53)	oncogene	amplification	Hu	SCC
[79]	*p53, p16/CDKN2* genes	TSG	mut. (point, delete, insert, frame-shifts)	Hu	SCC
[80]	bcl-2, p53 proteins	cell signal, TSG	mutation	Hu	SCC
[81]	Chromosomes 5q, 6p, 13q	?TSG	allelic loss, LOH	Hu	SCC
[82]	*p53, RB, APC, MCC, DCC*	TSG	LOH	Hu	SCC, EAC

Abbreviations: EAC, esophageal adenocarcinoma; Hu, human; LOH, loss of heterozygosity; SCC, esophageal squamous cell carcinoma; TSG, tumor suppressor gene.

proliferative cell, cyclin D1 binds to cyclin-dependant kinase 4 (Cdk4) and cyclin E with Cdk2. These assembled complexes aid in the phosphorylation of the Rb protein, thus rendering inactive this important R-point regulator. Both cyclin and c-erbB-2 genetic mutations appear important in the development of EAC [48,60,63,67]. In SCC, cyclin abnormalities may be important [72,79], but c erbB 2 abnormalities appear to play a lesser role.

Ignoring antiproliferative signals

Antiproliferative signals are often mediated by tumor suppressor gene products, such as Rb and APC proteins. Methods whereby tumor suppressor genes may be rendered silent include mutations (point or base substitutions), loss of heterozygosity (deletion of the chromosome region where the tumor-suppressor allele is located), or promoter hypermethylation (covalent attachment of methyl groups to the gene's promoter region, thus preventing transcription). Tumor suppressor gene products such as p16 and p53 proteins normally inhibit phosphorylation of *Rb*, but genetic alterations at these genes can bypass an otherwise normally functioning *RB* tumor suppressor gene. Both *RB* and *p53* mutations are found in EAC [43,46, 48–51,53,55,61] and SCC [72,79,80,82].

Aversion to apoptosis

Apoptosis is programmed cell death, and consists of extrinsic and intrinsic intracellular pathways that, when activated, can ultimately lead to cell death. The *Bcl* gene family regulates the balance of intracellular proapoptotic and antiapoptotic signals. Mutations favoring an abundance of antiapoptotic signals, such as amplification at *Bcl-2*, could overwhelm all other proapoptosis stimuli. Mutations in *p53* are also strongly antiapoptotic, because p53 protein is a potent initiator of apoptosis. *Bcl-2* mutation has been found in SCC [80], but its role in EAC is unknown.

Unlimited replication

Telomerase is a ribonucleoprotein reverse transcriptase that stabilizes and elongates telomere length. Telomeres are long segments of noncoding DNA repeats that act to protect the ends of chromosomes from unwanted degradation or fusion. Telomerase uses its own RNA template and adds telomeric sequences to chromosomal ends, thus maintaining telomere length. Normal DNA replication cannot fully copy the 3′ ends of chromosomes. As a result, about 50 to 200 base pairs of telomeric DNA are lost with each cell replication cycle. After several cell divisions, the telomere length cannot further protect chromosomal integrity, and triggers the cell to exit from the cell cycle. In the abnormal state, perpetual activation of telomerase activity translates into unlimited replication. Normal, noncancerous cells usually express very low levels of telomerase. Upregulation of telomerase has been found in EAC [58], although it may be a more common tumorigenic mechanism. To date, the difficulty in widely surveying for telomerase has been the lack of a technically simple assay.

Promoting neo-angiogenesis

The development of new blood vessels is critically important in supplying nutrients to a growing tumor. Communication with the bloodstream is needed for exchange of cytokines and hormone messengers between different parts of a single tumor, and is also the pathway of departure for metastatic tumor cells. Vascular endothelial growth factors (VEGF) stimulate endothelial cell proliferation and migration and are central to neo-angiogenesis. VEGF is up-regulated in Barrett's [40], a putative precursor of EAC, but its role in esophageal cancer development is still unclear.

Invasion and metastasis

Loss of cellular adhesion is a hallmark of metastasis. Plasma membrane cell–cell adhesion molecules such as the cadherin glycoproteins serve to anchor neighboring cells together. Cadherins attach to the intracellular actin cytoskeleton through β-catenin. Downregulation or dysfunctional E-cadherin or β-catenin proteins can ultimately lead to metastasis. Cell–cell adhesion appears abnormal in Barrett's and EAC [39]; less is known about these abnormalities in SCC.

Era of genomics

Gene microarrays

At the completion of the US National Institutes of Health (NIH) Human Genome Project, the era of genomics research was officially born. Not surprisingly, the same advances in technology that brought forth the molecular biology techniques needed to complete the Human Genome Project also spawned a host of technologies ready to catapult scientific research onto an even higher level of sophistication. One such technique is gene microarray analysis, which allows querying simultaneously hundreds or even thousands of genes within a single sample preparation. Today, gene microarray technology transforms work that may have previously taken researchers years to complete into work that can be completed in a few months.

The first step in gene microarray analysis is appropriate sample selection and preparation—in oncological research, the samples of interest arc often the cancerous tissue and its corresponding normal or putatively premalignant counterparts. The tissue or cells of interest are then processed for total RNA, which is then reverse-transcribed into labeled cDNA probes. The labeled cDNA is hybridized to microarrays constructed of multiple spots of cDNA clones from known genes. After hybridization of the labeled cDNA to the microarray, the array is imaged and then analyzed using sophisticated computer software. Upregulated or downregulated genes can be determined relative to reference probes hybridized to the same microarray.

There is already intriguing microarray data in esophageal squamous cell carcinoma [83–91]. Working with esophageal SCC, researchers have been able to determine differential expression of oncogenes/tumor suppressor genes, such as *Fra-1* and *Neogenin*, and cell cycle-related genes, such as *Id-1* and *CDC25B* [84] in SCC tissues. Also, using microarray analysis, SCC gene expression can be followed temporally at different stages of neoplastic progression [86,87]. Naturally, the global nature of microarray experiments ultimately helps to narrow the scope of further laboratory investigation to those genes or categories of genes that may be of further interest [89–90]. Ultimately, the value of any cancer research is its potential impact on therapy. To illustrate this point, Kihara and colleagues [91] have already applied cDNA microarray techniques to predict sensitivity to adjuvant chemotherapy in advanced stage esophageal cancer patients. In EAC, microarray analysis research is just beginning [92–93]; however, early results show that the application of supervised methods of analysis, such as artificial neural networks and gene filtering, can permit the correct identification of Barrett's phenotype versus EAC phenotype with extreme accuracy [93].

Future directions: proteomics

Proteomics is the study of proteins, the ultimate products of expressed genes. Proteomics is also a powerful method of analysis which harnesses a set of tools that can identify upregulated or underexpressed proteins from the vantage point of a panoramic approach. Proteins extracted from tumor tissues can be compared with those from a reference tissue. Because there are often hundreds of proteins in any given sample, resolution of individual proteins can be accomplished either through solid or liquid phase techniques. Subsequent isolation and characterization of differentially expressed proteins, usually through sophisticated mass spectrometry, can therefore reveal potential targets for intervention, important surrogate markers of drug responses, and diagnostic markers capable of identifying esophageal cancer patients earlier, leading to improved outcomes. One study has already found that the glycoprotein, clusterin, is downregulated in SCC tissue and preoperative blood serum [94]. Results such as these are encouraging, but more interesting data will likely follow as work matures in the field of proteomics and esophageal cancer.

Summary

The incidence of esophageal adenocarcinoma is rising in the United States and Western countries. Significant differences exist between esophageal adenocarcinoma and squamous cell carcinoma in the molecular mechanisms responsible for the tumorigenesis process. State-of-the-art techniques such as gene microarrays and proteomics will greatly aid in the development of new therapies targeting specific molecular pathways, ultimately leading to improved survival in patients who have esophageal cancer.

References

[1] Jemel A, Murray T, Samuels A, et al. Cancer statistics, 2003. CA Cancer J Clin 2003;53:5–26.
[2] Cancer Facts & Figures. Atlanta (GA): American Cancer Society; 2003.
[3] El-Serag HB. The epidemic of esophageal carcinoma. Gastroenterol Clin N Am 2002;31: 421–40.

[4] Yang PC, Davis S. Incidence of cancer of the esophagus in the US by histologic type. Cancer 1988;61:612–7.

[5] Blot WJ, Devesa SS, Kneller RW, et al. Rising incidence of adenocarcinoma of the esophagus and gastric cardia. JAMA 1991;265:1287–9.

[6] Blot WJ, Devesa SS, Fraumeni JF. Continuing climb in rates of esophageal adenocarcinoma: an update. JAMA 1993;270:1320.

[7] Pera M, Cameron AJ, Trastek VF, et al. Increasing incidence of adenocarcinoma of the esophagus and esophagogastric junction. Gastroenterology 1993;104:510–3.

[8] Reed PI, Johnston BJ. The changing incidence of oesophageal cancer. Endoscopy 1993;25: 606–8.

[9] Daly JM, Karnell LH, Menck HR. National cancer database report on esophageal carcinoma. Cancer 1996;78:1820–8.

[10] Heitmiller RF, Sharma RR. Comparison of prevalence and resection rates in patients with esophageal squamous cell carcinoma and adenocarcinoma. J Thorac Cardiovasc Surg 1996; 112:130–6.

[11] Younes M, Henson DE, Ertan A, et al. Incidence and survival trends of esophageal carcinoma in the United States: racial and gender differences by histological type. Scand J Gastroenterol 2002;37:1359–65.

[12] Powell J, McConkey CC, Gillison EW, et al. Continuing rising trend in oesophageal adenocarcinoma. Int J Cancer 2002;102:422–7.

[13] Walther C, Zilling T, Perfekt R, et al. Increasing prevalence of adenocarcinoma of the oesophagus and gastro-oesophageal junction: a study of the Swedish population between 1970 and 1997. Eur J Surg 2001;167:748–57.

[14] Corley DA, Buffler PA. Oesophageal and gastric cardia adenocarcinomas: analysis of regional variation using the Cancer Incidence in Five Continents database. Int J Epidemiol 2001;30:1415–25.

[15] Ke L. Mortality and incidence trends from esophagus cancer in selected geographic areas of China circa 1970–1990. Int J Cancer 2002;102:271–4.

[16] Chang SS, Lu CL, Chao JY, et al. Unchanging trend of adenocarcinoma of the esophagus and gastric cardia in Taiwan: a 15-year experience in a single center. Dig Dis Sci 2002;47(4):735–40.

[17] Law S, Wong J. Changing disease burden and management issues for esophageal cancer in the Asia-Pacific region. J Gastroenterol Hepatol 2002;17:374–81.

[18] Shaheen N, Ransohoff DF. Gastroesophageal reflux, Barrett esophagus, and esophageal cancer. JAMA 2002;287(15):1972–81.

[19] Murray L, Watson P, Johnston B, et al. Risk of adenocarcinoma in Barrett's oesophagus: population-based study. BMJ 2003;327.534–5.

[20] Anderson LA, Murray LJ, Murphy SJ, et al. Mortality in Barrett's oesophagus: results from a population-based study. Gut 2003;52:1081–4.

[21] Heading RC. Barrett's oesophagus: epidemiology comes up with a surprise. Gut 2003;52: 1079–80.

[22] Spechler SJ. Screening for Barrett's esophagus. Rev Gastroenterol Disord 2002;2(Suppl 2): S25–9.

[23] Shaheen N. Is there a "Barrett's iceberg?" Gastroenterology 2002;123(2):636–7.

[24] Gerson LB, Shetler K, Triadafilopoulos G. Prevalence of Barrett's esophagus in asymptomatic individuals. Gastroenterology 2002;123:461–7.

[25] Corley DA, Levin TR, Habel LA, et al. Surveillance and survival in Barrett's adenocarcinomas: a population-based study. Gastroenterology 2002;122:633–40.

[26] Dulai GS, Guha S, Kahn KL, et al. Preoperative prevalence of Barrett's esophagus in esophageal adenocarcinoma: a systematic review. Gastroenterology 2002;122:26–33.

[27] Sontag SJ. Preventing death of Barrett's cancer: does frequent surveillance endoscopy do it? Am J Med 2001;111(Suppl 8A):137S–41S.

[28] Shaheen NJ, Crosby MA, Bozymski EM, et al. Is there publication bias in the reporting of cancer risk in Barrett's esophagus? Gastroenterology 2000;119:333–8.

[29] Colin-Jones DG, Langman MJS, Lawson DH, et al. Post-marketing surveillance of the safety of cimetidine: 12 month mortality report. BMJ 1983;286:1713–6.

[30] Colin-Jones DG, Langman MJS, Lawson DH, et al. Post-marketing surveillance of the safety of cimetidine: mortality during second, third, and fourth year of follow-up. BMJ 1985; 291:1084–8.

[31] Colin-Jones DG, Langman MJS, Lawson DH, et al. Post-marketing surveillance of the safety of cimetidine: 10 year mortality report. Gut 1992;33:1280–4.

[32] Bateman DN, Colin-Jones D, Hartz S, et al. Mortality study of 18,000 patients treated with omeprazole. Gut 2003;52:942–6.

[33] Hanahan D, Weinberg RA. The hallmarks of cancer. Cell 2000;100:57–70.

[34] Sirieix PS, O'Donovan M, Brown J, et al. Surface expression of minichromosome maintenance proteins provides a novel method for detecting patients at risk for developing adenocarcinoma in Barrett's esophagus. Clin Cancer Res 2003;9:2560–6.

[35] Dunn JR, Risk JM, Langan JE, et al. Physical and transcript map of the minimally deleted region III on 17p implicated in the early development of Barrett's oesophageal adenocarcinoma. Oncogene 2003;22:4134–42.

[36] Mork H, Scheurlen M, Al-Taie O, et al. Glutathione peroxidase isoforms as part of the local antioxidative defense system in normal and Barrett's esophagus. Int J Cancer 2003;105: 300–4.

[37] Sarris M, Konopka M, Lee CS. Differential expression of nm23 protein in the progression of oesophageal adenocarcinoma. Pathology 2003;35:37–41.

[38] Marchetti M, Caliot E, Pringault E. Chronic acid exposure leads to activation of the cdx2 intestinal homeobox gene in a long-term culture of mouse esophageal keratinocytes. J Cell Sci 2003;116:1429–36.

[39] Tselepis C, Perry I, Dawson C, et al. Tumour necrosis factor-α in Barrett's oesophagus: a potential novel mechanism of action. Oncogene 2002;21:6071–81.

[40] Auvinen MI, Sihvo EI, Ruohtula T, et al. Incipient angiogenesis in Barrett's epithelium and lymphangiogenesis in Barrett's adenocarcinoma. J Clin Oncol 2002;20:2971–9.

[41] Buttar NS, Wang KK, Leontovich O, et al. Chemoprevention of esophageal adenocarcinoma by COX-2 inhibitors in an animal model of Barrett's esophagus. Gastroenterology 2002;122:1101–12.

[42] Ryan BM, McManus R, Daly JS, et al. A common p73 polymorphism is associated with a reduced incidence of oesophageal carcinoma. Br J Cancer 2001;85(10):1499–503.

[43] El-Rifai W, Frierson HF, Moskaluk CA, et al. Genetic differences between adenocarcinomas arising in Barrett's esophagus and gastric mucosa. Gastroenterology 2001; 121:592–8.

[44] Lee JS, Oh TY, Ahn BO, et al. Involvement of oxidative stress in experimentally induced reflux esophagitis and Barrett's esophagus: clue for the chemoprevention of esophageal carcinoma by antioxidants. Mutat Res 2001;Sep 1:189–200.

[45] Brabender J, Lord RV, Danenberg KD, et al. Increased c-myb mRNA expression in Barrett's esophagus and Barrett's-associated adenocarcinoma. J Surg Res 2001;99: 301–6.

[46] Weston AP, Banerjee SK, Sharma P, et al. p53 protein overexpression in low grade dysplasia (LGD) in Barrett's esophagus: immunohistochemical marker predictive of progression. Am J Gastroenterol 2001;96:1355–62.

[47] Kandil HM, Tanner G, Smalley W, et al. Cyclooxygenase-2 expression in Barrett's esophagus. Dig Dis Sci 2001;46(4):785–9.

[48] Sarbia M, Tekin U, Zeriouh M, et al. Expression of RB protein, allelic imbalance of the RB gene and amplification of the CDK4 gene in metaplasias, dysplasias, and carcinomas in Barrett's esophagus. Anticancer Res 2001;21:387–92.

[49] Romagnoli S, Roncalli M, Graziani D, et al. Molecular alterations of Barrett's esophagus on microdissected endoscopic biopsies. Lab Invest 2001;81(2):241–7.

[50] Dunn JR, Garde J, Dolan K, et al. The evolution of loss of heterozygosity on chromosome 17 during the progression to Barrett's adenocarcinoma involves a unique combination of target sites in individual specimens. Clin Cancer Res 2000;6:4033–42.

[51] Woodward TA, Klingler PD, Genko PV, et al. Barrett's esophagus, apoptosis, and cell cycle regulation: correlation of p53, Bax, Bcl-2, and p21 protein expression. Anticancer Res 2000; 20:2427–32.

[52] Lord RVN, O'Grady RO, Sheehan C, et al. K-*ras* codon 12 mutations in Barrett's oesophagus and adenocarcinomas of the oesophagus and oesophagogastric junction. J Gastroenterol Hepatol 2000;15:730–6.

[53] Dolan K, Garde J, Walker SJ, et al. LOH at the sites of the *DCC, APC*, and *TP53* tumor suppressor genes occurs in Barrett's metaplasia and dysplasia adjacent to adenocarcinoma of the esophagus. Hum Pathol 1999;30:1508–14.

[54] van Lieshout EM, van Haelst UJ, Wobbes T, et al. Immunohistochemical localization of glutathione S-transferase α and π in human esophageal squamous epithelium, Barrett's epithelium and carcinoma. Jpn J Cancer Res 1999;90:530–5.

[55] Fein M, Peters JH, Baril N, et al. Loss of function of *Trp53*, but not *Apc*, leads to the development of esophageal adenocarcinoma in mice with jejunoesophageal reflux. J Surg Res 1999;83:48–55.

[56] Soldes OS, Kuick RD, Thompson II, et al. Differential expression of Hsp27 in normal oesophagus, Barrett's metaplasia and oesophageal adenocarcinomas. Br J Cancer 1999;79: 595–603.

[57] van Lieshout EM, Roelofs HM, Dekker S, et al. Polymorphic expression of the glutathione S-transferase *P1* gene and its susceptibility to Barrett's esophagus and esophageal carcinoma. Cancer Res 1999;59:586–9.

[58] Morales CP, Lee EL, Shay JW. In situ hybridization for the detection of telomerase RNA in the progression from Barrett's esophagus to esophageal adenocarcinoma. Cancer 1998;83: 652–9.

[59] Michael D, Beer DG, Wilker CW, et al. Frequent deletions of *FHIT* and FRA3B in Barrett's metaplasia and esophageal adenocarcinomas. Oncogene 1997;15:1653–9.

[60] Palanca-Wessels MC, Barrett MT, Galipeau PC, et al. Genetic analysis of long-term Barrett's esophagus epithelial cultures exhibiting cytogenetic and ploidy abnormalities. Gastroenterology 1998;114:295–304.

[61] Younes M, Ertan A, Lechago LV, et al. p53 protein accumulation is a specific marker of malignant potential in Barrett's metaplasia. Dig Dis Sci 1997;42(4):697–701.

[62] Kumble S, Omary MB, Cartwright CA, et al. Src activation in malignant and premalignant epithelia of Barrett's esophagus. Gastroenterology 1997;112:348–56.

[63] Barrett MT, Sanchez CA, Galipeau PC, et al. Allelic loss of 9p21 and mutation of the CDKN2/p16 gene develop as early lesions during neoplastic progression in Barrett's esophagus. Oncogene 1996;13:1867–73.

[64] Galipeau PC, Cowan DS, Sanchez CA, et al. 17p (p53) allelic losses, 4N (G₂/tetraploid) populations, and progression to aneuploidy in Barrett's esophagus. Proc Natl Acad Sci USA 1996;93:7081–4.

[65] Schneider PM, Casson AG, Levin B, et al. Mutations of p53 in Barrett's esophagus and Barrett's cancer: a prospective study of ninety-eight cases. J Thorac Cardiovasc Surg 1996; 111:323–33.

[66] Gleeson CM, Sloan JM, McGuigan JA, et al. Base transitions at CpG dinucleotides in the *p53* gene are common in esophageal adenocarcinoma. Cancer Res 1995;55:3406–11.

[67] Hardwick RH, Shepherd NA, Moorghen M, et al. c-erbB-2 overexpression in the dysplasia/carcinoma sequence of Barrett's oesophagus. J Clin Pathol 1995;48(2):129–32.

[68] Liu Y, Wang XH, Liu F, et al. Translocation of annexin I from cellular membrane to the nuclear membrane in human esophageal squamous cell carcinoma. World J Gastroenterol 2003;9(4):645–9.

[69] Li X, Lu JY, Zhao LQ, et al. Overexpression of ETS2 in human esophageal squamous cell carcinoma. World J Gastroenterol 2003;9(2):205–8.

[70] Nie Y, Liao J, Zhao X, et al. Detection of multiple gene hypermethylation in the development of esophageal squamous cell carcinoma. Carcinogenesis 2002;23(10):1713–20.

[71] Zhou J, Wang H, Lu A, et al. A novel gene, *NMES1*, downregulated in human esophageal squamous cell carcinoma. Int J Cancer 2002;101:311–6.

[72] Mathew R, Arora S, Khanna R, et al. Alterations in p53 and pRb pathways and their prognostic significance in oesophageal cancer. Eur J Cancer 2002;38:832–41.

[73] Wang Q, Lu J, Yang C, et al. CASK and its target gene Reelin were co-upregulated in human esophageal carcinoma. Cancer Lett 2002;179(1):71–7.

[74] Nakakuki K, Imoto I, Pimkhaokham A, et al. Novel targets for the 18p11.3 amplification frequently observed in esophageal squamous cell carcinomas. Carcinogenesis 2002;23(1): 19–24.

[75] Kitamura A, Yashima K, Okamoto E, et al. Reduced Fhit expression occurs in the early stage of esophageal tumorigenesis: no correlation with p53 expression and apoptosis. Oncology 2001;61:205–11.

[76] Paweletz CP, Ornstein DK, Roth MJ, et al. Loss of annexin I correlates with early onset of tumorigenesis in esophageal and prostate carcinoma. Cancer Res 2000;60:6293–7.

[77] Bahl R, Arora S, Nath N, et al. Novel polymorphism in $p21^{waf1/cip1}$ cyclin dependent kinase inhibitor gene: association with human esophageal cancer. Oncogene 2000;19:323–8.

[78] Shibagaki I, Tanaka H, Shimada Y, et al. *p53* mutation, *Murine Double Minute 2* amplification, and human papillomavirus infection are frequently involved but not associated with each other in esophageal squamous cell carcinoma. Clin Cancer Res 1995;1:769–73.

[79] Gamieldien W, Victor TC, Mugwanya D, et al. p53 and p16/CDKN2 gene mutations in esophageal tumors from a high-incidence area in South Africa. Int J Cancer 1998;78:544–9.

[80] Parenti AR, Rugge M, Shiao YH, et al. bcl-2 and p53 immunophenotypes in pre-invasive, early and advanced oesophageal squamous cancer. Histopathology 1997;31:430–5.

[81] Shibagaki I, Shimada I, Wagata T, et al. Allelotype analysis of esophageal squamous cell carcinoma. Cancer Res 1994;54:2996–3000.

[82] Huang Y, Boynton RF, Blount PL, et al. Loss of heterozygosity involves multiple tumor suppressor genes in human esophageal cancers. Cancer Res 1992;52:6525–30.

[83] Lu J, Liu A, Xiong M, et al. Gene expression profile changes in initiation and progression of squamous cell carcinoma of esophagus. Int J Cancer 2001;91:288–94.

[84] Hu YC, Lam KY, Law S, et al. Identification of differentially expressed genes in esophageal squamous cell carcinoma (ESCC) by cDNA expression array: overexpression of *Fra-1*, *Neogenin, Id-1*, and *CDC25B* genes in ESCC. Clin Cancer Res 2001;7:2213–21.

[85] Kan T, Shimada Y, Sato F, et al. Gene expression profiling in human esophageal cancers using cDNA microarray. Biochem Biophys Res Commun 2001;286:792–801.

[86] Zhou J, Zhao LQ, Xiong MM, et al. Gene expression profiles at different stages of human esophageal squamous cell carcinoma. World J Gastroenterol 2003;9(1):9–15.

[87] Wang HT, Kong JP, Ding F, et al. Analysis of gene expression profile induced by EMP-1 in esophageal cancer cells using cDNA microarray. World J Gastroenterol 2003;9(3):392–8.

[88] Xu SH, Qian LJ, Mou HZ, et al. Difference of gene expression profiles between esophageal carcinoma and its precancerous epithelium by gene chip. World J Gastroenterol 2003;9(3): 417–22.

[89] Zhi H, Zhang J, Hu G, et al. The deregulation of arachidonic acid metabolism-related genes in human esophageal squamous cell carcinoma. Int J Cancer 2003;106:327–33.

[90] Kawamata H, Furihata T, Omotehara F, et al. Identification of genes differentially expressed in a newly isolated human metastasizing esophageal cancer cell line, T.Tn-AT1, by cDNA microarray. Cancer Sci 2003;94:699–706.

[91] Kihara C, Tsunoda T, Tanaka T, et al. Prediction of sensitivity of esophageal tumors to adjuvant chemotherapy by cDNA microarray analysis of gene-expression profiles. Cancer Res 2001;61:6474–9.

[92] Selaru FM, Zou T, Xu Y, et al. Global gene expression profiling in Barrett's esophagus and esophageal cancer: a comparative analysis using cDNA microarrays. Oncogene 2002;21: 475–8.

[93] Xu Y, Selaru FM, Yin J, et al. Artificial neural networks and gene filtering distinguish between global gene expression profiles of Barrett's esophagus and esophageal cancer. Cancer Res 2002;62:3493–7.

[94] Zhang LY, Ying WT, Mao YS, et al. Loss of clusterin both in serum and tissue correlates with the tumorigenesis of esophageal squamous cell carcinoma via proteomics approaches. World J Gastroenterol 2003;9(4):650–4.

ELSEVIER
SAUNDERS

Surg Clin N Am 85 (2005) 555–567

SURGICAL
CLINICS OF
NORTH AMERICA

Current Staging of Esophageal Carcinoma

Amit N. Patel, MD, MS,
Percival O. Buenaventura, MD*

*Section of Thoracic Surgery, University of Pittsburgh Medical Center,
Suite C-800, 200 Lothrop Street, Pittsburgh, PA 15213, USA*

The incidence of esophageal carcinoma is rising rapidly, increasing by about 10% per year in the United States [1,2]. Cancer of the esophagus constitutes about 1.5% of newly diagnosed malignancies in the United States annually. Over the last decade, the incidence of newly diagnosed esophageal cancer in the United States is 13,900, and there are over 13,000 deaths anticipated in 2004 [1]. The incidence in the Western Hemisphere is estimated to be 5 per 100,000. Worldwide, the most common histology is squamous cell carcinoma; however in the West, adenocarcinoma has become the predominant histology. Of these newly diagnosed patients, the majority have either locally advanced disease or have distant metastases at presentation. The two most important prognostic indicators for esophageal cancer are depth of tumor penetration and nodal involvement [3–7]. The 5-year survival rate for patients with tumors remaining in the esophageal wall is approximately 40%, but overall survival is only 14% [8–10].

As with all other tumors, outcome for patients with esophageal cancer is strongly associated with the stage of the disease at diagnosis [8–11]. Although esophageal cancer is potentially curable in its earliest stages, there are no curative options for advanced-stage disease. Palliative treatments are available, and should be offered to patients with advanced disease. It is therefore imperative to identify patients with early-stage disease, so that curative therapy may be given [12–14]. Overall, 5-year survival for patients with Stage I disease is 50%; Stage II disease, 31%; Stage III disease, 20%; and Stage IV disease, 4%. In the small minority of patients with early disease limited to the mucosa of the esophagus and who undergo complete surgical resection, the 5 year survival can be as high as 90% [8–10].

---

* Corresponding author.
E-mail address: buenaventurapo@upmc.edu (P.O. Buenaventura).

0039-6109/05/$ - see front matter © 2005 Elsevier Inc. All rights reserved.
doi:10.1016/j.suc.2005.01.012

Because the esophagus is the only portion of gastrointestinal tract to lack a serosa, squamous cell carcinoma of the esophagus may spread by direct extension to the thyroid, larynx, tracheobronchial tree, aorta, pericardium, lungs, and diaphragm. Because the lymph node drainage of the esophagus extends from the neck through the mediastinum to the upper abdomen, including lesser curvature and celiac nodes, lymph node metastases may be found anywhere along the drainage pathway.

The primary means of diagnosis for esophageal cancer is by barium swallow or through upper endoscopy with biopsy of the esophageal lesion. CT is typically the next test performed, and is most valuable at detecting metastatic (M) distant disease, particularly in the liver, lungs, and periaortic lymph nodes. Endoscopic ultrasound (EUS) combines endoscopy with high-frequency ultrasonography to obtain detailed images of the tumor and surrounding structures. EUS is the most accurate technique for the locoregional tumor size (T) and nodal involvement (N) staging of esophageal cancer [15–18]. The recent availability of EUS-directed, fine-needle aspiration (FNA) has allowed a tissue diagnosis of lymph nodes both periesophageal and in the celiac axis. EUS-FNA can also sample liver metastases. Laparoscopic and thoracoscopic techniques can also be used to sample thoracic and celiac axis lymph nodes, which also may be sentinel nodes [19–21]. Positron emission tomography (PET) scanning with 18-fluorodeoxyglucose also is useful in detecting distant disease [22–25]. Optimal staging strategies for esophageal cancer combine EUS-FNA with CT scans. The role of PET scanning continues to be evaluated, and information regarding its utility should come soon from the results of a clinical trial being conducted by the American College of Surgeons Oncology Group. The preoperative assessment of patients and subsequent selection for the various treatment arms depends on accurate clinical and radiographic staging. To date, surgery alone remains the gold standard for early-stage esophageal cancer. Several studies have reported improved survival among patients undergoing induction chemotherapy, with or without radiotherapy, followed by surgical resection [12]. Contrary to these reports, a large North American intergroup effort comparing conventional chemotherapy and surgery with surgical resection alone [26] did not demonstrate a survival benefit with combined modality therapy.

The present staging system applies to all primary malignancies of the esophagus except sarcomas. T staging refers to the depth of invasion of tumor. Tis refers to carcinomas in situ that have not grown through the basement membrane. High-grade dysplasia is considered within this Tis grouping. T1 tumors have grown through the lamina propria of the epithelium and into the submucosa. T2 refers to tumors that have invaded the muscularis propria. There is no distinction between the two layers of muscle within the esophagus. T3 tumors have invaded beyond the muscular boundary of the esophagus and invade the surrounding fatty adventitial tissues. Of note, the esophagus lacks a serosal layer as it traverses through the neck, posterior mediastinum, and upper retroperitoneum. T4 tumors have invaded surrounding mediastinal or hiatal structures. The separation of T1 into T1a and T1b is justified by the differences observed in the frequency of lymph-node metastasis and related prognosis. It has been reported that T1a tumors have a 0% rate of lymph node metastasis and a 100% 5-year survival rate with treatment; whereas T1b tumors have a 25% to 47% occurrence of lymph node metastasis, resulting in an 86% 5-year survival without nodal metastasis, and 43% 5-year survival when nodal metastasis is identified in the surgical specimen [8–10].

At the present time, nodal staging refers only to presence or absence of disease in the regional lymph nodes around the esophagus. For the purposes of anatomic distinction, the regional lymph nodes of the esophagus have been classified as follows. The regional lymph nodes of the cervical esophagus include scalene, internal jugular, supraclavicular, and upper and lower cervical periesophageal lymph nodes. The regional lymph nodes of the intrathoracic esophagus include the upper and lower periesophageal and subcarinal lymph nodes. For tumors of the gastroesophageal junction, the regional lymph nodes include the lower esophageal (below the azygous vein), diaphragmatic, pericardial, left gastric, and celiac lymph nodes. The staging for esophageal lymph nodes has been revised to include subcategories as follows: N1a is one to three nodes involved; N1b is four to seven nodes involved, and N1c is more than seven nodes involved. Esophageal cancers with celiac axis nodal involvement have been classified as metastases (M1). Thus, careful attention should be paid to this area on CT imaging and during EUS evaluation. The separation of lymph nodes into the categories of N1a, N1b, and N1c in the TNM system has been justified by differences observed in prognosis and survival. For N1a tumors, the 2-year survival rate is 22%, 5-year survival rate is 11%, and median survival is 12 months. For N1b tumors, the 2-year survival rate is 18%, 5-year survival rate is 0%, and median survival is 9 months. For N1c tumors, the 2-year survival rate is 0%, 5-year survival rate is 0%, and median survival is 6 months [3,4,8–10].

Distant metastatic disease is denoted by M status. More recently, metastatic disease has been further subdivided into M1a and M1b. M1a designates tumors with metastases to nonregional periesophageal lymph nodes (cervical lymph nodes for upper thoracic esophageal tumors and celiac lymph nodes for lower thoracic esophageal tumors). M1b tumors are those with distant metastases to visceral organs or other distant nonperiesophageal lymph nodes. The TNM staging of esophageal cancer is summarized in Box 1 [27].

Currently, to evaluate the extent of the esophageal cancer involves radiographic, endoscopic, surgical, and molecular biologic tools. No single testing modality can optimally stage both local and distant disease. There have been many studies comparing the accuracy of the various imaging modalities (Table 1) [28–34]. The various modalities used to stage esophageal cancer are outlined below.

Box 1. AJCC staging of esophageal cancer

Stage grouping
  Stage 0 Tis N0 M0
  Stage I T1 N0 M0
  Stage IIA T2 N0 M0
  T3 N0 M0
  Stage IIB T1 N1 M0
  T2 N1 M0
  Stage III T3 N1 M0
  T4 Any N M0
  Stage IV Any T Any N M1
  Stage IVA Any T Any N M1a
  Stage IVB Any T Any N M1b

Definition of TNM
Primary tumor (T)
  TX Primary tumor cannot be assessed
  T0 No evidence of primary tumor
  Tis Carcinoma in situ
  T1 Tumor invades lamina propria or submucosa
  T2 Tumor invades muscularis propria
  T3 Tumor invades adventitia
  T4 Tumor invades adjacent structures
Regional lymph nodes (N)
  NX Regional lymph nodes cannot be assessed
  N0 No regional lymph node metastasis
  N1 Regional lymph node metastasis
Distant metastasis (M)
  MX Distant metastasis cannot be assessed
  M0 No distant metastasis
  M1 Distant metastasis
Tumors of the lower thoracic esophagus:
  M1a Metastasis in celiac lymph nodes
  M1b Other distant metastasis
Tumors of the midthoracic esophagus:
  M1a Not applicable
  M1b Nonregional lymph nodes or other distant metastasis
Tumors of the upper thoracic esophagus:
  M1a Metastasis in cervical nodes
  M1b Other distant metastasis

Table 1
Accuracy of esophageal cancer staging by modality

Modality	% Accuracy
Computed tomography—tumor depth	49–60
Computed tomography—nodal status	39–74
Endoscopic ultrasound—tumor depth	80–92
Endoscopic ultrasound—nodal status	45–100
MRI scan—nodal status	56–74
PET scan—nodal status	76–87
Thoracoscopy/laparoscopy—nodal status	89–92

Data from Patel AN, Preskitt JT, Kuhn JA, et al. Surgical management of esophageal carcinoma. BUMC Proceedings 2003;16:280–4.

Radiographic evaluation

Barium swallow

The radiographic evaluation begins with a barium swallow. It allows for the evaluation of degree of stricture and level of obstruction. Length of tumor and angulation of the esophageal lumen have been shown to be prognostic factors [35]. Barium swallow can visualize the local extent of disease, and may provide an assessment of the proximal stomach as a conduit for reconstruction after esophagectomy; however, for TNM staging, it is of limited use.

Computed tomography

CT is the most efficient way of screening for esophageal cancer with regards to both locoregional and metastatic disease. Although CT scan excels in detection of metastatic disease to solid organs, it lags behind the other modalities in overall sensitivity and specificity in the detection of local nodal disease. Whereas T staging by computed tomography can only be inferred from esophageal wall thickness by CT scan, endoscopic ultra-sonography can predict more accurately the level of submucosal and transmural involvement, and morphologic regional node characteristics worrisome for metastasis [36].

Normal esophageal wall thickness by CT scan criteria is less than 5 mm. T1–2 disease presents with esophageal thickness of 5 to 15 mm. T3 disease is generally thicker than 15 mm, with an irregular border, whereas locally advanced disease (T4) tumors demonstrate CT findings consistent with invasion of proximal mediastinal structures. The accuracy of detection of aortic, tracheobronchial, and pericardial invasion is greater than 90% with modern CT imaging. Additionally, CT scanning allows assessment of initial local tumor bulk, and is used for follow-up in patients who undergo definitive cytoreductive therapy with chemo/radiotherapy or induction therapy before possible surgical resection.

CT scan assessment of lymph node involvement is only fair at best. Most recent series place the overall accuracy of CT scan for N stage between 45% and 60% (see Table 1). Moreover, the accuracy of CT scanning for lymph node involvement varies with location. A review of the literature reveals 83% to 87% accuracy in the assessment of periesophageal abdominal nodes, but only 51% to 70% accuracy in assessing adenopathy in the chest associated with esophageal cancer [37].

Magnetic resonance imaging

Magnetic resonance imaging (MRI) has high contrast sensitivity, especially with regard to delineating margins between the adjacent esophagus and mediastinal fat, and potential invasion with surrounding mediastinal structures. In addition, images can be viewed in axial, sagittal, and coronal planes [38]. Despite this fact, it is infrequently used clinically in staging esophageal cancer. A recent study [28] looked at the accuracy of CT, EUS, and MRI in the same group of cancer patients, with regard to their predictive values at different nodal stations. MRI appeared to offer no significant advantage when both EUS and CT are available.

Positron emission tomography

Positron emission tomography (PET) is a noninvasive means of detecting primary, nodal, and distant metastatic disease by identifying areas of high glucose metabolism [22–25]. The most common tracer used is ^{18}F-deoxyglucose (FDG). It has been shown to be an effective tool for staging lung cancer and other malignancies. More recently, data on its usefulness with regard to esophageal cancer are accumulating.

The accuracy of PET scanning surpasses that of CT scan in staging esophageal cancer with regard to nodal disease and metastatic involvement. A recent series of 36 esophageal cancer patients [31] directly compared PET and CT with pathologic findings obtained after esophagectomy or during tissue sampling. PET accurately predicted nodal involvement in 76%, compared with 45% for CT scan. Additionally, PET identified five other distant metastases that were absent on CT, and serendipitously identified a lung primary.

In a study by Flamen and colleagues [24] comparing preoperative PET to CT and EUS in the locoregional staging of 74 patients with potentially resectable esophageal or GE junction cancer, PET was falsely negative in 4 patients with T1 tumors. Additionally, in those patients who underwent lymph node dissection at the time of esophagectomy, PET scanning was not as sensitive as EUS for the detection of lymph nodes (33% versus 81%, respectively), although PET had a higher specificity than EUS (89% versus 67%). The primary role of PET scans in esophageal cancer appears to be in the detection of distant metastases. In a combined experience of

94 patients, PET detected 22 patients with distant disease who had a negative CT scan. In a recent series, 35 potentially resectable esophageal cancer patients were assessed by PET scanning and standard radiographic survey [23]. Patients with locally advanced disease or those with obvious metastatic disease based on tissue confirmation or standard radiographic survey were excluded from the study. PET scan accurately detected occult distant disease in 7 out of 35 patients. These sites included liver (4), cervical lymph nodes (2), and lung (1). PET falsely identified bony metastases in 2 patients. A false-negative result was encountered in a 2-mm liver surface lesion that was found on laparoscopy. These results yield an accuracy of 91%, with sensitivity and specificity of 88% and 93%, respectively, for distant metastatic disease. In another series of 91 patients with esophageal cancer, PET scans were more accurate than CT at detecting distant metastases; however, the benefit of PET scanning compared with CT has not been consistently demonstrated in studies of esophageal cancer [38a]. At the current time, it appears that PET scanning is a valuable diagnostic test to detect metastatic disease. On occasion, a PET scan can aid in the diagnosis of those rare patients with obstructive lesions of the esophagus from which diagnostic endoscopic biopsies cannot be obtained. Nevertheless, further studies are needed to define the role of PET in the routine clinical management of patients with esophageal cancer. In patients without evidence of distant disease who are candidates for surgery, accurate locoregional staging is best done by EUS.

Endoscopoic ultrasonography

EUS provides a better evaluation of T stage when compared with other modalities [15–18]. EUS provides detailed images of the esophagus and surrounding structures. It combines endoscopy with high-resolution ultrasonography, either via dedicated echoendoscopes (7.5 MHz to 20 MHz) or by high-frequency ultrasound probes (12 MHz to 30 MHz) passed through the channel of the instrument. Tumor staging by EUS relies on accurate identification of the layers of the gastrointestinal wall, and subsequent determination of extent of tumor involvement. Successful identification of the five-layer EUS pattern of the gastrointestinal wall, with alternating hyperechoic and hypoechoic layers, is key for accurate staging. The first (hyperechoic) and second (hypoechoic) layers correspond to the mucosa. The third hyperechoic layer is the submucosa. The fourth hypoechoic layer is the muscularis propria, and is often the easiest layer to identify. With proper high-frequency ultrasound imaging, one can visualize the separation of the longitudinal and circular muscle layers by the characteristic hyperechoic interface. The fifth hyperechoic layer in the esophagus is the adventitia. EUS has two significant limitations, however. First, it is operator-dependent, and second, high-grade obstructing lesions cannot be traversed, and therefore cannot be evaluated. Up to 20% of patients with obstructing esophageal carcinoma cannot be evaluated by endoscopic ultrasonography. More recently, smaller caliber probes, such as the catheter miniature echo probe, are coming into use. In experienced hands, EUS accuracy of T stage varies from 85% to 90%. Image resolution is in the order of 0.2 mm. Accuracy increases with deeper tumor penetration; accuracy of predicting T1 lesions is at approximately 80%, T2 lesions at 90%, and T3 and T4 lesions at 95%. Overstaging may occur with inflammation surrounding the tumor, which has been reported in the literature [36]. The accuracy of endoscopic ultrasound to determine nodal involvement ranges from 65% to 86%. Esophageal cancers seen on EUS demonstrate a circumscribed or diffuse wall thickening, and appear as echo-poor or echo-inhomogeneous lesions. The result of tumor penetration into and through the esophageal wall destroys the distinct endosonographic layers. Malignant lymph nodes typically appear hypoechoic, with a round shape, discrete borders, and size greater than 1 cm. Lymph nodes that meet all four of these criteria have an 80% to 100% likelihood of malignancy; however, only approximately 35% of malignant nodes demonstrate all four criteria. FNA by EUS improves the accuracy of staging. There is a risk of false-positive FNA that is minimized if one avoids both placing the needle through the primary tumor and removing the stylet from the aspiration needle until the lymph node is penetrated. EUS can also be used to visualize much of the liver, and has recently been directed to the liver to detect and sample tissue, using FNA of liver lesions. A series of 167 liver FNA cases from 22 centers was reported, of which 11% were esophageal cancers [38b]. In this report, EUS confirmation of liver mass resulted in a change of diagnosis or management in more than 90% of patients. Complications were noted in six patients (4%), including undrained biliary sepsis/death (1), bleeding (1), fever (2), and pain (2). It can be concluded that EUS-guided liver FNA is a relatively safe procedure that can have a significant impact on the management of patients. EUS evaluation of the liver should be considered in the routine staging of upper gastrointestinal malignancies [12].

Surgical staging

Prognosis of esophageal cancer is dependent on surgical resectability locally and presence of nodal disease. Patients with T3 tumors or less and no nodal disease have reasonable survival when resected for cure, regardless of adjuvant therapy. The current methods of noninvasive staging of esophageal carcinoma are still far from optimal at detecting abdominal and thoracic lymph node metastases, however. Minimally invasive surgical staging is an invaluable adjunct to accurate staging of nodal disease and invasion of adjacent structures.

Minimally invasive surgical staging involves a combination of video-assisted thoracoscopy and laparoscopy [19,20]. Thoracoscopy is usually performed in the right chest with the patient in the full lateral decubitus position, unless noninvasive studies suggest disease in the left chest. The approach through the right chest allows access to the entire thoracic esophagus, paraesophageal tissues, and subcarinal nodes. Evaluation is facilitated by mobilizing the inferior pulmonary ligament and identifying the inferior pulmonary vein and nodal station. During exposure of the mid and upper esophagus, care should be taken not to injure the airway, which is most vulnerable at the membranous portion of the trachea and main stem bronchi. Identification of the aorta prevents inadvertent injury, especially during dissection of the lower esophagus. The thoracic duct, which has a variable course near the esophagus along its entire length, must be avoided to prevent potentially troublesome chylous leaks.

Laparoscopic staging is performed with the patient in the supine position with steep reverse Trendelenburg. Upon entry into the abdomen, visualization of the entire peritoneal surface is done to rule out carcinomatosis. The liver surface is visually inspected. The lesser sac is entered by incising the gastro-hepatic ligament. Nodes adjacent to the lesser curve and celiac axis can be sampled. Extensive involvement of tumor into the cardia or fundus of the stomach can be assessed and may preclude the use of stomach as an esophageal conduit.

Laparoscopic ultrasonography may be used for the evaluation of the liver parenchyma; however, laparoscopic ultrasonography may be limited in its ability to detect new parenchymal lesions previously undetected by routine CT of the abdomen. In our ongoing series of nearly 50 patients, only one metastasis was identified by laparoscopic ultrasound that was not previously suspected on other noninvasive diagnostic studies.

A series of minimally invasive staging [19] evaluated 45 patients with potentially resectable esophageal carcinoma. Thoracoscopy was technically possible in 42 out of 45, whereas laparoscopy was performed only in the last 20 patients. In addition, laparoscopic staging was used in conjunction with laparoscopic feeding jejunostomies in patients who present with obstruction. The results of staging were confirmed after histopathologic evaluation of esophageal resection specimens. The accuracy of thoracoscopy was 93%, whereas laparoscopy was accurate in 94% of cases.

In another recent study, minimally invasive staging was compared with endoscopic ultrasonography in 26 patients [33]. All patients underwent both thoracoscopy and laparoscopy. Minimally invasive staging was found to be superior in detecting lymph node metastases. Moreover, minimally invasive staging allowed evaluation of patients (5 of 26) whose obstructing lesions prevented adequate EUS evaluation. Thoracoscopy and laparoscopy upstaged nodal disease in 6 out 8 patients thought to be N0 by EUS. In these patients, the nodes measured less than 1 cm (range 0.2 to 1.0 cm). In addition, 4 patients were found to have previously undetected liver metastases, (EUS and conventional radiographic work-up). Of note, 3 patients who had no evidence of nodal disease in the abdomen were found to have nodal disease on thoracoscopy.

The precise roles of thoracoscopy and laparoscopy in the staging of esophageal cancer remain unknown at the present time. To address this issue, a prospective multi-institutional study is currently under way (Cancer and Leukemia Group B 9380) [20]. Between 75 and 100 patients will be accrued in the next 3 to 4 years. The surgical staging protocol (CALGB 9380) requires that at least three lymph nodes from thoracoscopy and one lymph node from laparoscopy be obtained. Other end points include the finding of unresectability (either because of advanced local disease [T4] or metastatic disease) and frozen section-proven nodal disease in at least one lymph node. The efficacy, accuracy, and cost of thoracoscopic and laparoscopic staging, as well as the possible savings attained from avoiding unnecessary esophagectomy, will be evaluated.

Molecular biology

It is common for patients with apparently localized disease and histologically negative nodes on resection to present with distant disease a few months or years after surgery. This may represent a sampling error of lymph nodes at the time of surgery, inadequate evaluation of nodes by the pathologist, or occult disease in the nodes that can only be detected by other histopathologic markers. The application of molecular biologic techniques may allow the recognition of micrometastases that are histologically negative, and could have important clinical implications for staging and treatment options [39–42].

A new technique of detecting carcinoembryonic antigen mRNA in lymph nodes and bone marrow aspirates has been described. The use of a carcinoembryonic antigen (CEA-specific) nested reverse transcriptase-polymerase chain reaction (RT-PCR) detects epithelial CEA mRNA in these hematologic tissues and correlates with occult metastasis.

A recent study of patients with both benign and malignant esophageal disorders used the same CEA-specific RT-PCR. Lymph nodes were evaluated in 30 patients with esophageal cancer and in 13 patients with either achalasia or gastroesophageal reflux disease, one of whom had Barrett's metaplasia [40–42]. All histologically positive lymph nodes were also found to be positive by the RT-PCR assay. All lymph nodes from patients with benign esophageal diseases had negative assays. Of 10 patients with esophageal cancer who had histologically negative nodes, 5 were positive by the RT-PCR assay. Of these 5 patients, 3 have subsequently developed recurrent disease (2 died of disease within 3 months). In the remaining 5 patients who were negative histologically and by RT-PCR, all are alive, with 1 patient subsequently developing recurrent disease. A positive CEA-specific RT-PCR assay portends a poor prognosis.

Summary

The rational treatment of esophageal cancer requires the complete evaluation and preoperative staging of this disease. As the incidence of esophageal cancer increases, more clinicians will face the difficult task of allocating the appropriate treatment course for these patients. Accurate esophageal cancer staging is critical if stage-dependent algorithms are used to direct appropriate therapies. Although all of the staging techniques discussed may potentially provide useful information, it is not possible to use all techniques in all patients, especially given the limited availability of resources. The optimal staging strategy has not yet been determined; the authors provide the general algorithm used in our institution. Ultimately, minimally invasive surgical approaches will allow surgeons to evaluate locoregional disease with little or no procedure-associated morbidity, much as mediastinoscopy is used in lung cancer staging. Although currently the use of molecular biologic techniques may only be investigational, it holds great promise in the future.

References

[1] Jemal A, Murray T, Samuels A, et al. Cancer statistics, 2003. CA Cancer J Clin 2003;53(1): 5–26.
[2] Blot WJ, Devesa SS, Kneller RW, et al. Rising incidence of adenocarcinoma of the esophagus and gastric cardia. JAMA 1991;265(10):1287–9.
[3] Lerut T, Coosemans W, Decker G, et al. Leuven Collaborative Workgroup for Esophageal Carcinoma. Extracapsular lymph node involvement is a negative prognostic factor in T3 adenocarcinoma of the distal esophagus and gastroesophageal junction. J Thorac Cardiovasc Surg 2003;126(4):1121–8.
[4] Demeester SR. Lymph node involvement in esophageal adenocarcinoma: if you see one, have you seen them all? J Thorac Cardiovasc Surg 2003;126(4):947–9.
[5] Vazquez-Sequeiros E, Wiersema MJ, Clain JE, et al. Impact of lymph node staging on therapy of esophageal carcinoma. Gastroenterology 2003;125(6):1626–35.
[6] Rice TW, Blackstone EH, Adelstein DJ, et al. Role of clinically determined depth of tumor invasion in the treatment of esophageal carcinoma. J Thorac Cardiovasc Surg 2003;125(5): 1091–102.
[7] Roder JD, Busch R, Stein HJ, et al. Ratio of invaded to removed lymph nodes as a predictor of survival in squamous cell carcinoma of the oesophagus. Br J Surg 1994;81:410–3.
[8] Enzinger PC, Mayer RJ. Esophageal cancer. N Engl J Med 2003;349(23):2241–52.
[9] Ries LAG, Eisner MP, Kosary C, et al, editors. SEER cancer statistics review, 1973–1999. Bethesda (MD): National Cancer Institute; 2002.
[10] Eloubeidi MA, Mason AC, Desmond RA, et al. Temporal trends (1973–1997) in survival of patients with esophageal adenocarcinoma in the United States: a glimmer of hope? Am J Gastroenterol 2003;98(7):1627–33.

[11] Iyer RB, Silverman PM, Tamm EP, et al. Diagnosis, staging, and follow-up of esophageal cancer. AJR Am J Roentgenol 2003;181(3):785–93.

[12] Patel AN, Preskitt JT, Kuhn JA, et al. Surgical management of esophageal carcinoma. BUMC Proceedings 2003;16:280–4.

[13] Rice TW, Blackstone EH, Rybicki LA, et al. Refining esophageal cancer staging. J Thorac Cardiovasc Surg 2003;125(5):1103–13.

[14] Rice TW, Adelstein DJ. Precise clinical staging allows treatment modification of patients with esophageal carcinoma. Oncology (Huntingt) 1997;11(Suppl 9):58–62.

[15] Tytgat GN, Tio TL. Esophageal ultrasonography. Gastroenterol Clin North Am 1991; 20(4):659–71.

[16] Chandawarkar RY, Kakegawa T, Fujita H, et al. Endosonography for preoperative staging of specific nodal groups associated with esophageal cancer. World J Surg 1996; 20(6):700–2.

[17] Preston SR, Clark GW, Martin IG, et al. Effect of endoscopic ultrasonography on the management of 100 consecutive patients with oesophageal and junctional carcinoma. Br J Surg 2003;90(10):1220–4.

[18] Mariette C, Balon JM, Maunoury V, et al. Value of endoscopic ultrasonography as a predictor of long-term survival in oesophageal carcinoma. Br J Surg 2003;90(11):1367–72.

[19] Krasna MJ, Jiao X, Mao YS, et al. Thoracoscopy/laparoscopy in the staging of esophageal cancer: Maryland experience. Surg Laparosc Endosc Percutan Tech 2002;12(4):213–8.

[20] Krasna MJ, Reed CE, Nedzwiecki D, et al. CALGB Thoracic Surgeons. CALGB 9380: a prospective trial of the feasibility of thoracoscopy/laparoscopy in staging esophageal cancer. Ann Thorac Surg 2001;71(4):1073–9.

[21] Kato H, Miyazaki T, Nakajima M, et al. Sentinel lymph nodes with technetium-99m colloidal rhenium sulfide in patients with esophageal carcinoma. Cancer 2003;98(5):932–9.

[22] Wren SM, Stijns P, Srinivas S. Positron emission tomography in the initial staging of esophageal cancer. Arch Surg 2002;137(9):1001–6 [discussion: 1006–7].

[23] Luketich JD, Schauer PR, Meltzer CC, et al. Role of positron emission tomography in staging esophageal cancer. Ann Thorac Surg 1997;64(3):765–9.

[24] Flamen P, Lerut A, Van Cutsem E, et al. Utility of positron emission tomography for the staging of patients with potentially operable esophageal carcinoma. J Clin Oncol 2000; 18(18):3202–10.

[25] Flanagan FL, Dehdashti F, Siegel BA, et al. Staging of esophageal cancer with 18F-fluorodeoxyglucose positron emission tomography. AJR Am J Roentgenol 1997;168: 417–24.

[26] Kelsen DP, Ginsberg R, Pajak TF, et al. Chemotherapy followed by surgery compared with surgery alone for localized esophageal cancer. N Engl J Med 1998;339(27):1979–84.

[27] AJCC Cancer staging manual. 6th Edition. New York: Springer-Verlag; 2002.

[28] Nakashima A, Nakashima K, Seto H, et al. Thoracic esophageal carcinoma: evaluation in the sagittal section with magnetic resonance imaging. Abdom Imaging 1997;22(1):20–3.

[29] Wallace MB, Nietert PJ, Earle C, et al. An analysis of multiple staging management strategies for carcinoma of the esophagus: computed tomography, endoscopic ultrasound, positron emission tomography, and thoracoscopy/laparoscopy. Ann Thorac Surg 2002; 74(4):1026–32.

[30] Wakelin SJ, Deans C, Crofts TJ, et al. A comparison of computerised tomography, laparoscopic ultrasound and endoscopic ultrasound in the preoperative staging of oesophago-gastric carcinoma. Eur J Radiol 2002;41(2):161–7.

[31] Yoon YC, Lee KS, Shim YM, et al. Metastasis to regional lymph nodes in patients with esophageal squamous cell carcinoma: CT versus FDG PET for presurgical detection prospective study. Radiology 2003;227(3):764–70.

[32] Drudi FM, Trippa F, Cascone F, et al. Esophagogram and CT vs endoscopic and surgical specimens in the diagnosis of esophageal carcinoma. Radiol Med (Torino) 2002;103(4): 344–52.

[33] Luketich JD, Schauer P, Landreneau R, et al. Minimally invasive surgical staging is superior to endoscopic ultrasound in detecting lymph node metastases in esophageal cancer. J Thorac Cardiovasc Surg 1997;114(5):817–21 [discussion: 821–3].

[34] Rasanen JV, Sihvo EI, Knuuti MJ, et al. Prospective analysis of accuracy of positron emission tomography, computed tomography, and endoscopic ultrasonography in staging of adenocarcinoma of the esophagus and the esophagogastric junction. Ann Surg Oncol 2003;10(8):954–60.

[35] Akiyama H, Kogure T, Itai Y. The esophageal axis and its relationship to the resectability of carcinoma of the esophagus. Ann Surg 1972;176(1):30–6.

[36] Saunders HS, Wolfman NT, Ott DJ. Esophageal cancer. Radiologic staging. Radiol Clin North Am 1997;35(2):281–94.

[37] Botet JF, Lightdale CJ, Zauber AG, et al. Preoperative staging of esophageal cancer: comparison of endoscopic US and dynamic CT. Radiology 1991;181:419–25.

[38] Wu LF, Wang BZ, Feng JL, et al. Preoperative TN staging of esophageal cancer: comparison of miniprobe ultrasonography, spiral CT and MRI. World J Gastroenterol 2003;9(2):219–24.

[38a] Luketich JD, Friedman DM, Weigel TL, et al. Evaluation of distant metastases in esophageal cancer: 100 consecutive positron emission tomography scans. Ann Thorac Surg 1999;68(4):1133–6; discussion 1136–7.

[38b] ten Berge J, Hoffman BJ, Hawes RH, et al. EUS-guided fine needle aspiration of the liver: indications, yield, and safety based on an international survey of 167 cases. Gastrointest Endosc 2002;55(7):859–62.

[39] Jiao X, Eslami A, Ioffe O, et al. Immunohistochemistry analysis of micrometastasis in pretreatment lymph nodes from patients with esophageal cancer. Ann Thorac Surg 2003; 76(4):996–9 [discussion: 999–1000].

[40] Mori M, Mimori K, Inoue H, et al. Detection of cancer micrometastases in lymph nodes by reverse transcriptase-polymerase chain reaction. Cancer Res 1995;55(15):3417–20.

[41] Gerhard M, Juhl H, Kalthoff H, et al. Specific detection of carcinoembryonic antigen-expressing tumor cells in bone marrow aspirates by polymerase chain reaction. J Clin Oncol 1994;12(4):725–9.

[42] Luketich JD, Kassis ES, Shriver SP, et al. Detection of micrometastases in histologically negative lymph nodes in esophageal cancer. Ann Thorac Surg 1998;66(5):1715–8.

SURGICAL
CLINICS OF
NORTH AMERICA

ELSEVIER
SAUNDERS

Surg Clin N Am 85 (2005) 569–582

Esophageal Palliation—Photodynamic Therapy/Stents/Brachytherapy

Neil A. Christie, MD*, Amit N. Patel, MD, MS,
Rodney J. Landreneau, MD

Division of Foregut and Thoracic Surgery, Shadyside Medical Center, University of Pittsburgh, 5200 Centre Avenue, Suite 715 Pittsburgh, PA 15232, USA

Early spread of esophageal cancer and absence of symptoms in patients who have early cancer results in the majority of patients presenting with incurable cancer. The primary treatment for patients who have metastatic disease or unresectable disease is palliation of dysphagia and maintenance of adequate oral nutrition [1,2]. Even after aggressive treatment with combinations of radiotherapy and chemotherapy, many patients present with locally recurrent or persistent symptomatic disease [3]. Malignant dysphagia, defined as difficulty with swallowing due to cancer, results from a partially or completely obstructed esophageal lumen and leads to malnutrition, aspiration, and sialorrhea. Frequent pulmonary infections may be caused by regurgitation of food, vocal cord paralysis, or tracheo-esophageal (TE) fistulae. Many patients who have advanced cancer are sufficiently debilitated to prevent safe palliation with surgery or chemotherapy and radiation. In such patients, endoluminal therapies can improve the quality of life by relieving dysphagia [1–3]. Such therapies include photodynamic therapy, esophageal brachytherapy, and esophageal expandable metal stents.

Photodynamic therapy

Photodynamic therapy (PDT) is a two-stage process. In the first stage, the photosensitzer porfimer sodium is administered intravenously. The next stage is 48 hours after the initial injection. Because of differences in tumor vascular supply and lymphatic clearance, the photosensitizer is selectively

* Corresponding author.
E-mail address: christiena@upmc.edu (N.A. Christie).

0039-6109/05/$ - see front matter © 2005 Elsevier Inc. All rights reserved.
doi:10.1016/j.suc.2005.02.001   *surgical.theclinics.com*

retained in the tumor at 48 hours. Flexible endoscopy is then performed to visualize the tumor, and light is delivered to the tumor through a flexible gastroscope with an optical fiber (Fig. 1). The photosensitizer absorbs light energy, and through a photochemical reaction produces tumoricidal reactive oxygen species. The PDT tumor cytotoxicity occurs over hours to days after light application. A repeat endoscopy 48 to 72 hours after the initial treatment is usually undertaken to assess tumor response, for debridement of necrotic tumor, and for a second light application. The palliation of dysphagia is usually evident in 5 to 7 days [4]. Some patients may have temporary worsening of dysphagia caused by tumor edema before necrotic tissue separation. Porfimer sodium is administered intravenously at a dose of 2 mg/kg over 3 to 5 minutes. The monochromatic light (630 nm wavelength) dose administered is usually 300 to 400 joules/cm tumor with treatment times of 10 to 20 minutes required to deliver the light [5].

McCaughn et al [6] reported 77 patients who had inoperable esophageal cancer. Forty patients had failed conventional therapy (chemotherapy, surgery, external beam radiation, brachytherapy, or Nd:YAG laser). Patients were treated with 300 J/cm tumor with a repeat endoscopy 24 to 72 hours after the initial treatment. Tumors regressed and swallowing improved in all patients. Mean survival was 6.3 months. Many patients had prolonged survival, particularly those who had clinical Stage I tumors (Figs. 2, 3).

Moghissi and colleagues [7] reported 65 patients who had inoperable esophageal cancer and who were treated with PDT; 89% had previous treatment. Dysphagia was relieved in all patients and there was no mortality. Mean survival was 7.7 months, and was influenced by performance status at time of presentation and stage of disease.

Marcon [8] reported experience in 83 cases of esophageal cancer, 60% of whom had recurred after previous radiotherapy or surgery. The average length of survival reported was 4 months, with patients who had less advanced cancer experiencing longer survival. The average duration of improvement in swallowing was 6 weeks, and 40% of patients required retreatment for tumor ingrowth.

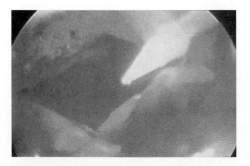

Fig. 1. Endoscopic view of light application for photodynamic therapy using flexible fiber.

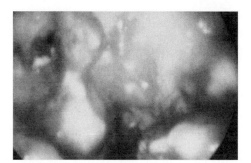

Fig. 2. Endoscopic view of tumor before photodynamic therapy.

Luketich and associates [5] reported results in 77 patients who had inoperable obstructing esophageal cancer treated with PDT, 43% of whom had undergone previous treatment with radiation or chemotherapy. The mean dysphagia score at 4 weeks improved in 91% of patients. PDT controlled bleeding in 6 of 6 patients who had bleeding. Twenty nine patients (38%) required more than one PDT course, and 7 patients required placement of an expandable metal stent for recurrent dysphagia. The mean dysphagia free interval was 11 weeks, and the median survival was 5.9 months.

In the Luketich series, complications were reported as esophageal stricture 4.8%, candida esophagitis 3.2%, symptomatic pleural effusion 3.2%, and skin photosensitivity reaction 10%. Three of 77 patients developed perforation in 125 treatments. Two perforations were treated with covered esophageal stents and one with diversion surgery. Thirty-day mortality was 3.9% (from aspiration pneumonia and from perforation). Other common morbidities reported after PDT included substernal pain, odynophagia, transient worsening of dysphagia, fever, and leukocytosis.

Patients who have had previous chemoradiation or radiation and brachytherapy may be particularly at risk of serious complications. Sanfilippo and colleagues [9] reported an epidural abscess, a TE fistula, and

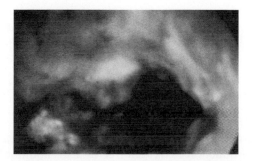

Fig. 3. Endoscopic view of tumor after photodynamic therapy.

esophageal fistulisation with the pulmonary artery and massive bleeding in three patients who had been pretreated with external-beam radiotherapy and brachytherapy.

Photofrin is a skin sensitizer, and patients must be educated about the precautions necessary to avoid skin reactions during the 4- to 6-week period of photosensitivity associated with photofrin. These precautions include avoidance of direct sunlight and use of opaque clothing and sunglasses. Commercially available sunscreens do not protect against skin injury, because they block ultraviolet light but not the damaging infrared light. Graded exposure to light promotes photobleaching and reduces the duration of photosensitivity [10].

PDT has been reported for esophageal obstruction secondary to tumor ingrowth and overgrowth of expandable metal stents [11]. PDT is not damaging to stents due to its nonthermal nature. The Luketich series [5] included 12 patients who were treated for tumor ingrowth or overgrowth through a previously placed esophageal stent, and an improvement in dysphagia score was seen in all of this subset of patients.

Before the advent of PDT, Nd:YAG laser had been used for the palliation of malignant dysphagia from obstructing esophageal cancer. Reports of success vary from 69% to 83% [2,12]. PDT was compared with Nd:YAG laser for palliation of esophageal cancer in a randomized multicenter study of 218 patients. Improvement in dysphagia was similar in both groups. Fewer treatment sessions were needed in the PDT group, but dysphagia was seen to recur at approximately 1 month in both groups. There was a higher rate of minor side effects in the PDT group (skin photosensitivity 19%, nausea 8%, fever 16%, pleural effusion 10%); however, the procedural perforation rate was 7% in the Nd:YAG group compared with only 1% in the PDT group. PDT was technically easier to apply and better tolerated by patients during the procedure. Tumors that were long, flat, angulated, and infiltrating were more easily treated with PDT [13].

Heier and coworkers [14] compared PDT with Nd:YAG laser in the management of obstructing esophageal cancer in a randomized trial of 52 patients (32 PDT patients and 20 Nd:YAG). Both modalities relieved dysphagia, but PDT resulted in a longer duration of response (84 versus 57 days). PDT was associated with an improved Karnofsky performance status at 1 month. Ninety-five percent of patients either had no dysphagia or dysphagia limited to solids 1 week after treatment, and 84% had no dysphagia or dysphagia limited to solids at 1 month. Marcon [8] commented that PDT is especially favorable for upper one-third esophageal cancers, tumors greater than 8 cm in length, and infiltrative tumors; and that it was superior to Nd:YAG in these circumstances.

Advantages of PDT over Nd:YAG laser relate to the nonthermal photochemical process of tumor ablation. Because PDT causes necrosis by light-stimulated production of oxygen free radicals and not by heat, the risk of perforation is theoretically lower. The depth of penetration and tumor necrosis after PDT is limited to approximately 5 mm. This limited depth provides a safety factor, and also likely contributes to the lower rate of perforation [15].

PDT is also useful for superficial tumors that are potentially respectable for cure, but that occur in patients who are otherwise poor operative candidates.

Corti and coauthors [16] treated 62 medically inoperable patients who had early-stage (in-situ, T1, and T2) and local recurrences that were not evident radiologically outside of the esophagus. They were injected with 5 mg/kg photofrin and treated with 200 to 300 J/cm tumor A complete response was seen in 37% (23/62) of patients with PDT alone. External beam therapy (64 Gy) was applied to incomplete responders to PDT, and complete response was seen in 82% (51/62) patients who received PDT with or without external beam therapy. Complete response was 44% in T in-situ and T1, 28% in T2, and 0% for local recurrence. The complete response was durable in 52% (median follow-up 32 months; range 3–90). Median time to progression was 49 months with T in situ/T1, 30 months with T2, and 14 months with local recurrence.

Sibille et al [17] in France treated 123 patients who had T1 and T2 adeno and squamous carcinomas. Complete response was seen in 87% at 6 months. The overall 5-year survival was 25%, but disease-specific survival was 75%, confirming the efficacy of PDT in appropriately selected patients. Tian and associates [18] treated 13 patients who had early squamous cell carcinoma of the esophagus . Using balloon cytology follow-up, 12 out of 13 patients had negative cytology results over 21 to 32 months.

Disadvantages of PDT include the requirement for expensive equipment, the relatively long waiting-time period between the time of drug injection and treatment, the high cost of the photosensitizing agents, and skin photosensitivity. Photosensitzers cost approximately $4000 per treatment. If subsequent retreatment is needed weeks or months after the initial therapy, additional doses of photosensitizer are required.

Advantages of PDT include safe and rapid reestablishment of an esophageal lumen, and improvement in patients' nutritional status and overall condition without limiting future treatment options, such as chemo-radiation or surgery. PDT also has numerous antitumor effects in addition to direct tumor necrosis, including cytokine and interleukin-associated inflammatory response, destruction of tumor vasculature, induction of apoptosis, and immune system stimulation [19].

Brachytherapy

Brachytherapy enables patients to obtain the benefits of radiation to decrease or obliterate the local tumor burden, without the harmful effects of collateral damage resulting from external beam radiation. Current brachytherapy catheters involve emission of high doses of radiation very close to the catheter. Within a very short distance, the dose exponentially decreases. This results in very little damage to the surrounding tissue. Although the role of brachytherapy for cure is limited, with only a few case reports in the literature, when used for palliation brachytherapy results in a 50% to 80% improvement in dysphagia. Sharma and associates [20] evaluated 58 patients who received palliative brachytherapy (38 patients) or combination external beam radiation and brachytherapy (20 patients). Median dysphagia-free survival was 10 months, but there was an overall complication rate of 30%. A recent randomized study [21] demonstrated that high-dose fractionated brachytherapy in 232 patients resulted in improvement in dysphagia, with few complications of stricture or fistulas (10%).

Other approaches to deliver effective brachytherapy have recently been developed. A novel approach to current brachytherapy options using Iridium 192 (Ir-192) is the addition of hyperthermia. A small in-vitro study [22] found a higher depth of penetration for tumoricidal effect when Ir-192 plus 42°C to 44°C was present. The researchers found that the depth of penetration was 5 to 10 mm beneath the esophageal mucosa. Recently, self-expanding, radionuclide-impregnated stents have been developed. They have been able deliver a higher dose of local radiation over a longer period of time. The key to this therapy is to determine a safe dose of radiotherapy without fear of transmural necrosis or perforation of the esophageal wall [23].

Brachytherapy enables relatively safe treatment of dysphagia and a decrease in tumor burden for nonresectable esophageal cancer. Further enhancement in delivery techniques may allow wider application of the therapy.

Expandable metal stents

Expandable metal stents are made of metal alloys, and are compressed and restrained on a delivery device. After positioning, expansion occurs, and the stents embed themselves in the tumor and surrounding tissue with radial pressure, and are eventually incorporated into the wall of the organ (Fig. 4).

Raijman and coworkers [24] reported experience in 101 metal esophageal stents. Dysphagia score was improved in all patients. Success in treating esophago-respiratory fistulae was seen in all patients. Overall complication rate was 38%. Life-threatening complications were seen in 7.9%, but there were no deaths. Sensation of well-being and quality of life was improved in 82% of patients. No worse outcome was noted in patients who had undergone previous chemoradiation.

Cwikiel and coauthors [25] reported experience in 100 expandable metal stents. A substantial reduction of dysphagia was noted. Effectiveness was independent of location, length, or diameter of stricture. A higher compli-

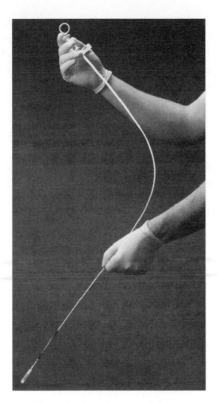

Fig. 4. Expandable metal stent delivery system.

cation rate was noted for treatment of strictures at the upper esophagus (53%) versus the mid or lower esophagus.

O'Sullivan and colleagues [26] reported 138 stents in 121 patients. Improvement in dysphagia was seen in 95% of patients. Average survival time after stent placement was 24 weeks. Reintervention was required in 26 patients.

There can be significant morbidity related to stent placement. Intraprocedural complications include those associated with conscious sedation, aspiration, malpositioning of the stent, and esophageal perforation. The smaller diameter of expandable metal stents before deployment makes aggressive dilation of the esophagus before or after deployment unnecessary, and the risk of perforation is lower with metal stents compared with plastic stents [27]. Because expandable metal stents are not meant to be removed, a major pitfall to be avoided is improper placement. The Ultraflex stent (Boston Scientific) may be moved proximally by grasping the string and pulling back. Other stents are harder to move. The radial force of the Wallstent (Boston Scientific, Boston, Massachusetts) is greater than that of the Gianturco Z-stent (Cook, Minneapolis, Minnesota), which is greater than that of the nitinol Ultraflex stent. Except for the Gianturco Z-type stent, all stents shorten up to 20% with expansion. Proper identification of the proximal and distal tumor margins is essential, and submucosal injection of radio-opaque contrast with a variceal needle, mucosal clips, or external markers has been described [28].

Immediate postprocedural complications may include chest pain, bleeding, foreign body sensation, and tracheal compression with resultant airway compromise and respiratory arrest. Tumors in the upper esophagus must be assessed very carefully, including use of bronchoscopy, to evaluate the presence of tracheal compression. Placement of expandable metal stents for very proximal esophageal lesions is technically difficult, because of the proximity of the stent to the upper esophageal sphincter and the lack of an uninvolved proximal margin, increasing the risk of foreign body sensation [29]. Continuous expansion pressure may result in chronic thoracic pain. Late complications include distal stent migration, formation of an esophageal fistula, bleeding, chronic reflux and aspiration pneumonitis, and stent occlusion. Obstruction can occur from tumor ingrowth in uncovered portions, tumor overgrowth, food impaction, stent migration, and angulation of the stricture causing the distal opening to impinge upon the esophageal wall or gastric wall (Fig. 5) [28]. Pressure necrosis by the expandable metal stent may result in gastrointestinal bleeding, perforation, or TE fistula. If the stent becomes occluded by tissue overgrowth or ingrowth, a second stent may be placed, or photodynamic therapy may be used to treat stent occlusion [5]. Polyurethane or silicone covered stents, used to prevent tumor ingrowth, do not become embedded, and thus migration is possible (Fig. 6). Partially covered stents are now generally used to prevent tumor ingrowth and still permit anchoring of the stent. Adam et al [30] evaluated 60 patients who had obstructing esophageal cancer: 23 were

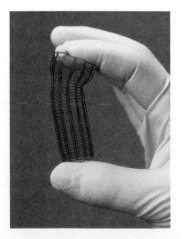

Fig. 5. Uncovered expandable metal stent.

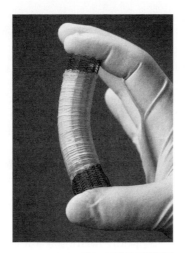

Fig. 6. Covered expandable metal stent.

treated with a covered stent, 19 with an uncovered stent, and 18 with laser ablative therapy. Six of 23 (26%) of covered stents migrated, whereas no uncovered stents migrated. Tumor ingrowth occurred in 5 of 19 (26%) of patients who had uncovered stents. Metallic stent endoprostheses gave better palliation of dysphagia than laser. There was equivalent short-term palliation with covered versus uncovered stents. Reintervention was necessary in 10 of 23 (43%) of patients who had covered stents, 5 of 19 (26%) who had uncovered stents, and 18 of 18 (100%) of patients treated with laser. Uncovered metallic stents did not migrate from their original position, whereas plastic-covered endoprostheses migrated in 6 patients (completely migrated into the stomach in 2 patients). The plastic covering is outside the metallic mesh, thus decreasing the friction between the stent and the esophageal wall. All the instances of migration occurred in patients who had low esophageal tumors. One should consider use of uncovered stents when the distal end extends into the stomach, because they are prone to migration.

Tumors at the esophagogastric (EG) junction create special problems. As short a stent as possible should be chosen and seated firmly in the tumor. Crossing the EG junction increases the risk of migration and reflux. When stents cross the EG junction, acid suppression and antireflux measures such as head of bed elevation are recommended. Expandable metal stents are best suited for midesophageal lesions.

Morbidity has been reported as perforation 6%, hemorrhage 3.5%, aspiration pneumonia 0.2%, and tube dislocation 15%. Late complications have been reported as obstruction 9.5%, dislocation 8%, pressure necrosis and fistulisation 3%. Mortality after a perforation runs 27% to 50%. Approximately 0.5% to 2.0% of patients who undergo the procedure die as a direct result of placement of an expandable metal stent [5,28]. Although expandable metal stents decrease the rate of early complications, late complications may be significant.

Several studies strongly suggest that the rates of delayed esophageal complications caused by expandable metal stents are higher in patients who have previously been treated with radiation, chemotherapy, or both. These complications are presumably due to stent-induced pressure within devitalized esophageal tissue. Unfortunately, patients who have recurrent or persistent dysphagia or a TE fistula after chemoradiation therapy often have no alternative to a stent for palliation of their symptoms. Kinsman and associates [31] reported increased complications occurring in patients who had a history of prior radiation therapy or chemotherapy compared with those who had no prior radiation or chemotherapy.

Compared with plastic stents, expandable metal stents offer an increased ease of insertion, because large-bore dilation is not required. The metal stent lumen is larger than the rigid state, and should have less food impaction (plastic tubes have internal diameters of 10–2 mm and external diameters of 14–17 mm). Metal stent placement can be done with intravenous sedation.

Knyrim and coworkers [27] reported a trial comparing expandable metal stents with conventional plastic prostheses. Complications related to device placement and functioning were significantly less in the metal stent group. A much longer hospitalization period was required in the plastic stent group. Roseveare and coauthors [32] evaluated expandable metal stents versus plastic Atkinson tubes in a randomized trial. Overall, the complications were similar. Patients who had Gianturco stents had better palliation of dysphagia, maintained their weight longer, enjoyed their food more, and survived longer. Median survival was 41 days following rigid stent insertion, and 96 days after expandable stent insertion. Nicholson and colleagues [33] found metal stents to be cost-effective, based on a decreased need for reinterventions and hospitalizations compared with conventional therapy. Depalma et al [34] also evaluated plastic stents versus expandable metal stents. Dysphagia scores improved significantly and similarly in both groups. Complications and mortality related to implantation were significantly less frequent with metal stents than with plastic prostheses (mortality 15.8% versus 0%). Both groups had obstruction by food, tube migration was only with plastic prostheses, and tumor ingrowth was only with metal stents. Davies and associates [35] evaluated Atkinson tubes versus metal expandable stents. Atkinson tubes were placed with a perforation rate of 17% and a length of stay of 10 days, compared with 41 metal stents placed with a perforation rate of 2.4% and a length of stay of 3 days. All patients reported an improvement in dysphagia after prosthesis insertion. There was no difference in median survival with 72 days after Atkinson tube and 91 days after metal stent.

Despite the substantially higher cost of expandable metal stents as compared with traditional rigid plastic esophageal stents, there are substantial overall cost savings resulting from the reduction in the number of days of hospitalization due to complications. Expandable metal stents, when compared with rigid prostheses, are easier and safer to place, open to a greater diameter, and perhaps decrease overall costs and morbidity. Owing to their relative lack of longitudinal flexibility, rigid stents cannot bend easily to fit around a curvature. They are difficult to stent at the EG junction.

Dallal and coworkers [36] looked at the relative efficacy of thermal ablative therapy versus expandable metal stents in the palliation of obstructing esophageal cancer. Thermal ablation therapy had a median survival of 125 days versus only 68 days for stent ($P < 0.05$). The median length of stay and cost, however, were greater for patients treated with thermal ablation. The median change in dysphagia score was zero in both groups at one month. Complications of this laser therapy include TE fistulae, bleeding, and perforation. Drawbacks include the fact that multiple treatments (two or three sessions) are frequently necessary to producer satisfactory relief of dysphagia, and that extrinsic or submucosal lesions cannot be treated with laser. Laser is most effective for exophytic short segment strictures, and can be useful for proximal lesions in which expandable metal stents are not feasible. Though proximal cervical tumors can be treated with stents, a general contraindication to stenting is a tumor within 3 cm of the cricopharyngeus. The discomfort and potential airway compression associated with proximal stents favor treatment with laser therapy first.

An advantage of expandable metal stents over other endoscopic palliative methods is that they can be used to treat dysphagia due to compression caused by cancer, although the improvement in dysphagia is less than for patients who have esophageal cancer. Stents are particularly useful for long asymmetric or tortuous strictures, tumors leading to extrinsic compression, or esophago-respiratory fistulae.

Esophageal expandable metal stents are used to treat TE fistulae due to cancer. TE fistulae develop in patients who have advanced esophageal cancer and lung cancer, and lead to continuous aspiration of saliva. TE fistula is the only condition in which covered expandable metal stents may increase survival as compared with other therapies. In a study of 29 patients who had TE fistulae [37] (9 as a complication of a previous stent), 26 of 29 closed successfully with stenting, and 3 of 9 with a previous stent were not fully closed. Dysphagia rate improved to 1.3 from 3.8, pneumonia improved in 83%, and dysphagia improved in 100%. Mean survival time was 127 days.

TE fistulae require tight sealing. Some favor a coated Schneider Wallstent because of funnel-shaped proximal end. The nitinol Ultraflex stents flange is more flexible, less flared, and has allowed "wisps" of contrast to flow between the flange and the esophageal wall.

Although essentially all stented patients have an improvement in swallowing, only 10% to 50% eat solids, and 50% to 70% are restricted to a semisolid diet. Patients who have esophageal stents must modify their diets to prevent large boluses of food from being impacted within the stent.

Considerations after stent placement are to avoid large solid food boluses by cutting food into small pieces and chewing well. Food should be accompanied by ample liquids.

Future directions with expandable metal stents are those that emit radiation or release chemotherapeutic agents.

Summary

The optimal treatment for malignant dysphagia should be safe, effective, cost-effective, and have minimal morbidity. Photodynamic therapy, brachytherapy, and esophageal stenting all represent viable options for the palliation of malignant dysphagia. Characterization of the patients and their tumors allows individualization of the treatment and the selection of the optimal treatment for each individual patient. Institutional resources and expertise also are significant factors in treatment. Further comparative studies may help further delineate the relative merits of these treatments and the optimal treatment of patients with malignant obstruction.

References

[1] Reed CE. Comparison of different treatments for unresectable esophageal cancer. World J Surg 1995;19:828–35.
[2] Ponec RJ, Kimmey MB. Endoscopic therapy of esophageal cancer. Surg Clin North Am 1997;77(5):1198–217.
[3] Adler DG, Baron TH. Endoscopic palliation of malignant dysphagia. Mayo Clin Proc 2001; 76(2):731–8.
[4] Bown SG, Millson CE. Photodynamic therapy in gatroenterology. Gut 1997;41(1):5–7.
[5] Luketich JD, Christie NA, Buenaventura PO, et al. Endoscopic photodynamic therapy for obstructing esophageal cancer: 77 cases over a two year period. Surg Endosc 2000;14:653–7.
[6] McCaughan JS, Ellison EC, Guy JT, et al. Photodynamic therapy for esophageal malignancy: a prospective twelve-year study. Ann Thorac Surg 1996;62:1005–110.
[7] Moghissi K, Dixon K, Thorpe JA, et al. The role of photodynamic therapy in inoperable oesophageal cancer. Eur J Cardiothorac Surg 2000;17:95–100.
[8] Marcon NE. Photodynamic therapy and cancer of the esophagus. Semin Oncol 1994;21(6): 20–3.
[9] San Filippo NJ, Hsi A, DeNittis AS, et al. Toxicity of photodynamic therapy after combined external beam radiotherapy and intraluminal brachytherapy for carcinoma of the upper aerodigestive tract. Lasers Surg Med 2001;28.278–81.
[10] Pass HI. Photodynamic therapy in oncology: mechanisms and clinical use. J Natl Cancer Inst 1993;85(6):443–56.
[11] Scheider DM, Siemens M, Cirocco M, et al. Photodynamic therapy for the treatment of tumor ingrowth in expandable metal stents. Endoscopy 1997;29:271–4.
[12] Overholt BF. Laser and photodynamic therapy of esophageal cancer. Semin Surg Oncol 1992;191–203.
[13] Lightdale CJ, Heier SK, Marcon NE, et al. Photodynamic therapy with porfimer sodium versus thermal ablation therapy with Nd:YAG laser for palliation of esophageal cancer: a multicenter randomized trial. Gastroint Endosc 1995;42:507–12.

[14] Heier SK, Rothman KA, Heier LM, et al. Photodynamic therapy for obstructing esophageal cancer: light dosimetry and randomized comparison with Nd:YAG laser therapy. Gastroenterology 1995;109:63–72.

[15] Barr H, Dix AJ, Kendall C, et al. Review article: the potential role for photodynamic therapy in the management of upper gastrointestinal disease. Aliment Pharmacol Ther 2001;15: 311–21.

[16] Corti L, Skarlatos J, Boso C, et al. Outcome of patients receiving photodynamic therapy for early esophageal cancer. Int J Radiat Oncol Biol Phys 2000;47(2):419–24.

[17] Sibille A, Lambert R, Souquet JC, et al. Long-term survival after photodynamic therapy for esophageal cancer. Gastroenterology 1995;108:337–44.

[18] Tian ME, Qui SL, Ji Q. Preliminary results of hematoporphyrin derivative laser treatment for 13 cases of early esophageal carcinoma. Adv Exp Med Biol 1985;193:21–5.

[19] Dougherty TJ, Gomer CJ, Henderson BW, et al. Photodynamic therapy. J Natl Cancer Inst 1998;90:889–905.

[20] Sharma V, Mahantshetty U, Dinshaw KA, et al. Palliation of advanced/recurrent esophageal carcinoma with high dose-rate brachytherapy. Int J Radiat Oncol Biol Phys 2002;52:310–5.

[21] Sur RK, Levin CV, Donde B, et al. Prospective randomized trial of HDR brachytherapy as a sole modality in palliation of advanced esophageal carcinoma—an international atomic energy agency study. Int J Radiat Oncol Biol Phys 2002;53(1):127–33.

[22] Furuta M, Tsukiyama I, Kano Y. Simultaneous intraluminal thermobrachytherapy: an in vitro study. Jpn J Cancer Res 2001;92(8):904–9.

[23] Won JH, Lee JD, Wang HJ, et al. Self-expandable covered metallic esophageal stent impregnated with beta-emitting radionuclide: an experimental study in canine esophagus. Int J Radiat Oncol Biol Phys 2002;53(4):1005–13.

[24] Raijman I, Siddique I, Ajani J, et al. Palliation of malignant dysphagia and fistulae with coated expandable metal stents: experience with 101 patients. Gastrointest Endosc 1998;48: 172–9.

[25] Cwikiel W, Tranberg K, Cwikiel M, et al. Malignant dysphagia: palliation with esophageal stents—long term results in 100 patients. Radiology 1998;207(2):513–8.

[26] O'Sullivan GJ, Grundy A. Palliation of malignant dysphagia with expanding metallic stents. J Vasc Interv Radiol 1999;10(3):346–51.

[27] Knyrim K, Wagner H, Bethge N, et al. A controlled trial of an expansile metal stent for palliation of esophageal obstruction due to inoperable cancer. N Engl J Med 1993;329: 1302–7.

[28] Reed C. Pittfalls and complications of esophageal prosthesis, laser therapy, and dilation. Chest Surg Clin N Am 1997;7(3):623–36.

[29] Kozarek RA, Ball TJ, Patterson DJ. Metallic self-expanding stent application in the upper gastrointestinal tract: caveats and concerns. Gastrointest Endosc 1992;38:1–6.

[30] Adam A, Ellul J, Watkinson AF, et al. Palliation of inoperable esophageal carcinoma: a prospective randomized trial of laser therapy and stent placement. Radiology 1997;202: 344–8.

[31] Kinsman KJ, DeGregorio BT, Katon RM, et al. Prior radiation and chemotherapy increase the risk of life-threatening complications after insertion of metallic stents for esophagogastric malignancy. Gastrointest Endosc 1996;43:196–203.

[32] Roseveare CD, Patel P, Simmonds N, et al. Metal stents improve dysphagia, nutrition and survival in malignant esopghageal stenosis: a randomized controlled trial comparing modified Gianturco Z-stents with plastic Atkinson tubes. Eur J Gastroenterol Hepatol 1998; 10:653–7.

[33] Nicholson DA, Haycox A, Kay CL, et al. The cost-effectiveness of metal oesophageal stenting in malignant disease compared with conventional therapy. Clin Radiol 1999; 54:212–5.

[34] DePalma GD, diMatteo E, Romano G, et al. Plastic prosthesis versus expandable metal stents for palliation of inoperable esophageal thoracic carcinoma: a controlled prospective study. Gastroint Endosc 1996;43(5):478–82.

[35] Davies N, Thomas HG, Eyre-Brook IA. Palliation of dysphagia from inoperable oesophaegal carcinoma using Atkinson tubes or self-expanding metal stents. Ann R Coll Surg Engl 1998;80:394–7.

[36] Dallal HJ, Smith GD, Grieve DC. A randomized trial of thermal ablative therapy versus expandable metal stents in the palliative treatment of patients with esophageal carcinoma. Gastrointest Endosc 2001;54(5):549–57.

[37] Kishi K, Takeuchi T, Sonomura T, et al. Treatment of a malignant esophageal fistula with a Gore-Tex-covered flexible nitinol stent. Cardiovasc Intervent Radiol 1997;20:63–6.

ELSEVIER
SAUNDERS

Surg Clin N Am 85 (2005) 583–592

SURGICAL
CLINICS OF
NORTH AMERICA

Ivor Lewis Esophagogastrectomy

Francis C. Nichols III, MD, Mark S. Allen, MD,
Claude Deschamps, MD*, Stephen D. Cassivi, MD,
Peter C. Pairolero, MD

*Division of General Thoracic Surgery, Mayo Clinic College of Medicine,
200 First Street SW, Rochester, MN 55905, USA*

Resection of the esophagus remains a challenge to general thoracic surgeons, even with modern surgical techniques [1]. Surgical treatment for carcinoma of the esophagus is further complicated because the patients are often elderly, obese, and have associated cardiopulmonary disease. Even the choice of which operation to perform is not simple, because there are a variety of "standard" operations for esophageal resection. One of the current standard operations for esophageal disease was presented on January 10, 1946, when Ivor Lewis gave the Hunterian Lecture to the Royal College of Surgeons in London [2,3]. At the time of this lecture, successful resections of the esophagus with primary anastomosis were a rarity. Operative procedures that entered the thoracic cavity were fraught with danger because anesthesia was primitive, antibiotics were basic, and sophisticated post-operative monitoring was yet to come. Nevertheless, Lewis described an operation in which the esophagus was resected via a thoracic approach in two stages. The first stage was done through an abdominal incision, and freed the stomach, basing it on the right gastric and right gastroepiploic arteries. He also placed a jejunostomy tube during this first stage for nutritional support. The second stage was done 1 to 2 weeks later, and involved resecting the esophagus and performing an anastomosis between the esophagus and stomach in the chest. Despite the simplicity of the pre- and postoperative care of the time, the operation was successful in five of seven patients. The details of the technical aspects of the Ivor Lewis esophagogastrectomy have changed since the original description, but the basic concept has remained the same.

Although different approaches have been described for the surgical resection of esophageal cancer, there is no statistical evidence, either in

---

* Corresponding author.
E-mail address: deschamps.claude@mayo.edu (C. Deschamps).

retrospective comparative series or in prospective randomized trials, that shows a significant difference in outcome. The authors use an Ivor Lewis approach for patients who have distal esophageal and esophagogastric junction carcinomas for several reasons [4–7]. This approach allows complete visualization of all perigastric and periesophageal lymph tissue. It also allows direct visualization and dissection of the thoracic esophagus, thus virtually eliminating the uncommon but potentially disastrous damage to adjacent structures that can occur with transhiatal esophagectomy. We favor the Ivor Lewis approach over the left thoracoabdominal because construction of the anastomosis high in the right chest is technically easier than performing an anastomosis high in the left chest. The procedure remains an excellent technique for patients who have mid and distal esophageal carcinomas. Indications for performing an Ivor Lewis esophagogastrectomy, other than esophageal carcinoma, include high-grade dysphagia in Barrett's esophagus, destruction of the lower two thirds of the esophagus by caustic ingestion, complex strictures following multiple antireflux operations, end-stage motility disorders, and rarely, a perforated esophagus. The Ivor Lewis approach is not indicated for high thoracic or cervical esophageal carcinomas, and can be difficult to perform in patients who have had a previous right thoracotomy.

The authors employ prophylactic cephalosporins (Ancef), subcutaneous heparin, and intraoperative venous compression boots. With the patient supine, an upper midline abdominal incision is made, usually extending alongside the xyphoid. The abdomen is explored. If there is carcinoma in the liver or in unresectable retroperitoneal nodes, the abdomen is closed.

Technical aspects

Setup and incision

To help improve exposure for the thoracic portion of the procedure, a double-lumen endotracheal tube is placed. A retracting device called a Mayo third arm is positioned to allow elevation of the costal arch and improve exposure to the hiatus. The patient is placed supine on the table, and prepared from the chin to the pubis in case a transition to a transhiatal approach is indicated after the exploration. An upper midline incision is begun just to the left of the xyphoid process and extended just cephalad to the umbilicus. Abdominal exploration is performed, carefully assessing for metastatic disease to the liver, peritoneum, and periaortic areas. The retractors are then placed, lifting the costal arch, and the patient is placed in a reverse Trendelenburg position. A Balfour abdominal spreader is placed near the caudal end of the incision to enhance exposure [8].

Assessing local resectability

Once metastatic disease is ruled out, local resectability is assessed. The gastroesophageal junction is mobilized to determine if the tumor is adherent to or invading the vertebral column, aorta, or pericardium. The left lobe of the liver is mobilized and retracted laterally, and the pharyngoesophageal ligament is divided. With blunt dissection, being careful not to transgress the tumor, the esophagus is circled with a Penrose drain. A portion of the crus and diaphragm can be resected with the tumor if necessary. Using manual palpation, adherence to mediastinal structures is assessed. If the tumor is mobile, the resection is begun.

Mobilization of the stomach

The portion of the esophagus that is removed is replaced with a gastric tube made from the greater curvature of the stomach. The goal of the abdominal portion of the operation is to mobilize the stomach. With the stomach retracted cephalad and the colon caudad, the lesser sac is entered through the mesocolon, below the right gastroepiploic arcade. The omentum is then divided, carefully preserving the right gastroepiploic vessels. The short gastric vessels are divided, initially using silk ligatures and hemoclips but later with the Harmonic Scalpel LCS (Ultra Cision, Smithfield, Rhode Island). The gastroduodenal pedicle is freed from the duodenum, so that with eventual elevation of the gastric tube, there is no connection to the colon. The stomach is then mobilized from the spleen, taking all short gastric vessels until the hiatus is reached. No attempt is made to leave extra tissue with the short gastric vessels. With the greater curve of the stomach lifted cephalad and the pancreas and celiac axis retracted caudad, the left gastric artery and vein are exposed, ligated, and divided. All nodal tissue found along the cephalad border of the pancreas is swept up with these vessels. The remaining tissue along the aorta cephalad to the hiatus is freed with the specimen. The stomach is then retracted laterally, allowing division of the hepatic branches of the vagal nerves and associated vessels. The stomach is confirmed to be free from the hiatus to the pylorus by passing the Penrose drain in ring fashion over the stomach tube. The hiatus is enlarged to four fingerbreadths by dividing a portion of the right crus, so that there is no ledge effect that may cause future gastric outlet obstruction. The lesser curve area is prepared by dividing all of the blood vessels to the level between the third and fourth branches of the left gastric artery (Fig. 1). The resulting bare area is where the stomach tube ends up in the chest. A pyloromyotomy (Fig. 2) or a pyloroplasty (Fig. 3) is performed to conclude the abdominal portion of the operation. Abdominal wall closure is then performed.

Right thoracotomy

The patient is placed in the left lateral decubitus position and the right lung collapsed. A fourth interspace incision is made over the fifth rib. This allows excellent access to the apex of the chest, so that a high anastomosis

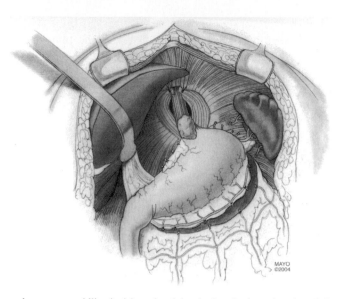

Fig. 1. Through an upper midline incision, the abdominal cavity is explored, and the stomach is mobilized as described in the text. Note that the short gastric vessels have been divided, the right gastroepiploic artery has been preserved, and the lesser curve has been denuded between the third and fourth branches of the left gastric artery. (Courtesy of the Mayo Clinic Foundation, Rochester, MN; with permission.)

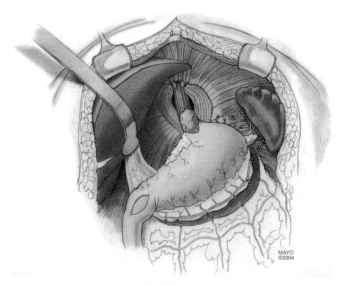

Fig. 2. A pyloromyotomy is attempted routinely. The pylorus muscle is divided under direct vision using Pott scissors. (Courtesy of the Mayo Clinic Foundation, Rochester, MN; with permission.)

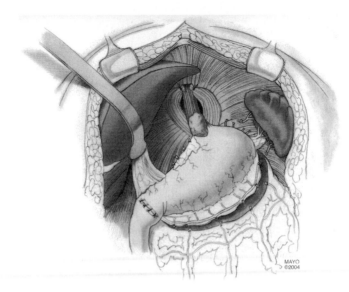

Fig. 3. If the pyloromyotomy results in a mucosal breach or there has been chronic scarring of the pylorus because of previous peptic ulcer disease, a pyloroplasty is performed. The closure is done in two layers, with interrupted 000 silk sutures. (Courtesy of the Mayo Clinic Foundation, Rochester, MN; with permission.)

can be performed. Exploration of the chest is performed, looking for any metastatic disease.

Mobilization of the esophagus

The mediastinal pleura overlying the esophagus is divided laterally along the herniazygos vein, across the hiatus, then back cephalad along the pericardium and to the azygos vein (Fig. 4). The entire envelope of tissue around the esophagus, including lymph nodes, fatty tissue, and the thoracic duct, is freed by developing a plane along the aorta. The thoracic duct is doubly clipped and divided. A Penrose drain is placed around the esophagus for traction. Separate lymph nodes are sampled from the low para-esophageal, inferior pulmonary ligament, subcarinal, and high para-esophageal/paratracheal areas. The azygos vein is ligated and divided at the level of the hemiazygos, disconnecting it from the superior vena cava. The stump on the superior vena cava is oversewn with a 3-0 polypropylene suture. A pleural flap is incised up to the apex of the chest in an inverted-J fashion. The proximal esophagus is then freed to the apex of the chest, staying close to the wall of the esophagus to avoid injury to both the right and left recurrent laryngeal nerves. When the esophagus has been freed to the apex of the thoracic cavity, a Satinski clamp is placed at this level, and the esophagus is divided 1.5 cm caudad to the clamp. The surgical margins are sent for frozen-section inspection.

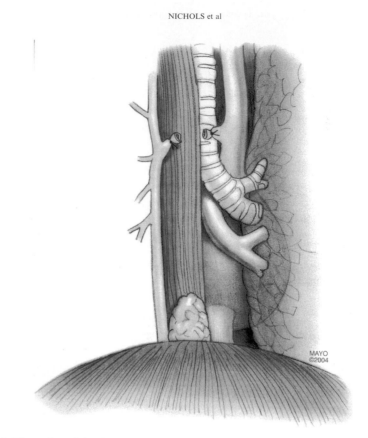

Fig. 4. Through a right thoracotomy approach, the azygos vein has been transected. The esophagus is mobilized from the hiatus up the apex of the chest, as described in the text. (Courtesy of the Mayo Clinic Foundation, Rochester, MN; with permission.)

Preparation of gastric tube and esophagogastric anastomosis

The stomach is transposed through the hiatus into the chest. Hemostasis is carefully achieved along the posterior mediastum where the esophagus was removed. Once the proximal esophageal margin is pathologically cleared, a gastric tube is made based on the greater curvature of the stomach. The fundus of the stomach is stretched out, and the distance to the anastomosis is measured along the greater curve. At this point, a linear stapler is placed transversely to make a 5-cm cut. A stomach tube is then fashioned by additional stapler applications parallel to the greater curvature to a site at the bare area on the lesser curve (Fig. 5). The fundus of the stomach is removed, along with a good portion of the lesser curve and the lymph nodes in this area. The staple lines of the stomach tube are oversewn with running 4-0 polypropylene. An end-to-side anastomosis is performed, placing the stomach tube posterior to the esophagus. A gastrotomy is made and a two-layer interrupted 3-0 polydioxanone (PDS) or silk anastomosis is performed (Figs. 6, 7). The anastomosis is covered with a mediastinal

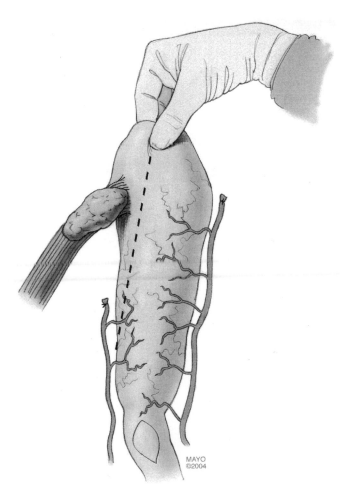

Fig. 5. The stomach has been pulled in the right chest cavity. The surgeon divides the stomach using a linear stapling device along the dotted line, trying to achieve a 5-cm distal margin. The stomach becomes a tube of about 4 cm in diameter. (Courtesy of the Mayo Clinic Foundation, Rochester, MN; with permission.)

pleural flap and the stomach tube secured to the mediastinum with interrupted 3-0 silk.

Chest wound closure

A nasogastric is placed down to the level of the hiatus. The incision is closed in the usual fashion after placement of one chest tube.

Postoperative care

The patient recovers in a monitored bed for one night. The nasogastric tube and chest tubes are removed on the third or fourth postoperative day.

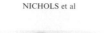

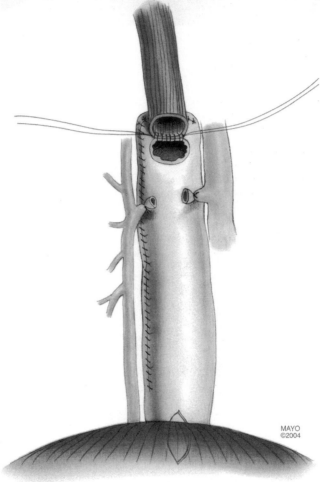

Fig. 6. The staple line on the stomach has been oversewn. The choice of sutures varies among surgeons. The authors use either silk or monofilament polyglyconate (Maxon) interrupted two layers anastomosis. (Courtesy of the Mayo Clinic Foundation, Rochester, MN; with permission.)

A water-soluble radiographic contrast swallow is performed on the sixth postoperative day, and if no leakage or obstruction is noted, the patient's diet is advanced to soft solids over the next 3 or 4 days.

Recent experience

More recently, the authors' group reviewed our experience with a group of patients where most were treated with surgery alone [9]. There were 196

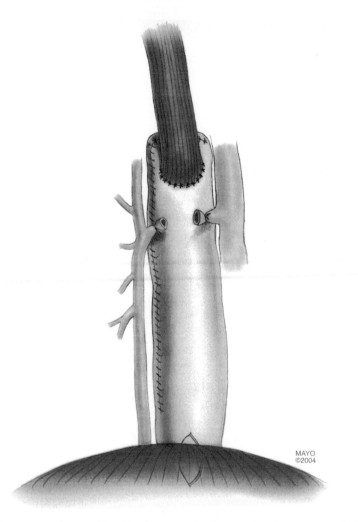

Fig. 7. The anastomosis second layer has been completed. Note that the anastomosis is located well above the azygos vein. (Courtesy of the Mayo Clinic Foundation, Rochester, MN; with permission.)

men (89.1%) and 24 women. Median age was 65 years (range, 29–85 years). Pathology was adenocarcinoma in 188 patients (85.4%), squamous cell carcinoma in 31 (14.1%), and leiomyosarcoma in 1 (0.5%). Postsurgical Stage was 0 in 10 patients, I in 19, IIa in 38, IIb in 28, III in 111, and IV in 14. Operative death occurred in three patients (mortality 1.4%), and complications in 83 (37.7%). Follow-up was 98.6% complete. Median survival for operative survivors was 1.9 years (range, 32 days to 8.7 years). Overall 5-year survival was 25.2%: for Stage 0, 80%; Stage I, 94.4%; Stage IIa, 36.0%; Stage IIb, 14.3%; Stage III, 10%, and Stage IV, 0%. We concluded that Ivor Lewis esophagogastrectomy for esophageal cancer was a safe operation; long-term survival was stage-dependent. The low survival associated with advanced cancers should encourage the search for effective neoadjuvant therapy.

Quality of life

Functional outcome following surgery is affected by age, sex, and type of resection. For those surviving 5 or more years, symptoms of reflux, dumping, and dysphagia are not uncommon. Even if long-term survival after esophagectomy for Stage I and II carcinoma is less than that expected in a normal population, quality of life after resection as assessed by the patients themselves is similar to the national norm [10].

Summary

In conclusion, an Ivor Lewis esophagogastrectomy is a safe surgical approach for esophageal cancer. The technique allows direct visualization and resection of most of the lymph node stations at risk. Survival is stage-dependent and, unfortunately, is low in advanced stages. The increased systemic recurrence warrants the continuing search for multimodality therapy. The authors hope that this series can serve as a baseline for comparison of new and more curative therapeutic options.

References

[1] Allen MS. Ivor Lewis esophagectomy. Semin Thorac Cardiovasc Surg 1992;4:320–3.
[2] Franklin FH. Ivor Lewis Lecture, 1975. The advancing frontiers of oesophageal surgery. Ann R Coll Surg Engl 1977;59:284–7.
[3] Lewis I. The surgical treatment of carcinoma of the oesophagus: with special reference to a new operation for growths of the middle third. Br J Surg 1946;34:18.
[4] King RM, Pairolero PC, Trastek VF, et al. Ivor Lewis esophagogastrectomy for carcinoma of the esophagus: early and late functional results. Ann Thorac Surg 1987;44:119–22.
[5] Lozac'h P, Topart P, Etienne J, et al. Ivor Lewis operation for epidermoid carcinoma of the esophagus. Ann Thorac Surg 1991;52:1154–7.
[6] Pera M, Cameron AJ, Trastek VF, et al. Increasing incidence of adenocarcinoma of the esophagus and esophagogastric junction. Gastroenterology 1993;104.510–3.
[7] Pera M, Trastek VF, Carpenter HA, et al. Barrett's esophagus with high-grade dysplasia: an indication for esophagectomy? Ann Thorac Surg 1992;54:199–204.
[8] Jaroszewski DE, Deschamps C, Gunderson LL, et al. Cancer of the esophagus. In: Kelly KA, Sarr MG, Hinder RA, editors. Mayo Clinic gastrointestinal surgery. Philadelphia: W.B. Saunders; 2004. p. 57–73.
[9] Visbal AL, Allen MS, Miller DL, et al. Ivor Lewis esophagogastrectomy for esophageal cancer. Ann Thorac Surg 2001;71(6):1803–8.
[10] McLarty AJ, Deschamps C, Trastek VF, et al. Esophageal resection for cancer of the esophagus: long-term function and quality of life. Ann Thorac Surg 1997;63(6):1568–72.

SURGICAL
CLINICS OF
NORTH AMERICA

ELSEVIER
SAUNDERS

Surg Clin N Am 85 (2005) 593–610

Transhiatal Esophagectomy

Jules Lin, MD[a], Mark D. Iannettoni, MD, MBA[b],*

[a]Department of Surgery, Section of Thoracic Surgery,
University of Michigan Medical Center, 2120 Taubman Center,
1500 E. Medical Center Drive, Box 0344, Ann Arbor, MI 48109, USA
[b]Department of Cardiothoracic Surgery, The University of Iowa Hospitals and
Clinics, 200 Hawkins Drive, Rm. 1602-JCP, Iowa City, Iowa 52242, USA

Transhiatal esophagectomy (THE) is being performed increasingly in the resection of benign and malignant esophageal disease and has several potential advantages over transthoracic esophagectomy, due to the avoidance of thoracotomy and intrathoracic anastomosis. This article discusses the indications, diagnostic evaluation, and operative techniques for transhiatal esophagectomy. Potential complications as well as the results from large clinical series are also discussed.

History

The first blunt transmediastinal esophagectomy without thoracotomy was reported by Denk in 1913 [1] using a vein stripper to avulse the esophagus in cadavers. In 1933, Turner [2] performed the first successful transhiatal esophagectomy for carcinoma. After the development of endotracheal anesthesia, however, transthoracic esophagectomy could be performed under direct vision, and transhiatal esophagectomy was only used occasionally.

In 1975, Orringer and Sloan [3] described the use of substernal gastric bypass and thoracic esophageal exclusion for palliation of dysphagia for incurable esophageal carcinoma. Although later results showed that this was not an effective palliative procedure and had a high morbidity [4], the results demonstrated that the stomach is able to reach above the level of the clavicles with proper mobilization for cervical esophagogastric anastomosis, and that cervical anastomotic leaks are usually less severe than disruption of an intrathoracic anastomosis. Based on these principles, Orringer and Sloan [5] reported a series in 1978 of 28 patients undergoing THE. The current

---

* Corresponding author.
E-mail address: mark-iannettoni@uiowa.edu (M.D. Iannettoni).

experience at the University of Michigan includes over 1200 patients who have undergone THE over the past 25 years [6,7] and has confirmed, along with the results of others [8–10], that few patients undergoing esophagectomy for benign or malignant disease require a thoracotomy. Operative techniques continue to be refined with the development of the side-to-side stapled cervical esophagogastric anastomosis, which has resulted in a significant decrease in anastomotic leaks—from 10% to 15% to less than 3%, a decreased need for anastomotic dilatation, and improved swallowing [11].

Indications and contraindications

All patients being evaluated for an esophagectomy for benign or malignant disease should be considered potential candidates for THE. Patients who have biopsy-proven distant metastatic disease are considered unresectable, because the risk of esophagectomy outweighs the short-term benefits in Stage IV patients, with a mean survival of only 6 months. Absolute contraindications include bronchoscopic evidence of tracheobronchial invasion in patients who have upper or middle esophageal carcinomas. THE is possible after radiation therapy, and with periesophageal adhesions from caustic injuries, previous operations, or achalasia [6,12,13]. Carcinomas of the cardia and proximal stomach can also be resected by THE, avoiding the intrathoracic anastomosis required after a traditional proximal hemigastrectomy.

Although CT scans are useful in determining metastatic disease, CT is not as reliable in assessing tissue invasion or regional lymph node status [14]. Endoscopic ultrasound (EUS) is more accurate in determining the depth of tumor invasion and regional lymph node dissemination, especially when combined with fine-needle aspiration [15,16]. Thoracoscopic and laparoscopic staging have also been reported [17,18], and positron emission tomography (PET) appears promising in selecting patients for esophagectomy [19,20]; however, the most important assessment is the surgeon's palpation through the hiatus and determination of esophageal fixation. If a safe transhiatal resection cannot be performed, one must be prepared to perform a thoracotomy.

Preoperative evaluation and management

Patients should undergo pulmonary physiotherapy and smoking cessation at least 2 weeks before THE. If weight loss and dehydration are severe because of high-grade esophageal obstruction, nasogastric feedings are started. Percutaneous gastrostomy or jejunostomy feeding tubes may interfere with gastric mobilization and are generally avoided. Patients should also be counseled on possible changes in their eating habits and digestive function. Although 90% of patients eventually have comfortable swallowing and eating, 50% to 60% may require early esophageal dilatations [6]. In addition, varying degrees of postvagotomy "dumping" symptoms are experienced by 26% to 49% of patients, although they are generally controlled with medications and decrease with time [6]. Although colonic bowel preparation is not routinely required, in patients who had previous gastric disease or surgery, a barium enema is performed to evaluate the colon as an esophageal replacement, along with a preoperative bowel preparation.

Anesthetic management

Continuous intra-arterial blood pressure monitoring is performed, because cardiac displacement during the mediastinal dissection may cause hypotension. Although the average blood loss is less than 1000 mL, two large-bore intravenous catheters should be placed in case rapid volume replacement is needed. An epidural catheter is routinely placed and improves postoperative pain control, leading to improvements in pulmonary function. A standard endotracheal tube is used, and can be advanced into the distal trachea or left bronchus if a tear occurs in the membranous trachea. In cases in which the patient has a history of prior esophageal surgery or upper or middle-third tumors, a double-lumen endotracheal tube is considered in case a thoracotomy is required. During the mediastinal dissection, close cooperation and communication between the surgeon and anesthesiologist are required to minimize hypotension.

Operative technique

Transhiatal esophagectomy has been described in detail elsewhere [21,22], and operative techniques are briefly summarized here.

Abdominal phase

The abdominal phase of the procedure is performed through a midline supraumbilical incision. After the triangular ligament is divided, the stomach is carefully examined for significant tumor involvement or scarring from previous surgery or disease. The right gastroepiploic artery is identified early and protected, especially with a history of previous abdominal surgery. The left gastroepiploic and short gastric vessels are ligated. The esophagogastric junction is mobilized, and the left gastric artery is ligated near its origin at the celiac axis. In carcinoma cases, the celiac lymph nodes are sent for pathological staging. Large celiac nodal metastases indicate incurable disease and are biopsied. The right gastric artery is protected as the dissection is continued along the lesser curvature. A Kocher maneuver is then performed to allow mobilization of the pylorus to the level of the xiphoid process. A pyloromyotomy is performed to decrease the incidence of postvagotomy delayed gastric emptying. Clips are placed at the level of the pyloromyotomy as markers for future radiographic studies of gastric emptying.

The distal 5 to 10 cm of esophagus is mobilized through the hiatus. The mobility of the esophageal tumor is then assessed to ensure that it is not fixed to the prevertebral fascia, aorta, or surrounding mediastinal structures. Deaver retractors inserted into the hiatus allow long right-angle clamps to be used to ligate the periesophageal tissues to the level of the carina under direct vision. A jejunostomy tube is placed before proceeding with the cervical phase.

Cervical phase

An oblique incision is made along the anterior border of the sternocleidomastoid muscle. Care must be taken to avoid retraction on the recurrent laryngeal nerve in the tracheoesophageal groove. The middle thyroid vein and inferior thyroid artery may be ligated as needed. After dissecting to the prevertebral fascia, blunt finger dissection is continued into the superior mediastinum. Sharp dissection is used along the anterolateral surface of the esophagus, staying posterior to the recurrent laryngeal nerve. The upper thoracic esophagus is mobilized almost to the level of the carina, using blunt dissection and keeping the fingers directly against the esophagus.

Mediastinal dissection

One hand is inserted through the diaphragmatic hiatus posterior to the esophagus while a half-sponge stick is placed through the cervical incision dissecting the esophagus off the prevertebral fascia (Fig. 1A). The blood pressure is carefully monitored to prevent prolonged hypotension, and a sump catheter is inserted through the cervical incision to evacuate blood from the posterior mediastinum. The anterior mobilization is performed from both the abdominal and cervical incisions, with the fingers directly against the anterior esophagus to avoid injury to the posterior membranous trachea. The esophagus is then held in the superior mediastinum, between the index and middle fingers of the hand inserted through the hiatus, and the remaining attachments are lysed with a downward motion (Fig. 1B). Subcarinal or subaortic periesophageal fibrosis can be finger fractured, or a partial upper sternotomy can be performed for improved exposure, as described by Waddell and Scannell [23]. The upper esophagus is then divided obliquely, leaving some redundancy, and the thoracic esophagus is delivered through the diaphragmatic hiatus. Using Deaver retractors, the posterior mediastinum is inspected through the hiatus for hemostasis. If the pleural cavities have been entered, which occurs in two thirds of cases, chest tubes are placed. The posterior mediastinum is packed to tamponade minor bleeding.

A partial proximal gastrectomy 4 to 6 cm distal to the tumor is performed using a GIA stapler (Fig. 2A). For benign disease or tumors of the middle esophagus, the amount of stomach resected is minimized to preserve

A   B

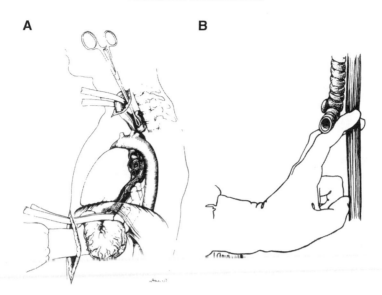

Fig. 1. (*A*) Esophageal mobilization from the prevertebral fascia. (*From* Orringer MB, Sloan H. Esophagectomy without thoracotomy. J Thorac Cardiovasc Surg 1978;76:643; with permission.) (*B*) A downward-raking motion is used to avulse the lateral periesophageal attachments. (*From* Orringer MB. Transhiatal blunt esophagectomy without thoracotomy. In: Cohn LH, editor. Modern techniques in surgery. Cardiovascular surgery, vol. 62. New York: Futura Publishing; 1983. p. 1; with permission.)

collateral circulation to the fundus. The staple line is then oversewn. The mobilized stomach is passed through the hiatus and delivered 4 to 5 cm above the clavicles, primarily by pushing the stomach up through the mediastinum (Fig. 2B). Traction sutures and suction devices to pull the stomach through the mediastinum are avoided to minimize trauma to the gastric tip. "Suspension sutures" to the prevertebral fascia are also avoided, due to the risk of vertebral osteomyelitis. The stomach is then palpated to ensure that there is no torsion.

The abdominal phase is then completed to avoid contamination with oral bacteria from the cervical esophagus. The diaphragm is reapproximated using silk sutures, so that the hiatus permits three fingers to pass alongside the stomach. The anterior gastric wall is approximated to the edge of the hiatus, and the triangular ligament is sutured over the hiatus using silk sutures to prevent hiatal hernia. The pyloromyotomy is covered with omentum.

Cervical esophagogastric anastomosis

A traction suture is placed in the anterior gastric wall to elevate the stomach into the wound. A 1.5 cm vertical gastrotomy is made in the anterior gastric wall, far enough below the gastric fundus to allow the Endo

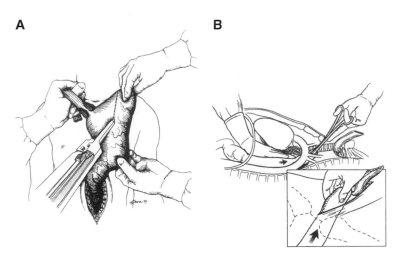

Fig. 2. (*A*) Partial proximal gastrectomy is performed by sequentially applying the GIA stapler. (*From* Orringer MB, Sloan H. Esophageal replacement after transhiatal esophagectomy without thoracotomy. In: Nyhus LM, Baker RJ, editors. Mastery of surgery. 2nd editon. Boston: Little, Brown; 1992. p. 569; with permission.) (*B*) The mobilized stomach is gently passed into the posterior mediastinum. A Babcock clamp is used to carefully grasp the stomach in the superior mediastinum, but the stomach is delivered primarily by pushing from below. (*From* Orringer MB, Marshall B, Iannettoni MD. Eliminating the cervical esophagogastric anastomotic leak with a side-to-side stapled anastomosis. J Thorac Cardiovasc Surg 2000;119:277; with permission.)

GIA (US Surgical, Norwalk, Connecticut) to be fully inserted into the stomach. The cervical esophageal staple line is then obliquely amputated, with enough redundancy to ensure a tension-free anastomosis and sent to pathology as the proximal esophageal margin (Fig. 3A). After placing two stay sutures to align the stomach and esophagus, the Endo GIA is inserted and closed (Fig. 3B, C). Before firing the stapler, two suspension sutures are placed on either side of the anastomosis. After firing the stapler, a nasogastric tube is placed across the anastomosis, and the anterior wall of the anastomosis is then completed in two layers (Figs. 4, 5). Clips are placed beside the anastomosis as radiographic markers, and the wound is closed over a drain.

Minimally invasive approaches

DePaula and associates [24] performed laparoscopic transhiatal esophagectomy in a series of 11 patients. Although technically feasible, there were no clear decreases in morbidity or mortality. Nguyen and coworkers [25] initially performed laparoscopic transhiatal esophagectomy, but switched to a combined laparoscopic and thoracoscopic approach for improved visibility. They compared a minimally invasive series to historical open transthoracic and transhiatal controls, and reported decreased intensive care usage, blood loss, operating times, and length of stay, although

A

B

C

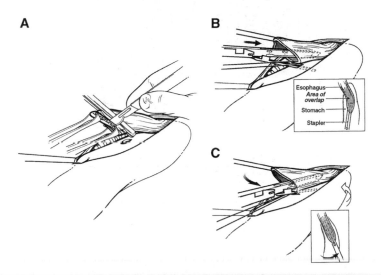

Fig. 3. (*A*) The esophageal staple line is amputated obliquely and submitted to pathology as the proximal margin. (*B*) The Endo GIA stapler is inserted with the thinner anvil into the stomach. (*C*) The stapler is rotated toward the patient's right ear as it is advanced, with care taken to keep the site away from the gastric staple line. (*From* Orringer MB, Marshall B, Iannettoni MD. Eliminating the cervical esophagogastric anastomotic leak with a side-to-side stapled anastomosis. J Thorac Cardiovasc Surg 2000;119:277; with permission.)

complication rates were similar. Glasgow and Swanstrom [26] described a hand-assisted approach, which may serve as a bridge to more advanced experience. Iannettoni and coauthors [27] reported a series of 3 patients using the robotic telemanipulator to perform an esophagectomy. Results were similar to open THE, although operative times were significantly longer, and the procedure will likely involve a learning curve. Three-dimensional visualization and multiarticulated arms may provide technical benefits, although this approach requires further evaluation. Minimally invasive esophagectomy is technically demanding, and further prospective studies are needed to determine if there are significant differences in costs, complication rates, and postoperative pain and recovery.

Postoperative care

A chest radiograph is obtained to evaluate for hemothorax, pneumothorax, or mediastinal widening suggestive of postoperative hemorrhage. Thoracic epidural anesthesia allows immediate extubation in most cases. Incentive spirometry is resumed, and ambulation is encouraged the evening after surgery. Postoperative ileus rarely lasts longer than 72 hours, and nasogastric drainage is usually less than 100 mL/shift by postoperative day 3. Jejunostomy tube feedings of 5% dextrose are started on postoperative day 3 at 30 mL per hour and increased to 60 mL per hour if well tolerated after

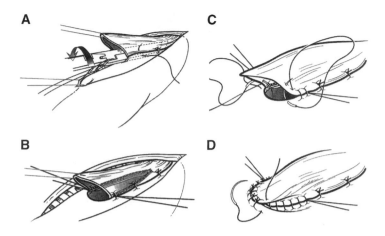

Fig. 4. (*A*) The jaws of the stapler are closed and two suspension sutures placed on either side. (*B*) The anastomosis is inspected for bleeding, and two corner sutures are placed. (*C*) The anterior wall of the anastomosis is completed using a running inner layer of 4-0 monofilament suture and (*D*) an outer interrupted layer. (*From* Orringer MB, Marshall B, Iannettoni MD. Eliminating the cervical esophagogastric anastomotic leak with a side-to-side stapled anastomosis. J Thorac Cardiovasc Surg 2000;119:277; with permission.)

12 hours. Half-strength tube feedings are started the next day, and full-strength feedings the day after that.

The nasogastric tube, Foley, epidural, and arterial catheters are removed by postoperative day 3 to 5. An oral liquid diet is started 24 hours after removal of the nasogastric tube, and tube feedings are decreased. A barium swallow is obtained on postoperative day 7 to confirm adequate gastric emptying and that the anastomosis is intact (Fig. 6). Patients are generally discharged on postoperative day 7. If oral intake is poor, nocturnal supplements are given by jejunostomy tube; however, in most cases patients are eating well, and the jejunostomy tube is removed 4 weeks postoperatively.

Complications of transhiatal esophagectomy

Intraoperative complications include pneumothorax, hemorrhage, and tracheal tear. Early complications that occur within 10 days include hoarseness or difficulty swallowing due to recurrent laryngeal nerve injury, disruption of the anastomosis, arrhythmias, chylothorax, and sympathetic pleural effusion. Early complications that occur in fewer than 1% of patients are epidural abscess, vertebral osteomyelitis, tracheogastric anastomotic fistula, pulmonary microabscesses from an internal jugular vein abscess, and gastric tip necrosis [28]. An inadequate gastric drainage procedure, narrowing of the hiatus, or tumor recurrence can also lead to delayed gastric

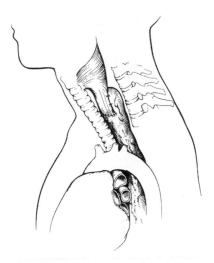

Fig. 5. The completed transhiatal esophagectomy and cervical esophagogastric anastomosis. Two suspension sutures are placed on either side of the anastomosis between the stomach and esophagus to prevent tension on the anastomosis. (*From* Iannettoni MD, Whyte RI, Orringer MB. Catastrophic complications of the cervical esophagogastric anastomosis. J Thorac Cardiovasc Surg 1995;110:1493; with permission.)

emptying. Late complications are relatively uncommon and include diaphragmatic hernia and cervical anastomotic stricture.

Hemorrhage

Aortic esophageal arteries are small branches and generally thrombose if avulsed during esophagectomy [29]. The average intraoperative blood loss is less than 1000 mL if patients are properly selected. Patients who have tumors fixed to the aorta or periesophageal tissues should not undergo THE. If intraoperative hemorrhage occurs, Deaver retractors are placed into the hiatus, a sump catheter is passed through the cervical wound, and the bleeding is identified and controlled. If the point of bleeding cannot be identified, the mediastinum is packed for 5 to 10 minutes with volume resuscitation. If the bleeding continues, the procedure is converted to a thoracotomy.

Tracheal tear

Upon identifying a tracheal tear, the endotracheal tube should be guided by the surgeon distal to the tear. If possible, the esophagectomy should be completed to achieve better exposure before repair. A partial upper sternotomy provides direct visualization of the upper trachea if necessary. Extensive tears involving the carina or mainstem bronchus may require a posterolateral thoracotomy. In these cases, the abdominal and cervical wounds are closed, and the patient is repositioned for a right thoracotomy. After repair, the patient is again placed supine, and the THE is completed.

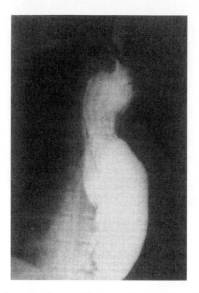

Fig. 6. Postoperative barium swallow with two clips marking the level of the cervical esophagogastric anastomosis. (*From* Orringer MB. Transhiatal esophagectomy without thoracotomy. In: Zuidema GD, Yeo CJ, Orringer MB, et al, editors. Shackelford's surgery of the alimentary tract, vol. 1. 5th edition. Philadelphia: WB Saunders Company; 2002. p. 423; with permission.)

Recurrent laryngeal nerve injury

Injury to the recurrent laryngeal nerve can result in hoarseness as well as cervical dysphagia and potentially serious aspiration pneumonia. This complication is preventable by avoiding the placement of retractors in the tracheoesophageal groove. Since initiating this policy, recurrent laryngeal nerve injury rarely occurs at the authors' institution.

Anastomotic leak

If a patient develops a fever greater than 101°F more than 48 hours postoperatively, a dilute barium swallow is obtained to evaluate for anastomotic leak. Gastrografin may result in chemical pneumonitis if aspirated, and is avoided. Anastomotic leaks are treated by opening the cervical wound at the bedside and initiating dressing changes. The patient can swallow water to wash out the wound. Once the amount of water exiting the leak is small, the patient begins a soft diet while applying pressure to the cervical wound. A 46-French Maloney dilator is passed at the bedside before discharge to decrease the chance of anastomotic stricture and to ensure that there is no distal obstruction [30]. The majority of leaks heal spontaneously in 2 to 3 weeks; however, approximately 50% of cases lead to anastomotic stricture and the need for chronic dilatation [30]. Anastomotic leaks rarely occur after postoperative day 10, and the acute morbidity is usually limited.

Chylothorax

Chest tube drainage greater than 200 to 400 mL per shift for greater than 48 hours should lead one to suspect a thoracic duct injury. Chest tube drainage will be serous until an oral diet of fats has been started. The diagnosis is confirmed by milky chest tube drainage after administering cream through the jejunostomy tube. Most patients are nutritionally compromised and do not tolerate the loss of protein rich chyle. Unless the leak improves within 3 to 5 days of elemental tube feedings, a thoracotomy should be performed with ligation of the thoracic duct.

Sympathetic pleural effusion

Sympathetic pleural effusion may occur during the first postoperative week, due to the mediastinal dissection. Asymptomatic, stable effusions are observed and generally resolve spontaneously. Symptomatic patients are treated with serial thoracentesis, and if the condition persists, injury to the thoracic duct should be considered.

Results of transhiatal esophagectomy

Katariya and colleagues [31] evaluated 23 series with a total of 1353 patients (99% esophageal cancer) published between 1981 and 1992. Complications included anastomotic leak (15.1%), recurrent laryngeal nerve injury (11.3%), cardiac complications (11.9%), splenectomy (2.6%), chylothorax (0.7%), and tracheal injuries (0.67%). Although pulmonary complications occurred in 50% of patients, a wide variety of complications were included, such as pneumothorax, pneumonia, and pleural effusions. Conversion to thoracotomy occurred in 1.3% of cases for hemorrhage, and 30-day mortality was 7.1%; however, 69.5% of the series included fewer than 50 patients and may not reflect the results of more experienced surgeons. Gandhi and Naunheim [32] evaluated eight series of 1192 patients reported between 1992 and 1994, including a series of 583 patients from the University of Michigan [7]. Complications included cardiac complications (16%), anastomotic leak (12%), pulmonary complications (12%), recurrent laryngeal nerve injury (9%), and hemorrhage (3%). The mortality rate was 6.7%.

The largest reported series of 1085 patients treated over 20 years was published by Orringer et al [6]. Twenty-six percent (285 patients) had benign disease, and 74% (800 patients) were treated for carcinoma (Table 1). Of the patients who had malignant disease, 225 patients (28%) had squamous cell carcinomas, and 555 (69%) had adenocarcinomas. Twenty-eight percent (226 patients) who had carcinoma were older than 71. THE was technically possible in 98.6% of cases, despite prior operations in 146 patients (50%) who had benign disease, history of perforations, and radiation treatment. Fifteen patients required thoracotomy for hemorrhage or esophageal fixation. Esophageal resection and reconstruction were performed at the

Table 1
Indications for transhiatal esophagectomy (1085 patients)

Diagnosis	No. of patients (%)
Benign conditions	285 (26)
Neuromotor dysfunction	93 (33)
Achalasia	70
Spasm/dysmotility	22
Scleroderma	1
Stricture	75 (26)
Gastroesophageal reflux	42
Caustic ingestion	19
Radiation	4
Other	10
Barrett's mucosa with high-grade dysplasia	54 (19)
Recurrent gastroesophageal reflux	21 (7)
Recurrent hiatus hernia	14 (5)
Acute perforation	14 (5)
Acute caustic injury	6
Other	8
Carcinoma of intrathoracic esophagus	800 (74)
Upper third	36 (4.5)
Middle third	177 (28.0)
Lower third thoracic and/or cardia	587 (73.5)

Data from Orringer MB, Marshall B, Iannettoni MD. Transhiatal esophagectomy: clinical experience and refinements. Ann Surg 1999;230:392–400.

same operation in all but 6 patients. Stomach was used for reconstruction in 96% (1040 patients), and is preferred for esophageal replacement because it is well-vascularized, usually has sufficient length to reach the neck, and is not prone to the redundancy that occurs with intestinal substitutes. It is also relatively easy to mobilize and requires only a single anastomosis. Colon was used in the remaining patients, due to gastric resection for caustic injury or ulcer disease. The stomach was placed in the posterior mediastinum in all but 20 patients who had retrosternal placement due to residual tumor or fibrosis.

Intraoperative blood loss averaged 795 mL in patients who had benign disease and 652 mL in patients who had carcinoma. With increasing experience and performing more of the esophageal dissection under direct vision, the intraoperative blood loss has been reduced to 360 mL for 114 consecutive cases between 1996 and 1997. Entry into the pleural cavity was found in 77% of cases. Injury to the membranous trachea occurred in 4 patients, and splenectomy was performed in 3% due to intraoperative injury. Duodenal or gastric perforation occurred during pyloromyotomy in fewer than 2% of patients, and was repaired and reinforced with omentum. Five patients required reoperation for mediastinal bleeding. Seven percent (74 patients) had recurrent laryngeal nerve injury, which persisted beyond 12 weeks in fewer than 1% (24 patients). By avoiding the placement of retractors in the tracheoesophageal groove, this complication has decreased to less than 3%. Thoracic duct injury occurred in fewer than 1% (18 patients), and 2% of patients had pneumonia.

Cervical anastomotic leak occurred in 13% (146 patients) and was more common after retrosternal placement, radiation therapy, and prior operation at the gastroesophageal junction, which may lead to impaired vascularization of the fundus. The cervical side-to-side stapled esophagogastric anastomosis has significantly decreased the anastomotic leak rate to 2.7% [11]. These results were confirmed by Casson and associates [33], who reported a leak rate that decreased from 22.6% to 7.9% after the initiation of a side-to-side semimechanical anastomosis. Fistulas healed spontaneously after opening the wound at the bedside with local wound packing in all but 9 patients, who required takedown of the anastomosis and cervical esophagostomy due to necrosis of the upper stomach. The hospital mortality rate was 4% (44 patients), and only 6 patients died of pulmonary insufficiency and 3 from intraoperative hemorrhage.

Functional results

Functional results were available with an average follow-up of 47 months in patients who had benign disease. With liberal usage of Maloney dilators for any degree of dysphagia, 77% (186 patients) had at least one esophageal dilatation; however, 65% (157 patients) were eating an unrestricted diet at their most recent follow-up, and only 4% (11 patients) had severe dysphagia requiring regular dilatations. Although gastroesophageal reflux is common with intrathoracic anastomoses, it is uncommon if the cervical anastomosis is performed correctly, with the anastomosis several centimeters from the top of the gastric fundus, forming an acute angle of entry. Sixty percent (146 patients) denied reflux symptoms. Thirty-two percent (77 patients) had occasional reflux when lying flat after eating, 7% (18 patients) had nocturnal reflux and had to sleep with the head of the bed elevated, and 1 patient had an aspiration-related pulmonary complication.

Postvagotomy cramping and diarrhea occurred in 49% (95 patients), but was temporary in most cases, resolving over the first postoperative year. At most recent follow-up, 61% (147 patients) denied cramping or diarrhea. Although 40% (95 patients) had some degree of diarrhea or cramping, only 7% were severe, and were controlled with medications. When functional results were rated from excellent (asymptomatic) to poor (symptoms requiring regular treatment), 29% had an excellent result, 39% good, 28% fair, and 4% had a poor result.

Patients who had carcinoma had a shorter survival, with a mean follow-up of 29 months. Eighty percent (575 patients) were free of dysphagia at the most recent follow-up, and only 2% (20 patients) had severe dysphagia requiring regular dilatation. Seventy-nine percent (571 patients) had no symptoms of reflux, 17% (124 patients) had mild reflux, 3.5% (25 patients) had nocturnal reflux, and 1 patient had an aspiration-related pulmonary complication. Seventy-four percent (530 patients) were free of postprandial diarrhea or cramping at the most recent follow-up. Twenty-six percent (191 patients) had some degree of "dumping" symptoms, although severe diarrhea was present in fewer than 1% (6 patients). The overall functional result was excellent in 54%, good in 28%, fair in 15%, and poor in 3%.

Survival of patients who have carcinoma

Of 764 survivors out of 800 patients who had carcinoma (31 patients were lost to follow-up), the 2-year survival was 47%, and 5-year was survival 23%. Five-year survival for lower-third cancers was 26%, 13% for middle-third tumors, and 24% for upper-third tumors (Fig. 7). Twenty-seven percent (217 patients) underwent neoadjuvant chemo- and radiation therapy [34,35]. Twenty-three percent (49 patients) had a complete pathologic response, with a 5-year survival of 48%. As expected, survival was associated with tumor stage. Adenocarcinomas were also associated with improved survival when compared with squamous cell carcinomas.

Summary

Controversy still remains regarding the appropriateness of THE as a cancer operation. Critics argue that without an en bloc mediastinal lymphadenectomy, THE does not provide accurate staging or the potential for a curative procedure [36–38]; however, operative margins are similar after

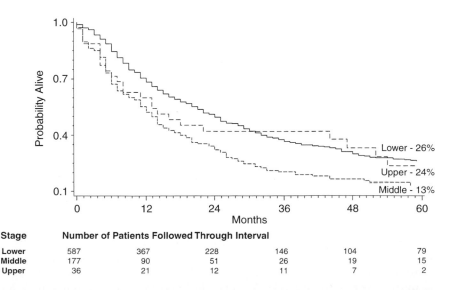

Stage	Number of Patients Followed Through Interval					
Lower	587	367	228	146	104	79
Middle	177	90	51	26	19	15
Upper	36	21	12	11	7	2

Fig. 7. Kaplan-Meier survival curves by tumor location after transhiatal esophagectomy for carcinoma. (*From* Orringer MB, Marshall B, Iannettoni MD. Transhiatal esophagectomy: clinical experience and refinements. Ann Surg 1999;230:392–400; with permission.)

Table 2
Early postoperative course in 220 patients randomly assigned to transhiatal esophagectomy or transthoracic esophagectomy with extended en bloc lymphadenectomy

Variable	Transhiatal esophagectomy (N = 106)	Transthoracic esophagectomy (N = 114)	P value
Postoperative complications—no. (%)			
Pulmonary complications[a]	29 (27)	65 (57)	<0.001
Cardiac Complications	17 (16)	30 (26)	0.10
Anastomotic leakage[b]	15 (14)	18 (16)	0.85
Subclinical	9 (8)	8 (7)	
Clinical	6 (6)	10 (9)	
Vocal-cord paralysis[c]	14 (13)	24 (21)	0.15
Chylous leakage	2 (2)	11 (10)	0.02
Wound infection	8 (8)	11 (10)	0.53
Ventilation time—days			<0.001
Median	1	2	
Range	0–19	0 76	
ICU-MCU stay—days[d]			<0.001
Median	2	6	
Range	0–38	0–79	
Hospital stay—days[e]			<0.001
Median	15	19	
Range	4–63	7–154	
In-hospital mortality—no. (%)	2 (2)	5 (4)	0.45

[a] Pulmonary complications include pneumonia and atelectasis.

[b] Subclinical anastomotic leakage was defined as leakage seen only on contrast radiography, and clinical anastomotic leakage as leakage resulting in a cervical salivary fistula.

[c] In most cases, vocal-cord paralysis was temporary.

[d] ICU = intensive care unit, MCU = medium care unit.

[e] The hospital stay was defined as the number of days from the day of operation to discharge.

Data from Hulscher JB, van Sandick JW, de Boen AG, et al. Extended transthoracic resection compared with limited transhiatal resection for adenocarcinoma of the esophagus. N Engl J Med 2002;347:1664.

transthoracic and transhiatal esophagectomy, and van Sandick and co-workers [39] reported that 73% of margins were microscopically negative [40,41]. In many cases, esophageal carcinoma appears to be a systemic disease at the time of diagnosis. According to Orringer and colleagues [6], 46% of patients have Stage III or IV disease at the time of operation, and Altorki and coauthors [37] found that 35% of patients thought to be potentially curable were found to have occult cervical lymph node disease after three-field lymph node dissection. In addition, survival after THE is similar to that reported after transthoracic esophagectomy [42–44] as well as radical esophagectomy with mediastinal lymphadenectomy [45]. The most important determinants of survival appear to be the biologic behavior of the tumor and the stage at the time of resection rather than the operative approach, and esophageal carcinoma will likely require systemic therapy for a cure.

Transhiatal esophagectomy has been used increasingly in the resection of benign and malignant disease, and has several potential advantages over transthoracic esophagectomy, including significantly decreased respiratory complications and mediastinitis due to the avoidance of thoracotomy and intrathoracic anastomosis. In a meta-analysis of fifty studies comparing transthoracic and transhiatal resection, Hulscher et al [46] found significantly higher early morbidity and mortality rates after transthoracic resections, which was confirmed in a later randomized study of 220 patients (Table 2) [47]. Survival after THE is also equivalent to or better than that seen after transthoracic esophagectomy, and transhiatal esophagectomy should be considered in all patients requiring esophagectomy for benign or malignant disease.

References

[1] Denk W. Zur Radikaloperation des osophaguskarfzentralbl [Radical operation for esophageal reconstruction]. Chirurg 1913;40:1065 [in German].

[2] Turner GG. Excision of thoracic esophagus for carcinoma with construction of extra-thoracic gullet. Lancet 1933;2:1315.

[3] Orringer MB, Sloan H. Substernal gastric bypass of the excluded thoracic esophagus for palliation of esophageal carcinoma. J Thorac Cardiovasc Surg 1975;70:836–51.

[4] Orringer MB. Substernal gastric bypass of the excluded esophagus—results of an ill-advised operation. Surgery 1984;96:467–70.

[5] Orringer MB, Sloan H. Esophagectomy without thoracotomy. J Thorac Cardiovasc Surg 1978;76:643–54.

[6] Orringer MB, Marshall B, Iannettoni MD. Transhiatal esophagectomy: clinical experience and refinements. Ann Surg 1999;230:392–400 [discussion: 3].

[7] Orringer MB, Marshall B, Stirling MC. Transhiatal esophagectomy for benign and malignant disease. J Thorac Cardiovasc Surg 1993;105:265–76 [discussion: 76–7].

[8] Barbier PA, Becker CD, Wagner HE. Esophageal carcinoma: patient selection for transhiatal esophagectomy. A prospective analysis of 50 consecutive cases. World J Surg 1988;12:263–9.

[9] Daniel TM, Fleischer KJ, Flanagan TL, et al. Transhiatal esophagectomy: a safe alternative for selected patients. Ann Thorac Surg 1992;54:686–9 [discussion: 9–90].

[10] Hankins JR, Miller JE, Attar S, et al. Transhiatal esophagectomy for carcinoma of the esophagus: experience with 26 patients. Ann Thorac Surg 1987;44:123–7.

[11] Orringer MB, Marshall B, Iannettoni MD. Eliminating the cervical esophagogastric anastomotic leak with a side-to-side stapled anastomosis. J Thorac Cardiovasc Surg 2000; 119:277–88.

[12] Orringer MB. Transhiatal esophagectomy for benign disease. J Thorac Cardiovasc Surg 1985;90:649–55.

[13] Orringer MB, Stirling MC. Esophageal resection for achalasia: indications and results. Ann Thorac Surg 1989;47:340–5.

[14] Quint LE, Glazer GM, Orringer MB, et al. Esophageal carcinoma: CT findings. Radiology 1985;155:171–5.

[15] Reed CE, Eloubeidi MA. New techniques for staging esophageal cancer. Surg Clin North Am 2002;82:697–710.

[16] Vickers J. Role of endoscopic ultrasound in the preoperative assessment of patients with oesophageal cancer. Ann R Coll Surg Engl 1998;80:233–9.

[17] Krasna MJ, Reed CE, Nedzwiecki D, et al. CALGB 9380: a prospective trial of the feasibility of thoracoscopy/laparoscopy in staging esophageal cancer. Ann Thorac Surg 2001;71: 1073–9.

[18] Luketich JD, Meehan M, Nguyen NT, et al. Minimally invasive surgical staging for esophageal cancer. Surg Endosc 2000;14:700–2.

[19] Block MI, Patterson GA, Sundaresan RS, et al. Improvement in staging of esophageal cancer with the addition of positron emission tomography. Ann Thorac Surg 1997;64:770–6 [discussion: 6–7].

[20] Luketich JD, Friedman DM, Weigel TL, et al. Evaluation of distant metastases in esophageal cancer: 100 consecutive positron emission tomography scans. Ann Thorac Surg 1999;68:1133–6 [discussion: 6–7].

[21] Orringer MB. Transhiatal esophagectomy without thoracotomy. In: Zuidema GD, Yeo CJ, Orringer MB, et al, editors. Shackelford's surgery of the alimentary tract, vol. 1. 5th edition. Philadelphia: WB Saunders Company; 2002. p. 407–42.

[22] Orringer MB. Resection of the esophagus. In: Shields TW, Locicero J III, Ponn RB, editors. General thoracic surgery, vol. 2. 5th edition. Philadelphia: Lippincott Williams and Wilkins; 2000. p. 1697–722.

[23] Waddell WR, Scannell JG. Anterior approach to carcinoma of the superior mediastinal and cervical segments of the esophagus. J Thorac Surg 1957;33:663.

[24] De Paula AL, Hashiba K, Ferreira EA, et al. Laparoscopic transhiatal esophagectomy with esophagogastroplasty. Surg Laparosc Endosc 1995;5:1–5.

[25] Nguyen NT, Schauer P, Luketich JD. Minimally invasive esophagectomy for Barrett's esophagus with high-grade dysplasia. Surgery 2000;127:284–90.

[26] Glasgow RE, Swanstrom LL. Hand-assisted gastroesophageal surgery. Semin Laparosc Surg 2001;8:135–44.

[27] Iannettoni MD, Chang A, Lee D. Total robotic esophagectomy (Surgical Motion Pictures). Presented at: The Society of Thoracic Surgeons Annual Meeting, San Diego, CA, February 1, 2003.

[28] Iannettoni MD, Whyte RI, Orringer MB. Catastrophic complications of the cervical esophagogastric anastomosis. J Thorac Cardiovasc Surg 1995;110:1493–500 [discussion: 500–1].

[29] Liebermann-Meffert DM, Luescher U, Neff U, et al. Esophagectomy without thoracotomy: is there a risk of intramediastinal bleeding? A study on blood supply of the esophagus. Ann Surg 1987;206:184–92.

[30] Orringer MB, Lemmer JH. Early dilation in the treatment of esophageal disruption. Ann Thorac Surg 1986;42:536–9.

[31] Katariya K, Harvey JC, Pina E, et al. Complications of transhiatal esophagectomy. J Surg Oncol 1994;57:157–63.

[32] Gandhi SK, Naunheim KS. Complications of transhiatal esophagectomy. Chest Surg Clin N Am 1997;7:601–10 [discussion: 11–2].

[33] Casson AG, Porter GA, Veugelers PJ. Evolution and critical appraisal of anastomotic technique following resection of esophageal adenocarcinoma. Dis Esophagus 2002;15: 296–302.

[34] Forastiere AA, Orringer MB, Perez-Tamayo C, et al. Preoperative chemoradiation followed by transhiatal esophagectomy for carcinoma of the esophagus: final report. J Clin Oncol 1993;11:1118–23.

[35] Orringer MB, Forastiere AA, Perez-Tamayo C, et al. Chemotherapy and radiation therapy before transhiatal esophagectomy for esophageal carcinoma. Ann Thorac Surg 1990;49: 348–54 [discussion: 54–5].

[36] Akiyama H, Tsurumaru M, Udagawa H, et al. Radical lymph node dissection for cancer of the thoracic esophagus. Ann Surg 1994;220:364–72 [discussion: 72–3].

[37] Altorki NK, Girardi L, Skinner DB. En bloc esophagectomy improves survival for Stage III esophageal cancer. J Thorac Cardiovasc Surg 1997;114:948–55 [discussion: 55–6].

[38] Hagen JA, Peters JH, DeMeester TR. Superiority of extended en bloc esophagogastrectomy for carcinoma of the lower esophagus and cardia. J Thorac Cardiovasc Surg 1993;106:850–8 [discussion: 8–9].

[39] van Sandick JW, van Lanschot JJ, ten Kate FJ, et al. Indicators of prognosis after transhiatal esophageal resection without thoracotomy for cancer. J Am Coll Surg 2002;194:28–36.

[40] Junginger T, Dutkowski P. Selective approach to the treatment of oesophageal cancer. Br J Surg 1996;83:1473–7.

[41] Roder JD, Busch R, Stein HJ, et al. Ratio of invaded to removed lymph nodes as a predictor of survival in squamous cell carcinoma of the oesophagus. Br J Surg 1994;81:410–3.

[42] Bolton JS, Sardi A, Bowen JC, et al. Transhiatal and transthoracic esophagectomy: a comparative study. J Surg Oncol 1992;51:249–53.

[43] Gluch L, Smith RC, Bambach CP, et al. Comparison of outcomes following transhiatal or Ivor Lewis esophagectomy for esophageal carcinoma. World J Surg 1999;23:271–5 [discussion: 5–6].

[44] Horstmann O, Verreet PR, Becker H, et al. Transhiatal oesophagectomy compared with transthoracic resection and systematic lymphadenectomy for the treatment of oesophageal cancer. Eur J Surg 1995;161:557–67.

[45] Skinner DB. En bloc resection for neoplasms of the esophagus and cardia. J Thorac Cardiovasc Surg 1983;85:59–71.

[46] Hulscher JB, Tijssen JG, Obertop H, et al. Transthoracic versus transhiatal resection for carcinoma of the esophagus: a meta-analysis. Ann Thorac Surg 2001;72:306–13.

[47] Hulscher JB, van Sandick JW, de Boer AG, et al. Extended transthoracic resection compared with limited transhiatal resection for adenocarcinoma of the esophagus. N Engl J Med 2002; 347:1662–9.

ELSEVIER
SAUNDERS

SURGICAL
CLINICS OF
NORTH AMERICA

Surg Clin N Am 85 (2005) 611–619

En-bloc Esophagectomy—The Three-Field Dissection

Nasser Altorki, MD

*Weill Medical College of Cornell University, 525 East 68th Street,
New York, NY 10021, USA*

Esophageal carcinoma is the third most common gastrointestinal malignancy, and among the ten most prevalent cancers worldwide [1]. Approximately 12,400 new patients will develop esophageal cancer annually in the United States, and more than 95% of them will succumb to their disease. The treatment options for esophageal cancer are varied, and include primary surgical resection, surgical resection after preoperative chemotherapy, preoperative chemoradiation, or nonoperative therapy using definitive chemoradiotherapy. Several randomized trials have failed to demonstrate the superiority of any one treatment strategy over all others [2–14]. For example, despite the promising pathological response rates reported after preoperative chemoradiotherapy, most randomized trials have shown that 5-year survival is no better than that achieved by surgery alone (Table 1). The same is true of nearly all randomized trials that examined the value of preoperative chemotherapy compared with primary surgical resection (Table 2). Dismayed by these results, an increasing number of medical oncologists currently advocate nonoperative treatment with chemoradiotherapy, and reserve the so-called "salvage esophagectomy" for those patients who have residual or recurrent intraluminal disease [15,16]. This position may appear justified, given that the results achievable by primary surgical resection, with or without preoperative therapy of any kind, are essentially identical to those reported after definitive chemoradiation alone [17,18]. For example, Herskovic et al [17] reported an intergroup randomized trial comparing radiotherapy with radiochemotherapy delivered with curative intent. The 5-year survival after combined modality therapy was 27%. Although this study did not examine a surgical question, the implication was clear. A more recently reported randomized trial [18] compared preoperative chemoradiation with primary chemoradiation in patients who had locally advanced

---

E-mail address: nkaltork@med.cornell.edu

Table 1
Preoperative CRT: phase III trials

Study	n	RT	Chemo	5-year survival	P value
Nygaard '92 [2]	88	35 Gy (seq)	CDDP-BL	9/17	NS
Le Prise '94 [11]	86	20 Gy (seq)	CDDP-B-VBL	13/19	NS
Walsh '96 [14]	113	40 Gy (con)	CDDP-FU	6/32 (3 yr)	0.01
Bosset '97 [5]	297	40 Gy (con)	CDDP	38/36 (3 yr)	NS
Urba '01 [13]	100	45 Gy (con)	CDDP-FU	33/18	NS
Burmeister '02 [12]	256	35 Gy	CDDP-FU	21.7/18.5	NS

Abbreviations: CDDP-BL, cisplatin-bleomycin; CDDP-B-VBL, cisplatin-vinblastine; CDDP-FU, cisplatin-fluorouracil; CDDP, cisplatin.

squamous cell carcinoma. Median survival was 19 months for the non-surgical arm and 17.7 months for the surgical arm. These studies raise the inevitable question about the role of surgery, if any, in esophageal cancer [19,20].

Why we fail

The primary argument for the poor results seen in the treatment of esophageal cancer by any modality is the fact that the great majority of patients develop metastatic disease, suggesting that the disease may have already disseminated at the time of diagnosis. Although this is undoubtedly the case in some patients, a careful analysis of the patterns of failure after surgical resection also suggests inadequate local control using current treatment modalities. For example, the locoregional failure rates reported in the surgery-alone arms of several randomized trials ranges between 30% and 45% [2–14]. In the large US trial reported in 1998 [6], locally recurrent or locally persistent disease was reported in 64% of patients. Interestingly, the addition of preoperative therapy of any kind did not meaningfully reduce this high local failure rate (Table 3). Although admittedly most patients will die from metastatic disease, it is doubtful that a favorable long-term outcome can be achieved in the absence of adequate local control.

Table 2
Preoperative chemotherapy phase III trials

Study	n	Survival surgery/preop chemo	Hazard ratio
Roth '88 [8]	39	5/25	0.79
Nygaard '92 [2]	91	9/3	1.1
Schlag '92 [3]	46	10 month	1.0
Law '97 [7]	147	44/31 (2 year)	0.69
Kok '97 [9]	36	18/11	-
Ancona '01 [10]	94	NS	1.0
Kelsen '98 [6]	428	20/20	1.0
Bancewicz '02 [4]	802	44/34 (2 year)	0.79

Table 3
Locoregional failure: phase III data

Study	Surgery only	Induction therapy
Urba '01 [13]	39%	19%
Kelsen '98 [6]	31% (+33% R_1)	32%
Law '97 [7]	45%	28%
Herskovic '92 [17]	66% (RT only)	43%

Abbreviations: R, microscopic residual disease; RT, radiation therapy.

En-bloc two-field esophagectomy

Standard techniques for esophageal resection, regardless of surgical access (transthoracic versus transhiatal), entail extirpation of the esophagus with its adjoining lymph nodes, without an attempt to perform a thorough lymphadenectomy of the mediastinum and upper abdomen. Additionally, the narrow confines of the posterior mediastinum present a significant challenge to the surgeon in obtaining a wider radial margin of resection, thus limiting the dissection to the esophageal adventitia and periesophageal fat. The concept of en-bloc resection, as originally proposed by Logan [21] and later reintroduced by Skinner [22], aims to maximize local tumor control by resecting the tumor-bearing esophagus within a wide envelope of surrounding tissues. Thus, for tumors of the middle or lower thoracic esophagus, the en-bloc specimen would include, in addition to the tumor-bearing organ, the pericardium anteriorly and both pleural surfaces laterally, as well as the thoracic duct and all other lympho-areolar tissue wedged posteriorly between the esophagus and the spine. Additionally, for tumors traversing the diaphragm, a 1-in cuff of diaphragm is excised circumferentially around the esophagus. The associated two-field lymphadenectomy includes en-bloc resection of all nodal groups between the tracheal bifurcation superiorly to the celiac axis inferiorly. The author's group previously reported our results after en-bloc esophagectomy performed in 111 patients who had esophageal carcinoma [23]. Overall 5-year survival was 40%. Stage-specific survival is shown in Table 4, and is notable for the 39% 5-year survival achieved in patients who had Stage III disease. An important finding was the remarkably low locoregional failure rate of

Table 4
Stage-specific survival after en-bloc esophagectomy

Stage	5-year survival	Median survival
I	78%	NR
IIA	72%	NR
IIB	0%	30 month
III	39%	53 month
IV	27%	20 month

Abbreviation: NR, not reached.

9%, which validates the basic concept of improved local control achieved by en-bloc resection.

En-bloc three-field esophagectomy

The concept of three-field lymph node dissection for esophageal cancer was developed by Japanese surgeons in the 1980s in response to the observation that as many as 40% of patients who had resected squamous cell esophageal cancer developed isolated cervical lymph node metastases [24]. A nationwide retrospective study was subsequently reported describing the findings and potential benefits of esophagectomy with three-field dissection [25]. The additional third field of dissection included excision of the nodes along both recurrent nerves as they course through the mediastinum and neck, as well as a modified cervical node dissection. The latter includes the nodes posterior and lateral to the internal jugular vein and an infraomohyoid node dissection bilaterally. Isono and colleagues [25] reported on 4600 patients who had undergone either two field (2800) or three-field (1800) node dissection. Previously unsuspected cervical nodal metastases, primarily in the recurrent nodes, were seen in approximately one third of patients. Furthermore, the study authors reported a significantly higher overall 5-year survival after three-field dissection than after two-field dissection. The relevance of these findings to a Western population afflicted primarily by esophageal adenocarcinoma was unknown. In 1994, the author's group [26] initiated our experience with esophagectomy and three-field lymph node dissection in patients who had squamous as well as adenocarcinoma of the esophagus. Patients were considered eligible for the procedure only if the tumor was present in the tubular esophagus. Tumors of the lower esophageal third were included only if they did not extend past the gastroesophageal junction (Siewert type 1). All patients underwent a thorough preoperative evaluation to exclude the presence of visceral metastases and to assess their ability to undergo the procedure from a cardiopulmonary standpoint. In 2002, our group reported our initial experience with 80 patients treated by this technique in order to determine the prevalence of unsuspected cervical nodal metastasis as well as the impact on overall and stage-specific survival [27].

Surgical procedure

All patients are explored through a right thoracotomy, followed by a laparotomy and cervical incision. In the thorax, the tumor-bearing esophagus is resected en-bloc within an envelope of adjoining tissues that includes both pleural surfaces laterally, the pericardium anteriorly (except in T_1a lesion), and all lymphovascular tissues wedged dorsally between the esophagus and the spine. The thoracic duct is included within the en-bloc resection throughout its course in the posterior mediastinum. For tumors traversing the esophageal hiatus, a 1-in cuff of diaphragm is resected circumferentially around the tumor. As described, the en-bloc resection necessarily includes a complete dissection of the middle and lower mediastinal nodes, including the periesophageal, parahiatal, subcarinal, and aortopulmonary window nodes. In the abdomen, an upper abdominal and retroperitoneal node dissection is performed, and includes resection of the celiac, splenic, common hepatic, left gastric, lesser curvature, and parahiatal nodes. Dissection of the third field is begun during the thoracic portion of the procedure and later completed through a collar neck incision. Dissection of the nodes in the superior mediastinum includes the nodes along the right and left recurrent laryngeal nerves throughout their mediastinal course. The paratracheal retrocaval compartment is not disturbed. The left recurrent nerve is exposed from the level of the aortic arch to the thoracic inlet. The nerve is dissected using a "no-touch" technique, and nodes along its anterior aspect are carefully excised. Notably, there is a paucity of nodal tissue along the left nerve in nearly all white patients. The right recurrent nerve is carefully exposed near its origin at the base of the right subclavian artery. The right recurrent nodal chain begins at that level and forms a continuous package that extends through the thoracic inlet to the neck. Again, the nerve is dissected using a strict no-touch technique. Through the cervical incision, the remainder of the recurrent nodes are dissected, as well as the lower deep cervical nodes located posterior and lateral to the carotid sheath. Thus, the third field includes a continuous anatomically inseparable chain of nodes that extends from the superior mediastinum to the lower neck. Finally, gastrointestinal reconstruction is achieved by advancing a greater curvature gastric tube to the neck for an esophagogastric anastomosis.

Postoperative care

Patients are cared for in an intensive care unit for 24 hours for fluid management and mechanical ventilation. Separation from mechanical ventilation is usually achieved in most patients by the morning after the procedure. Intense pulmonary hygiene is required, often with repeated bronchoscopy for the first 48 hours after extubation, because most patients develop a variable degree of bronchorrhea, which generally resolves on the third or fourth postoperative day. Oral intake is begun once anastomotic integrity is confirmed by a barium study on the sixth or seventh postoperative day.

Hospital mortality and morbidity

In a previously published series of 80 consecutive patients [27], there were three in-hospital deaths, for a hospital mortality of 3.75%. An additional patient died following discharge from massive hematemasis. The overall 30-day mortality was 5%. Nearly 50% of patients had an eventful post-operative course. Major complications occurred in 31% of patients and are listed in Table 5. Significantly, injury to the recurrent nerve occurred in only 7 patients, and was transient in 4. No patient required intubation or tracheostomy as a result of nerve injury.

Cervical nodal metastases

Twenty-nine patients (36.25%) had metastatic carcinoma in the cervicothoracic nodes, including 3 who also had celiac nodal disease. Thus, dissection of the third field yielded important staging information in 26 patients (32.5%). Metastases involved the right recurrent nodes in 22 patients, the left recurrent nodes in 1, and both groups in 4. Metastases to the deep cervical nodes were present in 4 patients, 2 of whom also had metastases in the recurrent nodes.

The frequency of cervicothoracic nodal disease was independent of cell type or tumor location within the esophagus (Table 6); however, the frequency of cervicothoracic nodal metastases was influenced by the nodal status within the abdomen or mediastinum. Forty-three percent (24/55) of patients who had node-positive disease in the abdomen or mediastinum also had nodal metastases in the cervicothoracic region. In contrast, among 30 patients who had node-negative disease in the abdomen and mediastinum, 4 (13%) had isolated metastases in the cervicothoracic nodes.

Perspective

There can no longer be any doubt that occult cervical nodal metastases are present in 30% to 40% of patients who undergo a presumably curative surgical resection. This high prevalence of occult residual disease is independent of either cell type or location of the tumor within the esophagus. Additionally, the prevalence of occult cervical nodal disease approaches

Table 5
Major complications after three-field dissection

Complication	%
Respiratory	26
Cardiac	15
Leaks	11
Infection	10
Recurrent nerve injury	8.75[a]
Other	8.75

[a] Three permanent, four transient (no tracheostomy in any).

Table 6
Prevalence of cervicothoracic nodes by cell type and tumor site

Cell type/tumor site	Prevalence
Adenocarcinoma	18/48 (37.42%)
Squamous carcinoma	11/32 (34.3%)
Lower third	18/55 (32.73%)
Middle third	10/17 (58.82%)
Upper third	1/8 (12.5%)

50% in those patients who have any mediastinal or abdominal nodal metastases; undoubtedly the great majority of patients. A possible clinical implication of these findings is that 50% to 60% of patients will be incompletely resected following a two-field dissection. The impact of such an incomplete resection on survival is controversial, but the bulk of the evidence suggests that R2 types of resections (residual gross disease) are associated with a distinctly poor prognosis, with essentially no survivors beyond 2 years [28,29]. Perhaps the least controversial aspect of three-field dissection is its ability to provide the most comprehensive staging information. In the author's experience, over 30% of patients were upstaged as a consequence of information obtained by three-field dissection. Although the majority of this stage shifting occurred from Stage III to Stage IV, occasionally patients are upstaged from Stages I and II to Stage IV disease. Clearly, the stage shift after three-field dissection results in improvement in stage-specific survival. For example, although our group previously reported the 5-year survival of Stage III patients to be 34% following two field en-bloc resection, Stage III survival was 54% after three-field dissection (Table 7) [27]. This apparent improvement in outcome is at least partly due to stage migration, because Stage III patients in the latter report represent a more homogeneous group [27]. Whether the procedure results in a survival benefit for patients who have Stage IV disease remains a crucial issue. Some surgeons, perhaps many, contend that the presence of metastases in the cervicothoracic region is essentially equivalent to systemic metastases, and that cure is simply not possible [30]. Data from our group [27], however, argue that such is not the case, particularly in patients who

Table 7
Stage-specific survival after three-field en-bloc esophagectomy

Stage	5-year survival
I	88%
IIA	84%
IIB	25%[a]
III	54%
IV	25%

[a] Three year.

have squamous cell carcinoma and cervical nodal disease, for whom the 5-year survival is 40%. Among 11 patients who had squamous cell carcinoma with positive cervicothoracic nodes, 3 are alive and free of disease at 3,5, and 6 years postoperatively. In contrast, patients who had Stage IV adenocarcinoma have discouraging 3- and 5-year survival rates of 30% and 15%, respectively. Although the author agrees that cure is an unlikely event, prolongation of survival is possible, and would represent a small but important achievement for these patients—a subset for whom novel adjuvant therapies are anxiously awaited.

References

[1] Stewart BW, Kleihues P. World cancer report. Lyon (France): IARC Press; 2003.
[2] Nygaard K, Hagen S, Hansen HS, et al. Pre-operative radiotherapy prolongs survival in operable esophageal carcinoma: a randomized, multicenter study of pre-operative radiotherapy and chemotherapy. The second Scandinavian trial in esophageal cancer. World J Surg 1992;16(6):1104–9 [discussion: 1110].
[3] Schlag PM. Randomized trial of preoperative chemotherapy for squamous cell cancer of the esophagus. The Chirurgische Arbeitsgemeinschaft Fuer Onkologie der Deutschen Gesellschaft Fuer Chirurgie Study Group. Arch Surg 1992;127(12):1446–50.
[4] Bancewicz J, Clark P, Smith D, et al. Surgical resection with or without preoperative chemotherapy in oesophageal cancer: a randomised controlled trial. Lancet 2002;359(9319): 1727–33.
[5] Bosset JF, Gignoux M, Triboulet JP. Chemoradiotherapy followed by surgery compared with surgery alone in squamous-cell cancer of the esophagus. N Engl J Med 1997;337(3): 161–7.
[6] Kelsen DP, Ginsberg R, Pajak TF. Chemotherapy followed by surgery compared with surgery alone for localized esophageal cancer. N Engl J Med 1998;339(27):1979–84.
[7] Law S, Fok M, Chow S. Preoperative chemotherapy versus surgical therapy alone for squamous cell carcinoma of the esophagus: a prospective randomized trial. J Thorac Cardiovasc Surg 1997;114(2):210–7.
[8] Roth JA, Pass HI, Flanagan MM. Randomized clinical trial of preoperative and postoperative adjuvant chemotherapy with cisplatin, vindesine, and bleomycin for carcinoma of the esophagus. J Thorac Cardiovasc Surg 1988;96(2):242–8.
[9] Kok T, Lanshot J, Siersema P. Neoadjuvant chemotherapy in operable esophageal squamous cell cancer: final report of a Phase III multicenter randomized controlled trial. in ASCO. 1997.
[10] Ancona E, Ruol A, Santi S, et al. Only pathologic complete response to neoadjuvant chemotherapy improves significantly the long term survival of patients with resectable esophageal squamous cell carcinoma: final report of a randomized, controlled trial of preoperative chemotherapy versus surgery alone. Cancer 2001;91(11):2165–74.
[11] Le Prise E, Etienne PL, Meunier M. A randomized study of chemotherapy, radiation therapy, and surgery versus surgery for localized squamous cell carcinoma of the esophagus. Cancer 1994;73(7):1779–84.
[12] Burmeister BH, Smithers BM, Fitzgerald L. A randomized Phase III trial of preoperative chemoradiation followed by surgery (CR-S) versus surgery alone (S) for localized resectable cancer of the esophagus. in ASCO. 2002. Orlando, FL.
[13] Urba SG, Orringer MB, Turrise A. Randomized trial of preoperative chemoradiation versus surgery alone in patients with locoregional esophageal carcinoma. J Clin Oncol 2001;19(2): 305–13.

[14] Walsh TN, Noonan N, Hollywood D. A comparison of multimodal therapy and surgery for esophageal adenocarcinoma. N Engl J Med 1996;335(7):462–7.

[15] Daly JM, Karnell LH, Menck HR. National Cancer Data Base report on esophageal carcinoma. Cancer 1996;78(8):1820–8.

[16] Daly JM, Fry W, Little A, et al. Esophageal cancer: results of an American College of Surgeons patient care evaluation study. J Am Coll Surg 2000;190(5):562–72 [discussion: 572–3].

[17] Herskovic A, Martz K, Al-Sarraf M, et al. Combined chemotherapy and radiotherapy compared with radiotherapy alone in patients with cancer of the esophagus. N Engl J Med 1992;326(24):1593–8

[18] Bedenne L, Michel P, Bouche O. Randomized Phase III trial in locally advanced esophageal cancer: radiochemotherapy followed by surgery versus radiochemotherapy alone (FFCD 9102). in ASCO. 2002. Orlando, FL.

[19] Coia LR. Esophageal cancer: is esophagectomy necessary? Oncology (Huntingt) 1989;3(4): 101–10 [discussion: 110–1; 114–5].

[20] O'Reilly S, Forastiere AA. Is surgery necessary with multimodality treatment of oesophageal cancer? Ann Oncol 1995;6(6):519–21.

[21] Logan A. The surgical treatment of carcinoma of the esophagus and cardia. J Thorac Cardiovasc Surg 1963;46.150–61.

[22] Skinner DB. En bloc resection for neoplasms of the esophagus and cardia. J Thorac Cardiovasc Surg 1983;85(1):59–71.

[23] Altorki N, Skinner D. Should en bloc esophagectomy be the standard of care for esophageal carcinoma? Ann Surg 2001;234(5):581–7.

[24] Isono K, Onoda S, Okuyama K, et al. Recurrence of intrathoracic esophageal cancer. Jpn J Clin Oncol 1985;15(1):49–60.

[25] Isono K, Sato H, Nakayama K. Results of a nationwide study on the three-field lymph node dissection of esophageal cancer. Oncology 1991;48(5):411–20.

[26] Altorki NK, Skinner DB. Occult cervical nodal metastasis in esophageal cancer: preliminary results of three-field lymphadenectomy. J Thorac Cardiovasc Surg 1997;113(3):540–4.

[27] Altorki N, Kent M, Ferrara C, et al. Three-field lymph node dissection for squamous cell and adenocarcinoma of the esophagus. Ann Surg 2002;236(2):177–83.

[28] Ellis Jr FH, Heatley G, Krasna M, et al. Esophagogastrectomy for carcinoma of the esophagus and cardia: a comparison of findings and results after standard resection in three consecutive eight-year intervals with improved staging criteria. J Thorac Cardiovasc Surg 1997;113(5):836–46 [discussion: 846–8].

[29] Lerut T, Leyn P, Coosemans W, et al. Surgical strategies in esophageal carcinoma with emphasis on radical lymphadenectomy. Ann Surg 1992;216(3):583–90.

[30] Orringer MB. Occult cervical nodal metastases in esophageal cancer: preliminary results of three-field lymphadenectomy. J Thorac Cardiovasc Surg 1997;113(3):538–9.

SURGICAL
CLINICS OF
NORTH AMERICA

ELSEVIER
SAUNDERS

Surg Clin N Am 85 (2005) 621–630

Multimodality Treatment of Esophageal Cancer

Ziv Gamliel, MD*, Mark J. Krasna, MD

Division of Thoracic Surgery, University of Maryland Medical Center,
22 South Greene Street, N4E35, Baltimore, MD 21201, USA

Patients who have esophageal cancer rarely present at an early stage of their disease. Symptoms do not usually arise until the tumor becomes large enough to cause obstruction, or when it invades adjacent structures. The lack of a serosal layer on the esophagus allows early tumor invasion into the trachea, aorta, and spine (T4). The length of time until the development of symptoms and the rich network of lymphatic drainage make lymph node involvement common at the time of presentation. As many as 30% of patients who have early (T1) lesions may have lymph node metastases [1]. Esophageal cancer can metastasize to virtually any organ in the body, and widespread distant metastases are almost always present at the time of death [2].

The prevalence of locally advanced disease and lymph node metastases at the time of presentation complicates the management of esophageal cancer in most cases. In addition to local control of the disease, systemic control must also be addressed. Modalities used for local control include surgical resection and radiotherapy. Systemic chemotherapy is used to treat metastatic disease. Although single modality regimens may be used, the aggressive management of esophageal cancer often involves combined modality therapy. Pretreatment staging is often helpful in selecting the most appropriate therapeutic approach.

Surgery

Despite ongoing advances in chemotherapy and radiotherapy, esophagectomy continues to play a vital role in the management of patients who

---

* Corresponding author. Division of Thoracic Surgery, University of Maryland Medical Center, 22 South Greene Street, N4E35, Baltimore, MD 21201.

E-mail address: zgamliel@smail.umaryland.edu (Z. Gamliel).

0039-6109/05/$ - see front matter © 2005 Elsevier Inc. All rights reserved.
doi:10.1016/j.suc.2005.01.011

have esophageal cancer. Intrathoracic esophagogastric anastomosis can be achieved via a left-chest-only approach or via a combined abdominal and right-chest (Lewis) approach. A cervical anastomosis can be achieved using a combined abdominal, right-chest and left-cervical (McKeown) approach or an abdominal, transhiatal and left-cervical (Orringer) approach [3]. The selection of operative approach depends upon the extent of disease and the physiologic status of the patient.

A Dutch prospective randomized trial [4] studied 220 patients who have adenocarcinoma of the mid-to-distal esophagus or adenocarcinoma of the gastric cardia involving the distal esophagus. Patients were randomized to undergo either transhiatal esophagectomy or transthoracic esophagectomy with extended en-bloc lymphadenectomy. Although perioperative morbidity was higher after transthoracic esophagectomy, there was no significant difference in in-hospital mortality. At 5 years, patients undergoing trans-thoracic esophagectomy had higher rates of disease-free survival (39% versus 27%) and overall survival (39% versus 29%), but these trends were not statistically significant.

Results of surgical resection for esophageal cancer are related to disease stage. With the exception of very early stage disease (T1N0), complete surgical resection of malignant tumors of the thoracic esophagus is best achieved via thoracotomy rather than the transhiatal approach. In Stage I (T1N0M0) disease, the majority of patients undergoing surgical resection alone will survive more than 5 years. Most patients presenting with dysphagia, however, are incurable by surgical resection alone. Such patients typically have occult systemic metastases (M1), involvement of regional lymph nodes (N1), or invasion of adjacent tissues (T3) or structures (T4). Overall, approximately 75% of patients present with locally advanced disease (T3 or T4). In all but the earliest stages of esophageal cancer (T1N0 or T2N0), both local and systemic recurrence of disease is common when surgical resection is performed as the sole treatment modality. In the presence of visceral metastasis or locally advanced tumor that is not completely resectable, the risks of esophagectomy are felt to outweigh the benefits.

Radiation

Treatment of esophageal cancer with radiotherapy alone is mainly useful for palliation of obstructive symptoms and permits a rapid return of swallowing and eating. Palliation can be achieved in up to 85% of patients with virtually no risk of treatment-related mortality and without serious morbidity. Palliation lasts a median of 5 to 10 months, and up to 20% of patients may remain free of dysphagia at 3 years [5]. Over half of patients will maintain swallowing ability until the time of their demise.

Curative radiotherapy as a lone modality requires total doses of at least 50 Gy. Patients who have noncircumferential tumors of the cervical esophagus less than 5 cm in length may have 5-year survival rates of up to 15%.

Carcinoma of the thoracic esophagus treated by radiotherapy alone has an associated 5-year survival rate of 6% to 9%.

Chemotherapy

Most patients who have esophageal cancer have disseminated disease at the time of diagnosis. As a result, systemic therapy often plays an important role in the management of esophageal cancer. Cisplatin is among the most active of single-agents, with a response rate of 32% in Phase II trials [6]. The addition of 5-fluorouracil to cisplatin is associated with significantly improved response rates. Combination chemotherapy is generally more effective than single-agent therapy in esophageal carcinoma. Only about 50% of patients respond to chemotherapy alone. Complete remissions may occur in 2% to 5% of patients.

Chemoradiation

In a prospective randomized trial [7], the Radiation Therapy Oncology Group (RTOG) compared chemoradiation of 50 Gy with concurrent 5-fluorouracil and cisplatin versus 64 Gy radiation alone. Radiation was given over 5 weeks. The first two cycles of chemotherapy were given concurrently with radiotherapy in weeks 1 and 5, followed by two additional cycles of chemotherapy in weeks 8 and 11. Significantly improved results in the chemoradiation group allowed the study to be stopped early. Patients receiving chemoradiation had improved median survival (12.5 versus 8.9 months), 1-year survival (50% versus 33%), and 2-year survival (38% versus 10%). A subsequent follow-up study [8] confirmed an improved 5-year survival (26% versus 0). Of note, chemotherapy could only be administered in 68% of patients as planned. Ten percent of patients in the chemoradiation group had life-threatening toxic effects, as compared with only 2% in the group receiving radiotherapy alone.

In another prospective randomized trial [9], the Eastern Cooperative Oncology Group compared the combined use of 5-fluorouracil, mitomycin C, and radiation therapy versus radiation therapy alone. Chemoradiation resulted in improved 2-year survival (27% versus 12%) and 5-year survival (9% versus 7%), as well as significantly improved median survival (14.8 versus 9.2 months). The same pattern of survival was noted in all subgroups, independent of surgical resection.

More recently, the RTOG published the results of a randomized prospective trial [10] in which patients received four monthly cycles of 5-fluorouracil and cisplatin and were randomized to receive concurrent radiotherapy with 64.8 Gy versus 50.4 Gy. The trial was stopped after an interim analysis due to excessive mortality in the high-dose arm. Although there were 11 treatment-related deaths in the high-dose arm compared with

2 in the standard-dose arm, 7 of the 11 deaths occurred in patients who had received 50.4 Gy or less. The higher radiation dose did not increase survival or local/regional control.

The management of esophageal cancer should be aimed at both systemic and local disease control. For patients who have esophageal cancer and who are not operative candidates, or who have clearly unresectable disease, nonoperative management should ideally include radiotherapy as well as cisplatin-based combination chemotherapy. Although the optimal total dose of radiation remains uncertain, 50 Gy appears to be reasonably safe and effective.

Preoperative radiation

A multicenter randomized controlled trial [11] conducted by the European Organization for Research and Treatment of Cancer (EORTC) involved the administration of 33 Gy in 10 fractions in the treatment arm, followed by esophagectomy within 8 days. There were no significant differences in resectability or operative mortality between the study arms. Although locoregional failure was significantly decreased from 67% to 46%, this was not associated with any survival benefit.

In a similar randomized trial [12] of 206 patients using 40 Gy, no significant difference was found in resectability or 5-year survival with preoperative radiation. Five-year survival was 50% in the subgroup of patients in whom preoperative radiotherapy achieved complete tumor sterilization. Local failure was significantly reduced from 41% to 34%. In contrast, a prospective, randomized controlled Norwegian study [13] of 186 patients using 35 Gy reported significantly improved 3-year survival with preoperative radiotherapy in patients who had squamous cell carcinoma and who were deemed resectable at the time of enrollment.

The rationale for using preoperative radiotherapy is to improve the resectability of marginally resectable tumors, reduce the risk of tumor spread during surgical manipulations, and treat tumor that extends beyond the surgical specimen. Preoperative radiation doses of 30 to 45 Gy have been reported to result in a 15% to 30% rate of tumor sterilization. Preoperative radiotherapy does not appear to adversely affect resectability or to increase surgical morbidity.

Postoperative radiation

In a French randomized controlled trial [14] of 221 patients who had squamous cell carcinoma of the lower two thirds of the esophagus, patients in the control arm underwent surgery alone. Patients in the treatment arm received postoperative radiotherapy doses of 45 to 55 Gy in daily fractions of 1.8 Gy. There was no significant difference in survival between the two groups. Among lymph-node negative patients, local recurrence rates were 10% in the postoperative radiotherapy group, compared with 35% with surgery alone.

A randomized controlled study from Hong Kong [15] reported on 130 patients who had undergone either palliative or curative resection for esophageal cancer. Patients randomized to the treatment arm of the study received postoperative radiotherapy doses of 49 to 52.5 Gy in daily doses of 3.5 Gy. The very high daily radiation dose used in this study was associated with a significantly decreased median survival when compared with surgery alone (8.7 months versus 15.2 months). No benefit in local control was noted in patients undergoing curative resection. Although postoperative radiotherapy was associated with improved local control in patients undergoing palliative resection left with gross residual disease, there was no survival benefit.

In a Chinese prospective randomized trial [16], 495 patients who had esophageal cancer and who had undergone surgical resection were randomized to receive postoperative radiotherapy or not. A midplane dose of 50 to 60 Gy was delivered in 25 to 30 fractions over 5 to 6 weeks. Compared with patients treated with surgery alone, patients treated with surgery followed by radiotherapy had higher overall 5-year survival (41.3% versus 31.7%), but this was not statistically significant. Among patients who were lymph-node positive, there was a trend toward significantly improved 5-year survival rates with surgery followed by radiation (29.2% versus 14.7%, $P = 0.07$). Among patients who had Stage III disease, 5-year survival was significantly improved with surgery followed by radiation (35.1% versus 13.1%).

Preoperative chemotherapy

There have been three randomized, controlled trials reported comparing preoperative chemotherapy followed by surgery with surgery alone for esophageal cancer. All three trials studied combinations of cisplatin and 5-fluorouracil. In an American study of 440 patients Kelsen et al [17] found no significant differences in 1-year (60%), 2-year (35%), or median survival (15–16 months); locoregional or distant recurrence rates; or perioperative morbidity and mortality between the two groups. No difference was found between squamous cell carcinoma and adenocarcinoma. Weight loss was a significant predictor of poor outcome.

A similar Italian study [18] of 96 patients who had esophageal squamous cell carcinoma reported a 40% response rate to preoperative chemotherapy and comparable rates of microscopically complete resection (74% versus 79%) in both treatment arms. Pathologic complete response was observed in 12.8% of patients receiving chemotherapy. Treatment-related mortality was 4.2% in each treatment arm. Responders to chemotherapy had significantly better 3-year and 5-year survival rates (74% and 60%) compared with nonresponders (24% and 12%) and patients undergoing surgery alone (46% and 26%). Survival was significantly improved for patients achieving a pathologic complete response, but not for those achieving a partial response.

In a British study [19] of 802 patients, the rate of microscopically complete resection was significantly higher for patients undergoing preoperative chemotherapy than for those undergoing surgery alone (60% versus 54%). Postoperative complication rates were similar in both groups (41% versus 42%). Patients undergoing preoperative chemotherapy enjoyed significantly improved median survival (16.8 versus 13.3 months) and 2-year survival (43% versus 34%). It should be noted that in this trial, clinicians could choose to give preoperative radiotherapy to all of their patients, irrespective of randomization.

Trimodality therapy

Both chemotherapy and radiotherapy have been reported to improve survival when administered preoperatively. The notion of "downstaging" esophageal cancer before surgical resection is appealing. Chemotherapy has been combined with radiotherapy in the neoadjuvant setting to improve the resectability of esophageal cancer and improve survival. Most reports of so-called "trimodality therapy" for esophageal carcinoma describe concurrent neoadjuvant chemoradiation using combinations of cisplatin and 5-fluorouracil while administering 30 to 45 Gy. Some have used additional postoperative chemotherapy. Most experienced centers report comparable results.

In an Irish study of 113 patients who had esophageal adenocarcinoma [20], patients were randomized to surgery alone versus trimodality therapy with neoadjuvant chemoradiation. Patients randomized to the trimodality group received two cycles of 5-fluorouracil/cisplatin given concurrently with 40 Gy, followed by surgery. Following neoadjuvant chemoradiation, the pathologic complete response rate was 25%. Trimodality was associated with significantly increased median survival (16 months versus 11 months) and 3-year survival (32% versus 6%). It should be noted that patients randomized to undergo surgery alone had a significantly higher incidence of lymph node involvement. Survival with surgery alone was lower than that reported in most other series.

A French trial of 282 patients who had squamous cell carcinoma of the esophagus [21] compared surgery alone versus two cycles of cisplatin chemotherapy and concurrent radiotherapy (total 37 Gy) followed 2 to 4 weeks later by surgical resection. In one of the largest randomized trials, trimodality therapy was associated with an increased rate of curative resection, longer local disease-free survival time, longer overall disease-free survival time, and fewer cancer-related deaths. Overall survival time, however, was 18.6 months in both treatment arms.

In an Italian Phase II study [22] of 111 patients who had squamous cell carcinoma of the thoracic esophagus, 72% underwent esophagectomy after completing concurrent neoadjuvant chemoradiotherapy with cisplatin/ 5-fluorouracil and 30 Gy. Pathologic complete response was seen in 21% of resected specimens, whereas minimal residual disease was seen in 17.5%. Six percent of resected specimens demonstrated residual tumor that did not extend beyond the submucosa. These 3 groups of so-called "good responders" had median, 2-year, and 5-year survivals of 24 months, 50%, and 35% respectively, compared with 13 months, 27%, and 11% in the remainder of the patients.

A similar French study [23] of 55 patients who had squamous cell carcinoma of the esophagus included those who had cancer of the upper esophagus. This study also used cisplatin/5-fluorouracil and increased the dose of radiation to 36 Gy. The full planned regimen of neoadjuvant chemoradiation was completed in only 67% of patients, but 96% underwent surgical resection. Twenty-two percent had a complete pathologic response with residual Stage I disease in 15% of patients. These so-called "responders" had 3-year and 5-year survivals of 58% and 53%, compared with overall 3-year and 5-year survivals of 39% and 33%.

A recently reported study [24] of 92 patients who had either adenocarcinoma or squamous cell carcinoma of the esophagus used protracted infusion of 5-fluorouracil in addition to cisplatin, and increased the dose of radiation to 44 Gy. Eighty-seven percent of patients underwent complete resection, and transhiatal resection was performed whenever possible. Pathologic complete response was seen in 33% of resected specimens, and was associated with 67% 5-year survival. Survival was similar for patients who had residual Stage I disease. Median survival was related to disease stage at the time of resection. Distant failure was 5 times more common than local recurrence of disease.

A meta-analysis [25] of 9 randomized controlled trials found that neoadjuvant chemoradiation was associated with significantly improved 3-year survival and reduced locoregional recurrence when compared with surgery alone. Although the rate of surgical resection was lower following neoadjuvant chemoradiation, the likelihood of complete (R0) resection was higher. There was a statistical trend toward higher treatment-related mortality with neoadjuvant chemoradiation. The improvement in 3-year survival was highly statistically significant with concurrent administration of chemotherapy and radiation, but not with sequential administration.

Pretreatment staging

For patients who have esophageal cancer, treatment outcome relates to disease stage. In addition to radiologic studies such as CT and positron emission tomography (PET), minimally invasive techniques have been used for pretreatment staging of esophageal cancer. Endoscopic ultrasonography has proven useful in staging the primary tumor as well as sampling of regional lymph nodes. The feasibility of thoracoscopy/laparoscopy for pretreatment staging in esophageal cancer was demonstrated by the Cancer and Leukemia Group B (CALGB) [26]. There were no deaths or complications among 113 patients, 73% of whom underwent thoracoscopic/laparoscopic staging successfully. With the correct use of minimally invasive surgical staging techniques, the incidence of false positive results is effectively zero. The rate of false negative results is lower than with standard radiologic methods.

A retrospective analysis of 45 patients who had esophageal cancer and who underwent pretreatment thoracoscopic/laparoscopic surgical staging followed by trimodality therapy was performed at our institution [27]. Patients received two cycles of 5-fluorouracil and cisplatin with 50.4 Gy concurrent radiation. Following neoadjuvant therapy, node-negative patients enjoyed a higher rate of complete pathologic response (59% versus 14%) and longer median survival (35 months versus 15 months). Patients whose nodes were cleared by chemoradiation had a 3-year survival of 40%, whereas patients who had persistent nodal disease all died within 2 years.

Summary

Stage specific management of non-small cell lung cancer is widely accepted. The use of pretreatment disease stage to guide therapy for esophageal cancer is an intellectually appealing concept. To date, there is a relative lack of data upon which one may base stage specific treatment decisions for esophageal carcinoma. This is because thorough pretreatment TNM staging is not universally practiced. As a result, stage-specific treatment varies widely. Based upon the available data, surgery alone may be appropriate for resectable, node-negative disease. In the case of clearly unresectable disease, definitive chemoradiation is indicated.

The value of neoadjuvant or adjuvant treatment modalities in the case of clearly resectable node-negative disease (T1N0 or T2N0) is questionable; however, in the presence of lymph node involvement (N1), or in the case of a marginally resectable primary tumor (T3 or T4), neoadjuvant chemoradiation is probably indicated. Although the achievement of a complete pathologic response following chemoradiation may obviate surgical resection, even microscopic residual cancer can result in local recurrence. To date, there is no reliable method of ascertaining a complete pathologic response before surgical resection. Therefore, when feasible, the addition of surgical resection following chemoradiation is warranted. Future treatment trials for esophageal cancer should include rigorous pretreatment staging protocols to elucidate stage-specific results of therapy.

References

[1] Roder JD, Busch R, Stein HJ, et al. Ratio of invaded to removed lymph nodes as a predictor of survival in squamous cell carcinoma of the oesophagus. Br J Surg 1994;81:410–3.

[2] Mantravadi R, Ladd T, Briele H, et al. Carcinoma of the esophagus: sites of failure. Int J Radiat Oncol Biol Phys 1982;8:1897.

[3] Sonett JR. Esophagectomy: the role of the intrathoracic anastomosis. Chest Surg Clin N Am 2000;10(3):519–30.

[4] Hulscher JBF, van Sandick JW, de Boer AGEM, et al. Extended transthoracic resection compared with limited transhiatal resection for adenocarcinoma of the esophagus. N Engl J Med 2002;347(21):1662–9.

[5] Caspers RJ, Welvaart K, Verkes RJ, et al. The effect of radiotherapy on dysphagia and survival in patients with esophageal cancer. Radiother Oncol 1988;12:15–21.

[6] Pancierre FJ, Leichman LP, Tilchen EJ, et al. Chemotherapy for advanced epidermoid carcinoma of the esophagus with single-agent cisplatin: final report on a Southwest Oncology Group study. Cancer Treat Rep 1984;68:1023–4.

[7] Herskovic A, Martz K, al-Sarraf M, et al. Combined chemotherapy and radiotherapy compared with radiotherapy alone in patients with cancer of the esophagus. N Engl J Med 1992;326:1593–8.

[8] Cooper JS, Guo MD, Herskovic A, et al. Chemoradiotherapy of locally advanced esophageal cancer: long-term follow-up of a prospective randomized trial (RTOG 85–01). Radiation Therapy Oncology Group. JAMA 1999;281(17):1623–7.

[9] Smith TJ, Ryan LM, Douglass HO Jr, et al. Combined chemoradiotherapy vs. radiotherapy alone for early stage squamous cell carcinoma of the esophagus: a study of the Eastern Cooperative Oncology Group. Int J Radiat Oncol Biol Phys 1998;42(2):269–76.

[10] Minsky BD, Pajak TF, Ginsberg RJ, et al. INT 0123 (Radiation Therapy Oncology Group 94–05) Phase III trial of combined-modality therapy for esophageal cancer: high-dose versus standard-dose radiation therapy. J Clin Oncol 2002;20(5):1167–74.

[11] Gignoux M, Roussel A, Paillot B, et al. The value of preoperative radiotherapy in esophageal cancer: results of a study by the EORTC. World J Surg 1987;11:426–32.

[12] Wang M, Gu XZ, Yin WB, et al. Randomized clinical trial on the combination of preoperative irradiation and surgery in the treatment of esophageal carcinoma: report on 206 patients. Int J Radiat Oncol Biol Phys 1989;16:325–7.

[13] Nygaard K, Hagen S, Hansen HS, et al. Pre-operative radiotherapy prolongs survival in operable esophageal carcinoma: a randomized, multicenter study of pre-operative radiotherapy and chemotherapy: the second Scandinavian trial in esophageal cancer. World J Surg 1992;16:1104–9.

[14] Teniere P, Hay JM, Fingerhut A, et al. Postoperative radiation therapy does not increase survival after curative resection for squamous cell carcinoma of the middle and lower esophagus as shown by a multicenter controlled trial. French University Association for Surgical Research. Surg Gynecol Obstet 1991;173(2):123–30.

[15] Fok M, Sham JS, Choy D, et al. Postoperative radiotherapy for carcinoma of the esophagus: a prospective randomized controlled study. Surgery 1993;113(2):138–47.

[16] Xiao ZF, Yang ZY, Liang J, et al. Value of radiotherapy after radical surgery for esophageal carcinoma: a report of 495 patients. Ann Thorac Surg 2003;75(2):331–6.

[17] Kelsen DP, Ginsberg R, Pajak TF, et al. Chemotherapy followed by surgery compared with surgery alone for localized esophageal cancer. N Engl J Med 1998;339(27): 1979–84.

[18] Ancona E, Ruol A, Santi S, et al. Only pathologic complete response to neoadjuvant chemotherapy improves significantly the long term survival of patients with resectable esophageal squamous cell carcinoma: final report of a randomized, controlled trial of preoperative chemotherapy versus surgery alone. Cancer 2001;91(11):2165–74.

[19] Medical Research Council Oesophageal Cancer Working Group. Surgical resection with or without preoperative chemotherapy in oesophageal cancer: a randomized controlled trial. Lancet 2002;359(9319):1727–33.

[20] Walsh TN, Noonan N, Hollywood D, et al. A comparison of multimodal therapy and surgery for esophageal adenocarcinoma. N Engl J Med 1996;335:462–7.

[21] Bossett JF, Gignoux M, Triboulet JP, et al. Chemoradiotherapy followed by surgery compared with surgery alone in squamous-cell cancer of the esophagus. N Engl J Med 1997; 337:161–7.

[22] Laterza E, de' Manzoni G, Tedesco P, et al. Induction chemo-radiotherapy for squamous cell carcinoma of the thoracic esophagus: long-term results of a Phase II study. Ann Surg Oncol 1999;6(8):777–84.

[23] Adham M, Baulieux J, Mornex F, et al. Combined chemotherapy and radiotherapy followed by surgery in the treatment of patients with squamous cell carcinoma of the esophagus. Cancer 2000;89(5):946–54.

[24] Kleinberg L, Knisely JP, Heitmiller R, et al. Mature survival results with preoperative cisplatin, protracted infusion 5-fluorouracil, and 44-Gy radiotherapy for esophageal cancer. Int J Radiat Oncol Biol Phys 2003;56(2):328–34.

[25] Urschel JD, Vasan H. A meta-analysis of randomized controlled trials that compared neoadjuvant chemoradiation and surgery to surgery alone for resectable esophageal cancer. Am J Surg 2003;185:538–43.

[26] Krasna MJ, Reed CE, Nedzwiecki D, et al. CALGB 9380: a prospective trial of the feasibility of thoracoscopy/laparoscopy in staging esophageal cancer. Ann Thorac Surg 2001;71(4): 1073–9.

[27] Suntharalingam J, Haas ML, Sonett JR, et al. Accurate lymph node assessment prior to trimodality therapy for esophageal carcinoma. Cancer J 2001;7(6):509–15.

ELSEVIER
SAUNDERS

Surg Clin N Am 85 (2005) 631–647

SURGICAL
CLINICS OF
NORTH AMERICA

Minimally Invasive Esophagectomy

Alberto de Hoyos, MD, Virginia R. Litle, MD,
James D. Luketich, MD*

*Division of Thoracic and Foregut Surgery and the Minimally Invasive Surgery Center,
University of Pittsburgh Medical Center, UPMC Presbyterian, Suite C-800,
200 Lothrop Street, Pittsburgh, PA 15213, USA*

The incidence of adenocarcinoma of the esophagus has increased in recent years in North America and Europe. Carcinoma of the esophagus remains a deadly disease, with an overall 5-year survival of only 5% to 10%. Stage-specific survival varies to some degree from series to series, primarily due to incomplete lymph node dissection and occult metastases that may be missed by conventional imaging. In most series of patients who undergo esophagectomy, the 5-year survival averages 30%; however, patients who have carcinoma of the esophagus arising in a columnar-lined esophagus (CLE, Barrett's carcinoma) and who are diagnosed with an in-situ or T1 lesion have 5-year survivals of from 90% to 100% [1].

Conventional esophagectomy is associated with significant morbidity and mortality rates; however, reductions in complication rates have been reported in centers with a high volume of esophageal surgery [2]. In an effort to further decrease the morbidity associated with esophagectomy, surgeons have reported the application of minimally invasive techniques for resection of the esophagus. In addition, a variety of benign conditions of the esophagus, such as achalasia and recalcitrant gastroesophageal reflux disease and its complications, may also eventually require esophagectomy for resolution of chronic incapacitating symptoms or to prevent progression to advanced carcinoma.

Current techniques of esophagectomy

Esophagectomy for carcinoma of the esophagus should include several objectives: complete resection of all disease, including removal of most of the esophagus; dissection of regional lymph nodes; and restoration of swallowing with placement of the gastric or intestinal anastomosis in the upper chest or in the neck [3,4].

---

* Corresponding author.
E-mail address: luketichjd@upmc.edu (J.D. Luketich).

0039-6109/05/$ - see front matter © 2005 Elsevier Inc. All rights reserved.
doi:10.1016/j.suc.2005.01.003   *surgical.theclinics.com*

Although the best approach to esophagectomy remains controversial, the two most frequently performed operations are the transthoracic (TTE) and the transhiatal esophagectomies (THE) [3,5]. The TTE (Ivor-Lewis) approach allows the surgeon to perform a wide mediastinal lymphadenectomy and provide adequate hemostasis. The anastomosis is constructed in the right chest, just above the divided azygos vein. The THE, or esophagectomy without thoracotomy, uses blunt transhiatal dissection of the esophagus, as popularized by Orringer [6], with the anastomosis constructed in the left neck. Other approaches include esophagectomy through a left thoraco-abdominal incision (Tanner) and a modification of the TTE—the three-field approach, with the addition of a left neck incision for a cervical anastomosis [7]. All of these surgical approaches require a laparotomy for mobilization and preparation of the gastric conduit.

Complication rates of esophagectomy vary between 30% and 80%, and average about 50%, depending on the series and the criteria used to define complications. Hospital mortality in most reported series is 5% to 10% for patients resected for cure [8]; however, in a recent review of the Medicare database [2], the mortality following esophagectomy from most centers was much higher, and ranged from 8% in high-volume centers to as high as 23% in centers performing a low volume of this complex operation. The factors that have traditionally guided the choice of approach have been largely surgeon preference and skills, concerns over the morbidity and mortality associated with each approach, and the ability to perform the appropriate lateral and longitudinal extent of resection. In fact, conventional approaches have attempted to either maximize the resection margin or to minimize the associated morbidity and complications. For example, the transthoracic approach provides excellent exposure to the mediastinum and facilitates an extensive lymphadenectomy, but is associated with the pain of a thoracotomy and the potential morbidity of related pulmonary complications and intrathoracic leak. On the other hand, the transhiatal approach, precluding an extensive mediastinal lymphadenectomy, avoids the risk of an intrathoracic leak, and may be associated with less pain and pulmonary morbidity. There is, nevertheless, still a significant morbidity and mortality associated with either approach.

The development of minimally invasive techniques has significantly reduced the pain and morbidity of many foregut procedures, and in some cases has made them technically easier to perform while maintaining sound surgical principles. With the recent advances in laparoscopic surgery, it has been possible to apply minimally invasive techniques to esophagectomy, as described below.

Minimally invasive esophagectomy

Advances in minimally invasive technology and surgical techniques have allowed surgeons to perform more complex procedures safely. Surgeons can now perform laparoscopic antireflux surgery [9], laparoscopic repair of giant paraesophageal hernia [10], laparoscopic or thoracoscopic myotomy for achalasia [11], laparoscopic and thoracoscopic staging for lung and esophageal cancer [12,13], and video-assisted thoracoscopic (VATS) lobectomy [14]. Although it is clear that not all minimally invasive operations yield results as good as open, in the authors' experience a thoracoscopic approach to a Belsey fundoplication was associated with an unacceptable recurrence at short-term follow-up, which led to our abandonment of this approach in favor of laparoscopic anti-reflux approaches, or an open thoracotomy if a Belsey fundoplication was necessary [15]. Similarly, other centers have reported suboptimal results for other complex minimally invasive operations, including laparoscopic repair of giant paraesophageal hernias, with higher recurrences and complications compared with open surgery [16,17]. The authors have been able to establish an effective approach to laparoscopic giant paraesophageal hernias, but did see significant difficulties in the early phases of the steep laparoscopic learning curve. With the limitations and successes gained in endoscopic surgery for benign conditions, surgeons have cautiously applied these techniques to resection of the esophagus for esophageal cancer. Techniques are listed in Box 1.

Initially, thoracoscopic esophagectomy was combined with a standard upper midline laparotomy and cervical anastomosis [18–21]. Subsequently, several authors demonstrated the feasibility and safety of a minimally invasive total laparoscopic approach, with transhiatal esophagectomy in combination with a cervical anastomosis [22–25]. This approach avoided the need for a laparotomy or thoracotomy; however, concerns with the completion of the thoracic mobilization, the technically difficult view of the upper esophagus during laparoscopy, and the inability to perform a complete lymph node dissection through this totally laparoscopic approach

---

Box 1. Endoscopic approaches to esophagectomy

- Thoracoscopic esophagectomy with laparotomy for gastric mobilization and cervical esophagogastrostomy
- Thoracoscopic esophagectomy with laparotomy for gastric mobilization and intrathoracic esophagogastrostomy
- Laparoscopic gastric mobilization, thoracotomy for esophagectomy with intrathoracic esophagogastrostomy
- Thoracoscopic esophagectomy, laparoscopic gastric mobilization, and cervical esophagogastrostomy
- Thoracoscopic esophagectomy, laparoscopic hand-assisted gastric mobilization
- Laparoscopic transmediastinal esophagectomy with cervical esophagogastrostomy

encouraged surgeons to apply their expertise with thoracoscopy to esophagectomy in combination with laparoscopy or laparotomy [26]. Several groups have reported their experience with this approach [26–28].

This article describes the authors' technique of minimally invasive esophagectomy (MIE) using a right VATS mobilization, followed by laparoscopic transhiatal esophagectomy, with a standard left-neck incision for anastomosis of the gastric conduit to the cervical esophagus [29,30].

Indications for minimally invasive esophagectomy

The authors have reported results of minimally invasive esophagectomy in 222 patients, and our experience is now approaching 500 cases [30]. Indications include esophageal cancer, columnar lined esophagus (Barrett's esophagus) with high-grade dysplasia, end-stage achalasia, recalcitrant esophageal strictures, and tracheo-esophageal fistulas. As we acquired experience and confidence with the procedure, we have extended our indications to include patients who have received neoadjuvant chemotherapy and radiation for locally advanced esophageal cancer [26,29,30].

Patient selection and preoperative work-up

All patients have a thorough history and physical examination to assess possible metastatic disease and comorbidities. Esophagoscopy is performed routinely to evaluate the esophageal pathology and confirm the presence and extent of carcinoma or Barrett's with high-grade dysplasia. Barium swallow is also performed. This simple and inexpensive contrast study allows the surgeon to view the anatomy preoperatively, and may uncover unsuspected obstacles such as large hiatal hernias, Zenker's diverticulum, and gastric abnormalities. Bronchoscopy is performed in patients who have carcinoma of the middle and upper thirds of the esophagus, in order to exclude airway involvement. Patients who have esophageal carcinoma undergo staging with endoscopic ultrasonography (EUS) and CT of the chest and abdomen. If the esophagogastroduodenoscopy, EUS, or CT scan findings suggest gastric extension, T4 local extension, or nodal metastases, we perform a staging laparoscopy, thoracoscopy, or both. CT of the brain and whole-body positron emission tomography (PET) scanning are used selectively.

Who is not a candidate for minimally invasive esophagectomy

Prior surgery involving the abdominal or thoracic cavity is rarely a contraindication to MIE. Patients who have bulky esophageal tumors or tumors involving surrounding structures should be carefully staged, and may need laparoscopy or thoracoscopy to determine their candidacy for surgery. In general, the authors would not operate on T4 tumors. A "hostile" abdomen from multiple previous laparotomies, massive ascites, previous major gastric resection, prior left pneumonectomy, or inability to tolerate single-lung anesthesia are also considered relative contraindications.

Operative technique

Anesthesia

Patients are intubated with a left double-lumen endotracheal tube for the thoracoscopic portion of the procedure. A radial artery catheter to monitor blood pressure and arterial blood gases is inserted. On the table, esophagogastroduodenoscopy is performed by the surgeon. Any concerns over resectability that have not been resolved by preoperative staging should be addressed by on-the-table laparoscopic staging. Single-lung ventilation is started as soon as possible to allow ample time for controlled atelectasis, which will facilitate entry into the chest and optimize visualization of the posterior mediastinal structures. For the laparoscopic portion of the procedure, the double lumen endotracheal tube is exchanged to a single lumen tube. All patients have a Foley catheter and antithrombotic sequential compression devices placed after intubation. All pressure points are adequately protected and antibiotic prophylaxis is administered.

The important technical elements of MIE are: (1) insertion of the thoracoscopic ports and complete en-bloc lymph node dissection of the mid and lower intrathoracic esophagus, (2)insertion of the laparoscopic ports and mobilization of the stomach with preservation of the right gastroepiploic arcade, (3) hiatal dissection, (4) pyloroplasty, (5) configuration of the gastric conduit and transhiatal mobilization, (6) creation of a cervical esophagogastric anastomosis, and (7) feeding jejunostomy.

Video-assisted thoracoscopic lobectomy: esophageal mobilization

With the patient in complete left lateral decubitus and with the table flexed at the hips, four thoracoscopic ports are introduced (Fig. 1). The surgeon stands posteriorly to the patient and the assistant stands anteriorly. The camera port (10 mm) is placed at the eighth intercostal space anteriorly. A 5-mm port is placed at the eighth or ninth intercostal space 2 cm posterior to the posterior axillary line, for the ultrasonic coagulating shears (US Surgical, Norwalk, Connecticut). Care is taken to avoid placing this port lower, which would make access to the upper chest difficult. Two additional ports are placed: one 5-mm port is placed posterior to the tip of the scapula, and one 10-mm port is placed at the fourth intercostal space at the anterior axillary line for retraction and counter-traction during the esophageal dissection. A single retracting Endo-stitch (US Surgical, Norwalk, Connecticut) is placed in the central tendon of the diaphragm and brought out of the inferior, anterior chest wall through a 1-mm skin nick. This suture allows downward traction on the diaphragm and excellent exposure of the distal esophagus, thus eliminating the need for an additional retractor.

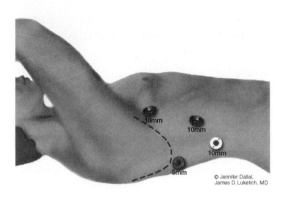

Fig. 1. Video-assisted thoracoscopic surgical port sites.

The inferior pulmonary ligament is divided to the level of the inferior pulmonary vein. The mediastinal pleura overlying the esophagus is then widely divided from the diaphragm up to the level of the azygos vein. The azygos vein is then divided using the Endo-GIA vascular stapler (Endo-GIA II, US Surgical, Norwalk, Connecticut). Care is taken to preserve the mediastinal pleura above the azygos vein. The authors believe that this pleura helps to maintain the gastric tube in a mediastinal location, and may also help seal the plane around the gastric tube near the thoracic inlet, thereby minimizing the downward extension of a cervical leak into the chest. Circumferential mobilization of the esophagus is performed up to the level of 1 to 2 cm above the carina, including all surrounding lymph nodes; periesophageal tissues and fat; and the plane along the pericardium, aorta, and contralateral mediastinal pleura, up to but not including the thoracic duct and azygos vein laterally (Fig. 2). The entire subcarinal node packet is

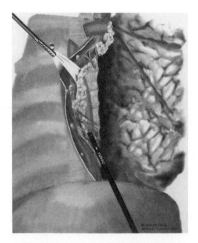

Fig. 2. Penrose drain around thoracic esophagus.

removed with the specimen; lymph nodes from the upper esophagus and adjacent to the recurrent nerve are only sampled. A Penrose drain is placed around the esophagus to facilitate traction and exposure. Care is taken to achieve hemostasis of the bronchial vessels supplying the lymph nodes. As the dissection proceeds toward the thoracic inlet, care is taken to stay near the esophagus, so as to avoid injury to the membranous trachea and the recurrent laryngeal nerves. The vagus nerves are typically divided above the level of the carina, and all periesophageal tissue is gently preserved above this level to avoid injury to the recurrent nerves, which are generally not visualized. Large Endoclips (Endot, Rockaway, New Jersey) are used during the dissection of the mid and lower esophagus on the chest wall side, to avoid lymphatic chylous leaks from branches of the thoracic duct and bleeding from aortoesophageal vessels posteriorly. After complete mobilization of the esophagus has been achieved, the Penrose drain is tucked into the thoracic inlet. The authors have found this to be helpful during the neck dissection and retrieval of and mobilization of the cervical esophagus. Regional anesthesia for up to 12 hours is achieved by injecting each intercostal space with 1 to 2 mL of 0.5% bupivacaine with epinephrine. The lung is gently inflated to search for any air leaks from the trachea and proximal bronchus. A single 28F chest tube is inserted through the camera port and positioned in the posterior mediastinum. All other port sites are closed in two layers with absorbable sutures.

Laparoscopy: gastric mobilization and preparation of the gastric conduit

In the supine position, five ports are placed on the anterior abdominal wall, in a similar orientation to our approach for laparoscopic Nissen fundoplication, but each slightly lower (Fig. 3). The surgeon stands on the patient's right and the assistant stands on the left. A 10-mm port is placed in the right epigastrium, using a blunt cut-down technique with entry into the peritoneum under direct vision. Pneumoperitoneum is then achieved in a routine fashion. Four additional 5-mm ports are placed in the following positions: bilateral subcostal, left epigastrium, and right flank. The left lobe of the liver is retracted upward to expose the esophageal hiatus using a Lapro-Flex retractor (Mediflex Surgical Products, Islandia, New York) and held in place with a self-retaining system placed on the left side of the table (Single flex arm system, Mediflex Surgical Products, Islandia, New York). With the patient in maximal reverse Trendelenburg position, the dissection begins with division of the gastro-hepatic ligament and exposure of the right crus of the diaphragm. The gastrocolic ligament is identified, and the dissection is performed lateral to the gastroepiploic arcade, using the ultrasonic coagulating shears. Dissection continues along the greater curve of the stomach, preserving the right gastroepiploic vessels (Fig. 4). The short gastric vessels are then divided using the ultrasonic coagulating shears or large Endoclips on the splenic side of the vessels. No clips are placed on

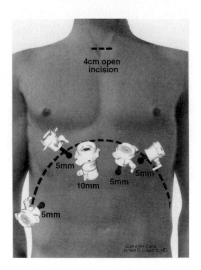

Fig. 3. Abdominal port sites for laparoscopy.

the gastric side, in order to avoid potential interference with endoscopic stapling devices during the construction of the gastric tube. The stomach is retracted superiorly, allowing lymph node dissection of the celiac and gastric vessels. During the entire procedure, the greater curve portion of the stomach that will constitute the ultimate gastric tube is only handled in an atraumatic fashion. The left gastric vessels are exposed and divided with the Endo-GIA II with vascular loads, near the celiac artery, after the lymph nodes in this area are dissected and removed.

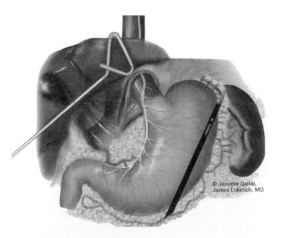

Fig. 4. Mobilization of greater curvature.

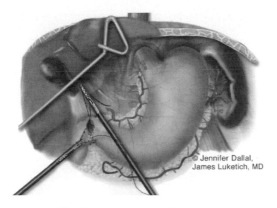

Fig. 5. Laparoscopic pyloroplasty.

A pyloroplasty is then performed using ultrasonic coagulating shears, and the defect is closed transversely in a Heinecke-Mikulicz fashion, using, on average, four to five 2-0 Endo-stitches (Fig. 5). A Kocher maneuver is performed by gentle dissection of the gastroduodenal attachments. The gastric tube is then constructed by dividing the stomach starting at the distal lesser curve, again preserving the right gastric vessels (Fig. 6). Multiple firings of the 4.8 mm Endo-GIA II stapler are used to achieve tubularization of the stomach. The authors currently prefer a gastric tube of 5 to 6 cm in diameter. The gastric tube and staple line are carefully inspected; any concerns over viability may require conversion to an open operation. The most cephalad portion of the gastric tube is then attached to the esophagogastric specimen using two Endo-stitch sutures (Fig. 7). The newly created gastric tube is then left in place, and attention is directed to the remaining laparoscopic portions of the operation. The gastric tube is again carefully examined for any bleeding staple lines or divided short gastric vessels and problems with viability before

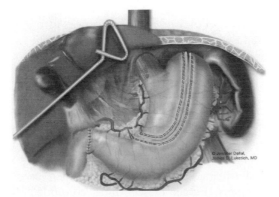

Fig. 6. Laparoscopic gastric tubularization.

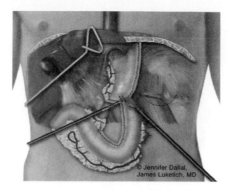

Fig. 7. Attachment of newly created gastric tube to resected specimen.

the pull-up. Extreme caution must be used when manipulating the gastric tube during mobilization and stapling to avoid trauma.

Next, the authors place an additional 10-mm port in the mid- to lower-right quadrants to facilitate placement of the feeding jejunostomy tube. The ligament of Treitz is identified by lifting the transverse colon, and a mobile loop of jejunum is identified approximately 25 to 30 cm distal to the ligament. The selected loop of jejunum is attached to the anterior abdominal wall using the Endo-stitch. A needle catheter kit (Compact Biosystems, Minneapolis, Minnesota) is inserted percutaneously into the peritoneal cavity, and under direct laparoscopic vision it is directed into the proximal loop of jejunum, taking care to avoid injury to the mesenteric vessels. The guidewire and catheter are threaded into the jejunum. The jejunum is tacked to the anterior abdominal wall with a total of three to four Endo-stitches around the entry site, and an additional stitch a few centimeters distally to prevent torsion of the jejunal limb. The feeding tube is secured to the skin with several 2-0 silk sutures and tested with air or saline to ensure patency.

The last step of the abdominal stage of the operation is the final dissection of the phrenoesophageal ligament, which opens the plane into the thoracic cavity. This step is performed last to minimize loss of pneumoperitoneum into the mediastinum or chest cavities. The authors also partially divide the right and left crura to widen the hiatus in order to prevent gastric-tube outlet obstruction.

Neck dissection: anastomosis

A 5-cm horizontal neck incision is made just above the suprasternal notch and slightly to the left. The platysma and strap muscles are divided with electocautery. One self-retaining retractor is used, but it is placed only on the skin and platysmal flap to minimize traction injury to the recurrent laryngeal nerve. Sharp and blunt dissection is then used to expose and mobilize the esophagus. Finger dissection is continued distally until the thoracic dissection plane is encountered. This is generally easily found, due to the high periesophageal dissection that was performed during thoraco-scopy. The Penrose drain encircling the esophagus is retrieved and used to assist in the delivery of the proximal esophagus and gastric remnant through the neck incision. As the esophagus and specimen are being retrieved, an assistant simultaneously performs laparoscopy to guide the pull-up of the newly created gastric tube, in order to assure that the correct orientation is maintained to avoid spiraling and to avoid any tension on the specimen as it passes through the hiatus. As the specimen is delivered into the neck, the gastric tube is carefully pulled into the neck area, and an assessment of length and viability is made. The sutures holding the gastric tube to the esophagogastric specimen are removed. Next, a careful mobilization of the very proximal cervical esophagus is performed to minimize distortion of the axis after construction of the anastomoses. We prefer to divide the proximal esophagus very near the cricopharyngeus using an auto purse-string device (US Surgical, Autosuture, Norwalk, Connecticut). The esophagus is transected distally and the esophagogastric specimen is examined and sent for frozen section margin assessment. An anastomosis is performed between the cervical esophagus and the gastric tube using a 25-mm EEA stapler (US Surgical, Autosuture, Norwalk, Connecticut). For this purpose, the selected anvil is lubricated and gently positioned inside the esophagus, and purse string is tied. A small gastrotomy is created in the tip of the gastric conduit, and the EEA stapler is advanced into position. The EEA is directed out the postero-lateral area of the gastric conduit several centimeters from the tip. Generally, there is ample length of gastric tube to easily perform this maneuver. The authors avoid an anastomosis directly on the lesser curve staple line, and also prefer to not come out in the direct line of the short gastrics on the greater curve, because the anastomotic vascular network is in this location. Once the anastomosis is created, the stapler is inspected for the presence of two complete tissue rings. A nasogastric tube is placed across the anastomosis and positioned within the distal portion of the intrathoracic stomach tube. The gastrotomy is closed with the Endo-GIA II stapler.

Attention is now directed to the laparoscopic view. The gastric tube is gently pulled downward as the neck anastomosis is directly visualized. Downward tension on the gastric tube is performed to deliver any redundancy lying within the thoracic cavity that may have developed during the cervial anastomosis. As the anastomosis is noted to move downward, this generally indicates that all excess intrathoracic gastric tube has been delivered intra-abdominally. The gastric tube is tacked to the diaphragm using three to four interrupted sutures. Care is taken to avoid trauma to the vascular supply of the gastric tube. Again, at this point, care is taken to attempt to align the stomach with the gastropiploic arcade near the left crus and the right gastric artery near the right crus. Tacking of the gastric tube is essential to prevent subsequent thoracic herniation of other intra-abdominal organs, most notably the transverse colon (Fig. 8). The neck incision and

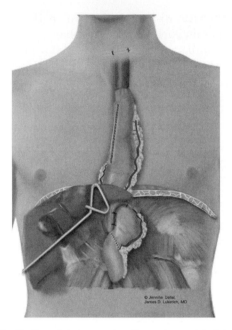

Fig. 8. Completed reconstruction using gastric tube.

abdominal port sites are irrigated with antibiotic solution and closed. The authors prefer to only close the neck incision very loosely with one or two interrupted sutures, so that if a leak occurs, it will be more likely to drain out of the cervical neck incision and not travel into the right chest.

Postoperative management

Patients are typically extubated in the operating room and kept in the intensive care unit overnight. Pain management is provided by patient controlled analgesia. Heparin 5000 units sq is administered as thromboembolic prophylaxis every 12 hours. Incentive spirometry and early ambulation are encouraged to prevent pulmonary complications. A barium contrast study is performed on postoperative day 3 or 4. If hoarseness is present, a modified swallow should be performed to assess for aspiration. The chest tube is removed and clear liquid diet started when the contrast study demonstrates no leak. Supplemental jejunal feedings are administered routinely for 2 weeks, and are generally cycled to run at night. No medications are administered through the needle catheter feeding tube, to avoid clogging. Daily inspection of the appropriate mark on the feeding tube is performed to avoid inadvertent dislodgment. Patients are routinely assessed by nutrition therapy and instructed in their diet. Generally, if no leak is present, patients are sent home on 1 to 2 ounces of full liquids every 2 hours and supplemented with nocturnal feeds. We have found that early oral diets in excess of this may lead to unnecessary early gastric tube dilatation and the potential for aspiration, and may contribute to gastric conduit ischemia. Routine outpatient follow-up is done at 2 to 3 weeks after discharge. At this time, if the limited oral diet is tolerated and no other complications are present, we advance to a soft diet and discontinue the jejunostomy feeds.

Complications

Intraoperative

Intraoperative complications have been uncommon in the authors' experience, but include potentially serious problems. These include bleeding requiring conversion to open procedure, injury to the airway, injury to the gastric conduit, injury to the hypopharynx or recurrent laryngeal nerve, or injury to other intrathoracic or intra-abdominal structures. A difficult laparoscopic dissection that in the judgment of the surgeon, is not proceeding in a timely manner, or is not proceeding safely, should be converted to an open approach. Several complications deserve special comment. During the thoracoscopy, care must be taken to perform gentle dissection in the area of the thoracic duct. The authors prefer to use Endoclips along duct branches to minimize the potential for postoperative chylothorax. When performing dissection of the esophagus near the posterior membranous bronchi and trachea, one cannot allow the ultrasonic shears or the electrocautery to come into contact, because immediate or delayed injury may occur. Aortoesophageal branches should be carefully identified and clipped to avoid bleeding. An aortoesopahgeal branch divided near the aorta that continues to bleed is a very difficult problem. It is generally not life-threatening, but visualization may be problematic, and it may be necessary to open to deal with this. At the completion of the thoracoscopy, a careful inspection for air leaks is performed using irrigation, and a final inspection for chyle or bleeding areas is important.

Postoperative

Minor postoperative complications include urinary retention, air leaks, pleural effusions, atrial fibrillation, and atelectasis, and occur in approximately 50% of patients. Major complications include anastomotic leaks, delayed gastric emptying, chylothorax, mediastinal or abdominal abscess, wound infections, pyloric leak, venous thromboembolisms, myocardial infarction, pneumonia, adult respiratory distress syndrome, port-site recurrence, and anastomotic stricture requiring dilatation.

Results at the University of Pittsburgh

The authors reported our initial experience with a combined approach to esophagectomy, including thoracoscopic mobilization of the esophagus, laparoscopic completion of esophagectomy, and transhiatal passage of the gastric conduit with a cervical anastomosis [26,29]. In subsequent reports, we updated our experience with over 220 undergoing MIE [30]. Indications for operation included esophageal carcinoma in 175 (78.8%) and high-grade dysplasia in patients who had CLE in 46 (21.2%). Neoadjuvant chemotherapy was used in 78 patients (35.1%), and radiation was used in 36 patients (16.2%). The mean operative time was 7.5 hours (range 4–13.6 hours). The mean intensive care unit stay was 1 day (range 0–60 days). The mean hospital stay was 7 days (range 4–73 days). Time to oral intake was 4 days (1–40). The mean follow-up was 19 months (1–68).

MIE was successfully completed in 206 patients (92.8%). Thoracotomy was required in 12 (5.4%) and laparotomy in 4 patients (1.8%). The 30-day operative mortality was 1.4% (n = 3). Causes of death included pneumonia, pericardial tamponade, and postoperative myocardial infarction. Anastomotic leak rate was affected by the size of the gastric tube. In those patients with our standard gastric tube of 5 to 6 cm, anastomotic leaks occurred in 10 of 164 patients (6.1%). In those patients in whom a narrow tube was used (3–4 cm), the leak rate was significantly higher ($P < 0.001$), occurring in 15 of 58 patients (26%).

Other series

DePaula and associates [22] were the first to report on a series of patients undergoing an esophagectomy without thoracotomy or laparotomy. They performed a total transhiatal esophagectomy laparoscopically with a single incision in the neck for the anastomosis. Although this proved to be a lengthy and very difficult operation, most procedures were successfully completed laparoscopically without operative mortality. Subsequently, Swanstrom and Hansen [24] reported their experience with total laparoscopic transhiatal esophagectomy in nine highly selected patients. One patient required thoracoscopy and intrathoracic anastomosis because of questionable viability of the gastric conduit. The mean operative time was 6.5 hours (range 4–10 hours), although these times shortened significantly with more experience. The mean hospital stay was 6.4 days (range 4–10 days). There were two intraoperative complications, poor gastric tube viability, and a liver laceration. No further intervention was required in these two cases. Five patients developed transient hoarseness, and one developed permanent hoarseness that required vocal cord augmentation. One patient had a cervical anastomotic stricture that required dilatation. There was no operative mortality, but there were three late deaths; two from metastatic cancer and one from cardiac disease.

Akaishi and associates [28] reported their experience with thoracoscopic esophagectomy. After a period of animal experimentation, they performed thoracoscopic esophagectomy in 39 patients who had squamous cell carcinoma of the esophagus. A standard upper midline laparotomy and a cervical anastomosis were used. All procedures were completed thoracoscopically and there was no operative mortality.

Nguyen et al [27] recently published their experience with MIE in 18 patients using a combined approach. They compared MIE with their previous experience with TTE (n = 16) and THE (n = 20). Minimally invasive esophagectomy was associated with shorter operative times, less blood loss, fewer transfusion requirement, and shortened intensive care unit and hospital stay. There was no significant difference in the incidence of anastomotic leak or respiratory complications among the three groups. Long-term survival data after MIE are not yet available. Prospective clinical trials will be required to define the role of this approach.

Oncologic perspectives

One of the most controversial aspects of treating esophageal cancer is the appropriate extent of resection to achieve the best outcome. An R0 resection is consistently identified as the most important prognostic factor for long-term survival. An R0 resection results in total removal of the tumor mass (primary and lymph nodes) with clear proximal, distal, and lateral margins. As with other laparoscopic operations for cancer, concern has been raised about the appropriateness of MIE for carcinoma of the esophagus. Concerns with MIE include inadequate staging, local recurrence due to inappropriate margins, completeness of nodal dissection, port-site recurrence, and tumor dissemination.

Oncologic principles are followed during MIE. Trocars are used routinely at all thoracic sites to prevent direct contact of the dissecting instruments with the chest wall. Intraoperative endoscopy is used liberally to identify the proximal and distal extent of the tumor before surgical resection. The addition of thoracoscopy has allowed better visualization of the surrounding esophageal tissues for nodal clearance, as demonstrated in the authors' experience. The esophagogastrectomy specimen is removed through the cervical incision instead of through a limited abdominal or thoracic port site. The mean number of nodes retrieved from MIE specimens is similar to the number retrieved from our open esophagectomies. Frozen section analysis is performed routinely to ensure absence of tumor at the proximal and distal resection margins. Refinements in minimally invasive technology and the increasing experience of surgeons with minimally invasive procedures have made possible en-bloc esophagectomy without thoracotomy or laparotomy.

Summary

Minimally invasive esophagectomy can be safely performed in selected cases in centers specializing in minimally invasive esophageal surgery. Potential benefits include lessened physiologic insult, with decreased hospital stay and a more rapid recovery to full activity. Drawbacks include the cost of the disposable instrumentation and the steep learning curve. As thoracic surgeons continue to acquire expertise with this procedure, improved results may be expected. Prospective trials with longer follow-up will be required to confirm any advantages of MIE over conventional approaches. Open surgical approaches should remain the standard operation for esophagectomy in most institutions.

References

[1] Lerut T, Coosemans W, Van Raemdonck D, et al. Surgical treatment of Barrett's carcinoma: correlations between morphologic findings and prognosis. J Thorac Cardiovasc Surg 1994; 107:1059–65.

[2] Birkmeyer JD, Siewers AE, Finlayson EV, et al. Hospital and surgical mortality in the United States. N Engl J Med 2002;346:1128–37.

[3] Wu PC, Posner MC. The role of surgery in the management of oesophageal cancer. Lancet Oncol 2003;2:481–8.

[4] Law S, Wong J. Use of minimally invasive oesophagectomy for cancer of the esophagus. Lancet Oncol 2002;3:215–22.

[5] Mllikan KW, Silverstein J, Hart V, et al. A 15-year review of esophagectomy for carcinoma of the esophagus and cardia. Arch Surg 1995;130:617–24.

[6] Orringer MB, Marshall B, Iannettoni MD. Eliminating the cervical esophagogastric anastomotic leak with a side-to-side stapled anastomosis. J Thorac Cardiovasc Surg 2000; 119:277–87.

[7] Lerut T, Coosemans W, De Leyn P, et al. Reflections on three field lymphadenectomy in carcinoma of the esophagus and gastroesophageal junction. Hepatogastroenterology 1999; 46:717–25.

[8] Mathisen DJ, Grillo HC, Wilkins EW, et al. Transthoracic esophagectomy: a safe approach to carcinoma of the esophagus. Ann Thorac Surg 1988;45:137–45.

[9] Bais JE, Bartelsman JF, Bonjer HJ, et al. Laparoscopic or conventional Nissen fundoplication for gastro-esophageal reflux disease: randomized clinical trial. The Netherlands Antireflux Surgery Group. Lancet 2000;355:170–4.

[10] Pierre AF, Luketich JD, Fernando HC, et al. Results of laparoscopic repair of giant paraesophageal hernias: 200 consecutive cases. Ann Thorac Surg 2002;74:1909–16.

[11] Luketich JD, Fernando HC, Christie NA, et al. Outcomes after minimally invasive esophageal myotomy for achalasia. Ann Thorac Surg 2001;72:1909–12.

[12] Sonett JR, Krasna MJ. Thoracoscopic staging for intrathoracic malignancy. In: Yim APC, Hazelrigg SR, Izzat MB, editors. Minimal access cardiothoracic surgery. Philadelphia: W.B. Saunders Co; 2000. p. 183–93.

[13] Luketich JD, Schauer P, Landreneau R, et al. Minimally invasive surgical staging is superior to endoscopic ultrasound in detecting lymph node metastasis in esophageal cancer. J Thorac Cardiovasc Surg 1997;114:817–23.

[14] Walker WS, Codispoti M, Soon SY, et al. Long-term outcomes following VATS lobectomy for non-small cell bronchogenic carcinoma. Eur J Cardiothorac Surg 2003;23:397–402.

[15] Nguyen NT, Schauer PR, Hutson W, et al. Preliminary results of thoracoscopic Belsey Mark IV antireflux procedure. Surg Laparosc Endosc 1998;8:185–8.

[16] Dahlberg PS, Deschamps C, Miller DL, et al. Laparoscopic repair of large paraesophageal hiatal hernia. Ann Thorac Surg 2001;72:1125–9.

[17] Diaz S, Brunt LM, Klingensmith ME, et al. Laparoscopic paraesophageal hernia repair, a challenging operation: medium-term outcome in 116 patients. J Gastrointest Surg 2003;7: 59–66.

[18] McAnena OJ, Rogers J, Williams NS. Right thoracoscopically assisted esophagectomy for cancer. Br J Surg 1994;81:236–8.

[19] Robertson GM, Lloyd DM, Wicks AC, et al. No obvious advantages for thoracoscopic two-stage oesophagectomy. Br J Surg 1996;83:675–8.

[20] Dexter SPL, Martin JG, McMahon MJ. Radical thoracoscopic esophagectomy for cancer. Surg Endosc 1996;10:147–51.

[21] Law P, Jok M, Chu KM, et al. Thoracoscopic esophagectomy for esophageal cancer. Surgery 1997;122:8–14.

[22] DePaula AL, Hashiba K, Ferreira EAB, et al. Transhiatal approach for esophagectomy. In: Tooli J, Gossot D, Hunter JG, editors. Endosurgery. New York: Churchill Livingstone; 1996. p. 293–9.

[23] Jagot P, Sauvanet A, Berthoux L, et al. Laparoscopic mobilization of the stomach for esophageal replacement. Br J Surg 1996;83:540–2.

[24] Swanstrom LL, Hansen P. Laparoscopic total esophagectomy. Arch Surg 1997;132: 943–9.

[25] Luketich JD, Nguyen N, Schauer P. Laparoscopic transhiatal esophagectomy for Barrett's esophagus with high grade dysplasia. JSLS 1998;2:75–7.

[26] Luketich JD, Nguyen NT, Weigel TL, et al. Minimally invasive approach to esophagectomy. JSLS 1998;2:243–7.

[27] Nguyen NT, Follette DM, Wolfe BM, et al. Comparison of minimally invasive esophagectomy with transthoracic and transhiatal esophagectomy. Arch Surg 2000;135: 920–5.

[28] Akaishi T, Kaneda I, Higuchi N, et al. Thoracoscopic en bloc total esophagectomy with radical mediastinal lymphadenectomy. J Thorac Cardiovasc Surg 1996;112:1533–41.

[29] Luketich JD, Schauer PR, Christie NA, et al. Minimally invasive esophagectomy. Ann Thorac Surg 2000;70:906–12.

[30] Luketich JD, Alvelo-Rivera M, Buenaventura PO, et al. Minimally invasive esophagectomy: outcomes in 222 patients. Ann Surg 2003;238:486–95.

ELSEVIER
SAUNDERS

SURGICAL
CLINICS OF
NORTH AMERICA

Surg Clin N Am 85 (2005) 649–656

Long-term Function and Quality of Life After Esophageal Resection for Cancer and Barrett's

Claude Deschamps, MD*, Francis C. Nichols III, MD,
Stephen D. Cassivi, MD, Mark S. Allen, MD,
Peter C. Pairolero, MD

*Division of General Thoracic Surgery, Mayo Clinic College of Medicine,
200 First Street SW, Rochester, MN 55905, USA*

Esophagectomy is the treatment of choice for cancer or high-grade dysplasia. Although the patients frequently experience symptoms postoperatively, their quality of life is most often comparable to that of a control population. This article provides details of postesopahegctomy symptomatology and examines how quality of life can be measured in these patients.

Function and quality of life after resection for carcinoma

Because the incidence of adenocarcinoma of the esophagus and esophagogastric junction is increasing, endoscopic surveillance for Barrett's disease will very likely lead to earlier cancer detection and resection, and possibly to improved long-term survival; however, little is known of the functional status and quality of life of long-term survivors after curative resection for esophageal carcinoma [1–10]. Clearly, a better understanding of the functional outcome and quality of life of long-term survivors is needed in this new era of health care. Appropriate tools to measure outcome, however, are limited, and development of such instruments will become increasingly important in the future if surgeons are to better plan preoperative counseling, surgical approach, and postoperative care.

The authors' group reviewed and analyzed both esophageal function and quality of life in patients who survived more than 5 years after resection of

---

* Corresponding author.
  E-mail address: deschamps.claude@mayo.edu (C. Deschamps).

esophageal carcinoma. Between January 1972 and December 1990, 359 patients underwent esophageal resection at the Mayo Clinic for Stage I or II (A and B) carcinoma of the esophagus. One hundred and seven of these patients (30%) survived 5 or more years. The records of these patients were analyzed for functional outcome and quality of life. Follow-up data were obtained from patients' most recent clinic visit and a two-part mail survey. Part one evaluated subjective digestive function as it relates to the esophagectomy patient. It specifically addressed the qualitative and quantitative estimate of dysphagia, the need for esophageal dilatation, the presence of heartburn, and the need for medication. The size and number of daily meals, presence of dumping symptoms, bowel habits, and weight change also were queried. Part two used the Medical Outcomes Study 36-Item Short-Form Health Survey (MOS SF-36) [11]. This national standardized questionnaire is a self-administered health assessment tool that permits group comparisons in eight conceptual areas: general health (health perception), daily activities (physical functioning), work (role—physical), emotional problems (role—emotional), social activities (social functioning), nervousness/depression (mental health), pain (bodily pain), and vitality (energy/fatigue). A numerical score is arrived at for the answers in each of the conceptual areas. Means and standard deviation of the numerical score were determined and compared with national norms matched for age and sex. The MOS SF-36 survey was constructed to measure population differences in physical and mental health status, the health burden of chronic disease, and the effect of treatments on general health status. It provides a common yardstick to compare those patients who have chronic health problems with those sampled from the general population. Evaluation of the patients' responses to the Health Status Questionnaire relative to a matched population (national norm) was done using the signed rank test.

The two-part written survey was sent to 80 patients believed to be alive at the beginning of this study. Complete data were available in 64 patients, for a response rate of 80%. The results of part one of the written survey were combined with information obtained from our outpatient clinic to provide information on all patients.

Clinical findings

There were 81 men and 26 women. At the time of esophagectomy, median age was 62 years (range, 30 to 81 years). The operation performed was an Ivor Lewis esophagogastrectomy in 77 patients (72%), transhiatal esophagectomy in 14 (13%), extended esophagectomy in 4 (4%), left thoracoabdominal esophagectomy in 4 (4%), partial esophagectomy and total gastrectomy in 3 (3%) and segmental esophageal resection in 5 (4%). Intestinal continuity was reestablished with the stomach in 99 patients (93%), small bowel in 4 (4%), and isoperistaltic left colon in 3 (3%). One patient (1%) had a primary end-to-end esophageal anastomosis after a segmental resection of the cervical esophagus. Overall, 87 patients (81.3%) had an intrathoracic anastomosis and 20 patients (18.7%) had a cervical anastomosis. A pyloromyotomy was done in 52 (49%) and a pyloroplasty in 36 (34%).

Functional outcome

Information on functional esophageal outcome was available in all 107 patients. Seventeen patients (16%) were entirely asymptomatic. Twenty-seven patients (25%) had dysphagia to solid food, 10 (9%) had pain on swallowing, 10 (9%) had dysphagia to a pureed diet, and 3 (3%) had dysphagia to liquids. Forty-six patients (43%) underwent at least one postoperative dilatation. Sixty-four patients (60%) had heartburn, which was intermittent in 58 and continuous in 6. Thirty-one patients (29%) required antacids for relief of heartburn. Forty patients (37%) ate smaller, more frequent meals. Fifty-two patients (49%) never regained lost weight following their operation, 27 (25%) maintained their initial preoperative weight, and 6 (6%) gained weight above their preoperative weight. Fifty-three patients (50%) experienced symptoms of postprandial dumping, including 26 (24%) who had diarrhea, 17 (16%) who had abdominal cramps, 8 (8%) who had nausea, 7 (7%) who had dizziness, and 6 (6%) who had diaphoresis.

Factors affecting late functional outcome were analyzed. Patients who had a cervical anastomosis had significantly less symptoms of reflux ($P < 0.05$) than those who had an intrathoracic anastomosis. Dumping symptoms occurred more frequently in younger patients ($P < 0.05$) and in women ($P < 0.01$). Neither the type of resection ($P = 0.82$) or the occurrence of a postoperative leak ($P = 0.56$) influenced the need for dilatation. The time interval since operation, tumor location, histology, adjuvant therapy, anastomotic leak, and type or absence of gastric drainage did not significantly affect late functional outcome.

Quality of life

Information on quality of life as assessed by the MOS SF-36 Health Survey Questionnaire was available in 64 patients (60%). A score was computed for each patient in each of the eight conceptual areas. Data are expressed as mean ($\pm$ standard deviation) for the group. Physical function scores were decreased significantly ($P < 0.01$) compared with the national norm. Ability to work, social interaction, daily activities, emotional dysfunction scores, and perception of health were similar to the national norm. Level of energy was decreased compared with the national norm, but the significance was borderline ($P = 0.05$). Our patients had higher scores in the area of mental health ($P < 0.05$).

Factors affecting quality of life were also analyzed. The occurrence of a postoperative anastomotic leak adversely affected the physical functioning and the health perception scores in our population ($P < 0.05$). Also, the need for postoperative dilatation adversely affected the social functioning score ($P < 0.01$). Age, sex, time interval since the surgery, location of lesion, histology, type of surgery, and adjuvant therapy did not significantly affect any of the eight conceptual areas measured by the quality of life questionnaire (Table 1).

Discussion

Patient's perspective on quality of life is crucial. We are in an era during which health care outcome will increasingly be evaluated from the patient point of view. J.D. Kirby, who founded the Oesophageal Patients Association, suggested nine elements of a good quality of life after esophagectomy. These are outlined in Box 1.

Health outcome is better measured by using general health measures and traditional biomedical tools (ie, disease-specific) synchronously. The authors prefer to combine a questionnaire aimed at upper and lower digestive functions with a quality-of-life survey.

Our data demonstrate that when queried, the majority of patients were symptomatic years after esophagectomy. Only a minority of our patients (16%) were completely symptom-free 5 or more years after esophageal resection. More than 50% complained of reflux symptoms, half had some degree of dumping, and 46% had difficulty with swallowing. Moreover, dumping was increased in younger patients and in women. These findings have been also reported by others. In contrast to our functional outcome findings, however, esophagectomy for cancer did not appear to influence

Table 1
Quality of life survey after esophagectomy for carcinoma

	Results of MOS SF-36	
Quality of life factors	Patient population	Normal population
Health perception	65.3 (19.7)	69.9 (5.3)
Physical functioning	70.9 (25.8)*	80.5 (9.4)
Role—physical	76.2 (36.6)	75.8 (12.7)
Role—emotional	87.2 (25.8)	86.4 (6.2)
Social functioning	86.5 (23.6)	88.4 (4.4)
Mental health	80.5 (14.8)*	78.3 (1.6)
Bodily pain	79.3 (22.2)	76.2 (5.2)
Energy/fatigue	56.5 (20.4)**	62.9 (3.5)

Scores are expressed as mean (standard deviation).
* $P < 0.05$ when compared to normal population matched for age and sex.
** $P = 0.05$.

Box 1. Nine elements of a good quality of life after esophagectomy

- To be able to eat adequately and enjoy it
- To be able to drink as desired, with moderate alcohol consumption
- To be able to do both of the above socially
- To have weight stability
- To be able to sleep comfortably in a normal position
- To be free of pain
- To be able to earn one's living
- To be able to participate in sports or hobbies
- To have unimpaired libido

From Kirby JD. Quality of life after oesophagectomy: the patient perspective. Dis Esophagus 1999;12:168–71; with permission.

---

quality of life. Our patients were comparable to the national norm in all except physical functioning, and actually scored significantly higher than the national norm in the area of mental health.

One significant finding in the authors' study revolves around the location of the anastomosis. The incidence of reflux is significantly reduced if the anastomosis is located in the neck; however, reduction in late reflux has to be balanced against an increased rate of fistula and recurrent nerve injury associated with the cervical anastomosis in the early postoperative period. Moreover, the occurrence of a postoperative leak had an adverse impact on quality-of-life scores that measure physical functioning and health perception. In addition, the need for dilatation postoperatively did adversely affect the social functioning score.

No standardized tool exists for evaluating quality of life in esophageal carcinoma, and the discrepancy in the results observed in the two parts of our study points to the difficulty in developing a valid questionnaire for a specific population of patients. Others have reported similar findings in which symptoms specific to esophageal disease correlated poorly with quality of life scores. One possible explanation for the poor correlation is that despite symptoms secondary to their surgery, most patients can function at home or work, and are happy to be alive and free of cancer. We found that functional outcome following surgery is affected by age, sex, and type of resection. For those surviving 5 or more years, symptoms of reflux, dumping, and dysphagia are not uncommon; however, quality of life after resection as assessed by the patients themselves is similar to the national norm.

Function and quality of life after resection for Barrett's who had high-grade dysplasia

The authors recently reviewed our group's experience with function and quality of life after esophagectomy for high-grade dysplasia in Barrett's esophagus [10,12–14]. From June 1991 through July 1997, 54 consecutive patients underwent esophageal resection for Barrett's esophagus with high-grade dysplasia (HGD) at the Mayo Clinic Rochester. Ivor Lewis esophagogastrectomy was performed in 34 patients (63%), transhiatal esophagectomy in 10 (18%), extended Ivor Lewis esophagogastrectomy in 8 (15%), and other procedures in 2. Follow-up data were obtained from the patients' clinical records and a two-part mail survey that was mailed to all 46 patients thought to be alive in August 1999. We used the same two-part written survey described earlier. All 46 two-part written surveys were returned, for a response of 100%. The follow-up was complete in all 54 patients. The median follow-up was 5.3 years (range, 6 months to 9 years).

Functional outcome

Long-term (greater than 2 years) functional outcome was available for 48 patients. Seven patients (13%) were entirely asymptomatic. Ten patients experienced no change in their weight. Thirty-one patients lost a median of 9 kg (range, 1–50 kg), and 7 patients gained a median of 2 kg (range, 1–5 kg). Thirty patients had no dysphagia. Mild, moderate, and severe dysphagia were seen in 15, 1, and, 2 patients respectively. Reflux was present in 36 patients (75%). The majority had minimal symptoms with medical management. Dumping was present in 8 patients (16.6%).

Long-term functional outcome was significantly affected by the level of the anastomosis. Patients who had a cervical anastomosis had significantly more dumping than those patients who had an intrathoracic anastomosis (33.3% versus 6.7%, $P = 0.04$). The authors were unable to detect any significant difference in dysphagia, reflux, or dumping with regards to age, gender, anastomotic location, or postoperative leaks.

Quality of life

Forty-four patients (82%) completed the MOS SF-36 Health Status Questionnaire. A score was competed for each patient for each of the eight conceptual areas. The results for our HGD patient population are outlined in Table 2. If the patients who had HGD only (ie, no cancer) are compared with the national norm, significant differences in role—physical and role—emotional are identified ($P < 0.03$). In both categories, the authors' patients find themselves to be better than the norm.

Table 2
Results of quality of life survey HGD patients*

Category	HGD patients	Normal population
Physical functioning	76.0 (27.0)	80.74 (10.0)
Role—physical	76.7 (38.2)**	75.4 (13.9)
Role—emotional	86.5 (6.7)***	86.0 (25.5)
Social functioning	83.9 (26.4)	88.1 (4.9)
Mental health	76.9 (17.1)	78.5 (1.2)
Bodily pain	79.6 (20.3)	76.4 (5.5)
Energy/fatigue	58.2 (19.6)	63.0 (4.4)
Health perception	62.8 (24.9)	69.6 (6.0)

* Scores are shown as the mean with the standard deviation in parentheses.
** Significance: $P = 0.02$ compared with normal population matched for age and gender.
*** Significance: $P = 0.03$.

When factors affecting quality of life were analyzed, the occurrence of an anastomotic leak adversely affected the social functioning scores in our population ($P = 0.02$). Age is significantly correlated with physical functioning ($r = -0.49$, $P = 0.0007$) and role—physical ($r = -0.33$, $P = 0.03$). As our patients become older, their physical function and physical performance at work are less than the norm. Time from surgery is significantly correlated with social functioning ($r = 0.34$, $P = 0.02$). The longer our patient population is out from surgery, the better is their social function. The authors were unable to detect any difference in the categories of bodily pain, health perception, energy/fatigue, role—emotional, and mental health with the age, gender, time from surgery, anastomotic leak, reflux, or dumping.

Discussion

Only 7 (13%) of our patients were truly symptom-free 2 or more years after esophagectomy. Thirty-eight percent of patients had swallowing difficulties, but in only 6% was this moderate to severe. Reflux was present in 68% of our patients. This, however, was well-controlled with medication in the majority of patients. Dumping was present in 15% of patients. Interestingly, in this patient group, neither dysphagia nor reflux was significantly related to the level of the anastomosis. In this group of patients, dumping was much greater in patients who had a cervical anastomosis compared with our patients who had carcinoma, in whom dumping was more common in younger patients and women. Although the functional outcomes were acceptable but less than ideal, esophagectomy had no measurable negative impact on these patients' quality of life. Although a postoperative leak adversely affected the social functioning score, it improved significantly as the time interval from surgery increased. In conclusion, the vast majority of these patients can experience a positive quality of life.

References

[1] Blazeby JM, Williams MH, Brookes ST, et al. Quality of life measurement in patients with oesophageal cancer. Gut 1995;37:505–8.

[2] Collard J-M, Otte J-B, Reynaert M, et al. Quality of life three years or more after esophagectomy for cancer. J Thorac Cardiovasc Surg 1992;104:391–4.

[3] De Leyn P, Coosemans W, Lerut T. Early and late functional results in patients with intrathoracic gastric replacement after oesophagectomy for carcinoma. Eur J Cardiothorac Surg 1992;6:79–85.

[4] Finley RJ, Lamy A, Clifton J, et al. Gastrointestinal function following esophagectomy for malignancy. Am J Surg 1995;169:471–5.

[5] Gelfand GAJ, Finley RJ. Quality of life with carcinoma of the esophagus. World J Surg 1994;18:399–405.

[6] Kuwano H, Ikebe M, Baba K, et al. Operative procedures of reconstruction after resection of esophageal cancer and the postoperative quality of life. World J Surg 1993;17:773–6.

[7] Suzuki H, Shichisaburo A, Kitamura M, et al. An evaluation of symptoms and performance status in patients after esophagectomy for esophageal cancer from the viewpoint of the patient. Am Surg 1994;608:920–3.

[8] van Knippenberg FCE, Out JJ, Tilanus HW, et al. Quality of life in patients with resected oesophageal cancer. Soc Sci Med 1992;35:139–45.

[9] McLarty AJ, Deschamps C, Trastek VF, et al. Esophageal resection for cancer of the esophagus: long-term function and quality of life. Ann Thorac Surg 1997;63:1568–72.

[10] Deschamps C, Nichols FC, Miller DL, et al. Function and quality of life after esophageal resection. In: Tilanus HW, Attwood SEA, editors. Barrett's esophagus. (Netherlands): Kluwer Academic Publishers; 2001. p. 387–92.

[11] Ware JE. SF-36 health survey. Manual and interpretation guide. Boston: Nimrod; 1993.

[12] Kirby JD. Quality of life after oesophagectomy: the patient perspective. Dis Esophagus 1999;12:168–71.

[13] Headrick JR, Nichols FC, Miller DL, et al. High-grade esophageal dysplasia: long-term survival and quality of life after esophagectomy. Ann Thorac Surg 2002;73:1697–703.

[14] Pera M, Trastek VF, Carpenter HA, et al. Barrett's esophagus with high-grade dysplasia: an indication for esophagectomy? Ann Thorac Surg 1992;54:199–204.

ELSEVIER
SAUNDERS

Surg Clin N Am 85 (2005) 657–663

SURGICAL
CLINICS OF
NORTH AMERICA

Index

Note: Page numbers of article titles are in **boldface** type.

Changing Your Address?

Make sure your subscription changes too! When you notify us of your new address, you can help make our job easier by including an exact copy of your Clinics label number with your old address (see illustration below.) This number identifies you to our computer system and will speed the processing of your address change. Please be sure this label number accompanies your old address and your corrected address—you can send an old Clinics label with your number on it or just copy it exactly and send it to the address listed below.

We appreciate your help in our attempt to give you continuous coverage. Thank you.

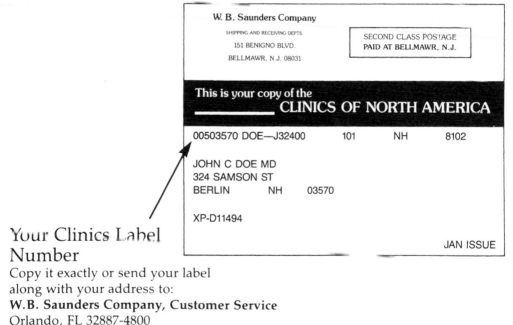

W. B. Saunders Company

SHIPPING AND RECEIVING DEPTS.
151 BENIGNO BLVD.
BELLMAWR, N.J. 08031

SECOND CLASS POSTAGE
PAID AT BELLMAWR, N.J.

This is your copy of the
_____ CLINICS OF NORTH AMERICA

00503570 DOE—J32400   101   NH   8102

JOHN C DOE MD
324 SAMSON ST
BERLIN   NH   03570

XP-D11494

JAN ISSUE

Your Clinics Label Number

Copy it exactly or send your label along with your address to:
W.B. Saunders Company, Customer Service
Orlando, FL 32887-4800
Call Toll Free 1-800-654-2452

Please allow four to six weeks for delivery of new subscriptions and for processing address changes.